Practical Theology Amid Environmental Crises

Practical Theology Amid Environmental Crises

Editors

Pamela R. McCarroll
HyeRan Kim-Cragg

MDPI • Basel • Beijing • Wuhan • Barcelona • Belgrade • Manchester • Tokyo • Cluj • Tianjin

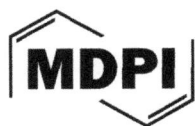

Editors
Pamela R. McCarroll
Emmanuel College of
Victoria University,
University of Toronto,
Toronto, ON, Canada

HyeRan Kim-Cragg
Emmanuel College of
Victoria University,
University of Toronto,
Toronto, ON, Canada

Editorial Office
MDPI
St. Alban-Anlage 66
4052 Basel, Switzerland

This is a reprint of articles from the Special Issue published online in the open access journal *Religions* (ISSN 2077-1444) (available at: https://www.mdpi.com/journal/religions/special_issues/ptaec).

For citation purposes, cite each article independently as indicated on the article page online and as indicated below:

LastName, A.A.; LastName, B.B.; LastName, C.C. Article Title. *Journal Name* **Year**, *Volume Number*, Page Range.

ISBN 978-3-0365-5793-9 (Hbk)
ISBN 978-3-0365-5794-6 (PDF)

Cover image courtesy of Photo by USGS on Unsplash.

© 2023 by the authors. Articles in this book are Open Access and distributed under the Creative Commons Attribution (CC BY) license, which allows users to download, copy and build upon published articles, as long as the author and publisher are properly credited, which ensures maximum dissemination and a wider impact of our publications.
The book as a whole is distributed by MDPI under the terms and conditions of the Creative Commons license CC BY-NC-ND.

Contents

About the Editors vii

Pamela R. McCarroll and HyeRan Kim-Cragg
Introduction to the Special Issue "Practical Theology Amid Environmental Crises"
Reprinted from: *Religions* 2022, *13*, 969, doi:10.3390/rel13100969 1

Mary Elizabeth Moore
Responding to a Weeping Planet: Practical Theology as a Discipline Called by Crisis
Reprinted from: *Religions* 2022, *13*, 244, doi:10.3390/rel13030244 7

Pamela R. McCarroll
Embodying Theology: Trauma Theory, Climate Change, Pastoral and Practical Theology
Reprinted from: *Religions* 2022, *13*, 294, doi:10.3390/rel13040294 21

Un-Hey Kim
Christian Planetary Humanism in the Age of Climate Crisis
Reprinted from: *Religions* 2022, *13*, 224, doi:10.3390/rel13030224 35

Mary E. Hess
Shifting Epistemologies, Shifting Our Stories—Where Might We Find Hope for a World on the Brink of Climate Catastrophe?
Reprinted from: *Religions* 2022, *13*, 625, doi:10.3390/rel13070625 45

Christine Tind Johannessen
Belonging to the World through Body, Trust, and Trinity: Climate Change and Pastoral Care with University Students
Reprinted from: *Religions* 2022, *13*, 527, doi:10.3390/rel13060527 65

Danielle Elizabeth Tumminio Hansen
The Body of God, Sexually Violated: A Trauma-Informed Reading of the Climate Crisis
Reprinted from: *Religions* 2022, *13*, 249, doi:10.3390/rel13030249 83

Ryan Williams LaMothe
Climate Emergency as Revelation: The Tragedy and Illusion of Sovereignty in Christian Political Theologies
Reprinted from: *Religions* 2022, *13*, 524, doi:10.3390/rel13060524 95

Tallessyn Zawn Grenfell-Lee
Unshakeable Hope: Pandemic Disruption, Climate Disruption, and the Ultimate Test of Theologies of Abundance
Reprinted from: *Religions* 2022, *13*, 404, doi:10.3390/rel13050404 109

Jeane C. Peracullo and Rosa Bella M. Quindoza
The Environmental Activism of a Filipino Catholic Faith Community: Re-Imagining Ecological Care for the Flourishing of All
Reprinted from: *Religions* 2022, *13*, 56, doi:10.3390/rel13010056 123

Leah D. Schade
Who Is My Neighbor? Developing a Pedagogical Tool for Teaching Environmental Preaching and Ethics in Online and Hybrid Courses
Reprinted from: *Religions* 2022, *13*, 322, doi:10.3390/rel13040322 139

HyeRan Kim-Cragg
Preaching Addressing Environmental Crises through the Use of Scripture: An Exploration of a Practical Theological Methodology
Reprinted from: *Religions* **2022**, *13*, 226, doi:10.3390/rel13030226 . . . . **151**

Panu Pihkala
Eco-Anxiety and Pastoral Care: Theoretical Considerations and Practical Suggestions
Reprinted from: *Religions* **2022**, *13*, 192, doi:10.3390/rel13030192 . . . . **163**

Joyce Ann Mercer
Children and Climate Anxiety: An Ecofeminist Practical Theological Perspective
Reprinted from: *Religions* **2022**, *13*, 302, doi:10.3390/rel13040302 . . . . **183**

About the Editors

Pamela R. McCarroll
Vice Principal, Associate Professor of Practical Theology, Emmanuel College of Victoria University in the University of Toronto. Her present research focuses on ecofeminist, decolonizing approaches to practical theology that serve Earth and intersectional justice. She also publishes in the area of spiritual care and chaplaincy, and has written or edited books on the theology and phenomenology of hope in addition to practical and contextual theology. She is a Certified Supervisor with CASC and ordained in the Presbyterian Church of Canada.

HyeRan Kim-Cragg
Principal, Timothy Eaton Church Professor of Preaching, Emmanuel College of Victoria University in the University of Toronto. Committed to an interdisciplinary approach to homiletics in practical theology, her research addresses topics related to biblical interpretation, postcolonial theories, feminist homiletics and liturgy, migration, and decolonizing practices. She has published twelve books, including *Postcolonial Preaching* (2021) and *Interdependence: A Postcolonial Feminist Practical Theology* (2018). Hailing from the Presbyterian Church in the Republic of Korea, she has been actively involved in the United Church of Canada for the last three decades.

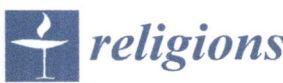

Editorial

Introduction to the Special Issue "Practical Theology Amid Environmental Crises"

Pamela R. McCarroll * and HyeRan Kim-Cragg *

Emmanuel College of Victoria University, University of Toronto, Toronto, ON M5S 1K, Canada
* Correspondence: pam.mccarroll@utoronto.ca (P.R.M.); hyeran.kimcragg@utoronto.ca (H.K.-C.)

Citation: McCarroll, Pamela R., and HyeRan Kim-Cragg. 2022. Introduction to the Special Issue "Practical Theology Amid Environmental Crises". *Religions* 13: 969. https://doi.org/10.3390/rel13100969

Received: 13 September 2022
Accepted: 21 September 2022
Published: 13 October 2022

Publisher's Note: MDPI stays neutral with regard to jurisdictional claims in published maps and institutional affiliations.

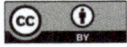

Copyright: © 2022 by the authors. Licensee MDPI, Basel, Switzerland. This article is an open access article distributed under the terms and conditions of the Creative Commons Attribution (CC BY) license (https://creativecommons.org/licenses/by/4.0/).

By most accounts, the world we live in has entered the epoch of the Anthropocene, the period in which human activity has irrevocably altered the geology, biosphere and climate of the planet. Not only do humans experience the impacts of environmental crises in their daily lives, but people's dreams for the future are also haunted by the spectre of ecological apocalypse. Some suggest that compared to other fields and disciplines, practical theology so far has offered little to the interdisciplinary conversations on climate and the environmental crises (McCarroll 2020; Miller-McLemore 2020). This Book seeks to change that perception.

Practical Theology, broadly speaking, has been described as a field that privileges, engages and transforms *human* experience and practices with its guiding motif of the living *human* web (Miller-McLemore 2018), and its focus on *human* suffering, flourishing and justice. The human-centered givens of the field highlight its anthropocentric ethos. No doubt, this ethos has contributed to the delay in fulsome engagement with the environmental crisis through the research, teaching and practice of practical theology. Indeed, when we as co-editors consider the methodological, theological and practical implications of shifting the field away from human-centeredness and towards earth-centeredness, it can be quite overwhelming (see also McCarroll 2020; LaMothe 2021; Pihkala 2018). Practical theology also prioritizes *context* or *situatedness* as it seeks to discern the divine presence and call in the very midst of life. Unlike some other theological disciplines, it engages realities of inequities, oppression and the struggle for justice as it carves out pathways to renewed ways of living and being in the world. It is notable that despite its focus on context and situatedness, the dire realities of our context of environmental crises have yet to be fulsomely taken up in the field even as these realities press in upon all of life at the micro, meso and macro levels of being.

While over the last decade within the field there has been an increase in the amount of research produced on the topic, other than a few exceptions within specific guilds (see Clinebell 1996; Moore 1998; Ayers 2019), this literature is spread across several journals and books and can be challenging to find (Kim-Cragg 2018; McCarroll 2020; Miller-McLemore, forthcoming). A quick look at the tables of contents over the last five years of our field's premier journals (*International Journal of Practical Theology* and *Practical Theology*) demonstrates the extent to which concern about environmental and climate crises has been peripheral to practical theology. From a total of two hundred and forty-two research articles, only four focus on climate change and the environmental crisis. These numbers suggest that, while there is some awareness of the theme, it is hardly a focus for research (see Williams 2018; McCarroll 2020; Ayers 2021; Marlow 2022). Thankfully, some practical theology associations recently have begun to identify climate change as an emerging priority. For example, the 2022 meetings of the *Association for Practical Theology* hosted a roundtable on climate change, chaired by Bonnie Miller-McLemore and Jennifer Ayers, which generated much inspiration and dialogue with practical theologians across several guilds. Also, the 2023 meetings of the *International Academy of Practical Theology* will focus on practical theology in the Anthropocene. Additionally, within various guilds of the field, there are some signs that interest is beginning to build.[1]

Even as these signs are promising, it is clear, that there is yet to be a sustained conversation in the field on the theme of the climate and environmental crises. We believe this book, *Practical Theology Amid Environmental Crises*, will make a significant contribution and mark the beginning of a generative and creative conversation. The volume brings together the voices of many around the world who have begun to wrestle with the realities and implications of climate and environmental crises for their own research, teaching and practices from their various social locations. In bringing these voices together, we seek not only to model a collaborative and interactive conversation and contribute to the larger multi/interdisciplinary conversation, but to begin to discern the primary contours and themes of the conversation within the field.

In envisioning this project, we as co-editors first identified some key leaders in the various guilds of practical theology whose research demonstrated interest in the area. We then put out a call for papers more widely. We invited research that "**contributes to practical theological approaches to the multilayered environmental crises**". We sought out submissions to help construct a sustained conversation on climate change in the practical theological literature and to contribute to the ongoing interdisciplinary conversation regarding the environmental crises. We identified a need for papers that engage practical theology from intersectional perspectives with a concern for justice and for work that reimagines the field beyond its anthropocentric foundations. We encouraged researchers to retrieve earth-centered resources through texts and practices from the various sub-disciplines of practical theology and identified our interest in action-based, narrative and other practical theological approaches that highlight human embeddedness, dependence and interconnectivity within and as a part of creation. The call went out and we were positively overwhelmed by the response. We cannot be more pleased with this final product. Not only does the enthusiasm of our contributors and the quality of their work suggest that a sustained conversation is emerging through this publication, but the volume also demonstrates depth, insight and creativity, offering much toward continuing the conversation.

When we inductively explore the content of the chapters of the volume, we are not surprised to see concentrations on methodology, theology and practice. In some cases, practices are starting points that generate theological and methodological reflection. In other cases, authors present critical and constructive theological-methodological content that leads to renewed practices. In still other cases, authors share what we will call eco-practical theological models and narratives that invite the reader into new forms of practice and imagination. In all cases, authors seek to address realities of living in the context of environmental and ecological change and instability and to consider this in relation to theology and practices of people of faith and their respective communities. We are delighted to have most of the guilds of the discipline represented within our authorship—religious education, preaching and worship, community and congregational leadership, pastoral and spiritual care. Throughout the book there are several repeated themes that emerge including a focus on embodiment and materiality, on specific populations such as children, youth, students and women, on the impacts of ecological emotions such as eco-anxiety and climate trauma, on the interconnections between Earth justice and social justice, and between the climate crisis and colonialism. The book is rich with convergences, but also includes creative tensions between and among issues represented in the chapters.

In terms of the flow of content in the book, we have ordered the chapters into three distinct groupings or sections following one after the other. The first section is made up of chapters one to four, each of which is addressed to the field of practical theology as a whole and focuses on the intersections of methodology, epistemology, theology and practice. The second section includes chapters five to eight. Each of these chapters present theological reflections on lived experiences of climate and environmental crises, and through this lens reimagine some key theological concepts and practices. The third section includes chapters nine to thirteen. These final chapters look toward the future by presenting models and approaches for renewed eco-integrated practice, teaching and research across the different guilds.

Addressing Intersections of Methodology, Epistemology, Theology and Practice

In each of the first four chapters, the authors identify how the climate crisis demands a complete re-imagining of the givens of the field of practical theology—the methodologies, epistemologies and theologies central to its research, teaching and practice. Each chapter is addressed to the field as a whole and calls for change in response to the climate crisis. Chapter one, by Mary Elizabeth Moore, identifies the extent to which practical theology has always been concerned with change and explores the how the climate crisis demands radical change across the field. Drawing from eco-theologians and other ecological thinkers, from Indigenous wisdom and from the wisdom of the Earth itself, the chapter identifies challenges, practices and alternative worldviews and concludes by offering up life practices to direct and re-shape life and the field toward climate justice. In chapter two, Pamela McCarroll examines the literature on climate trauma in terms of its interpretation of public discourse, denial and (in)action in relation to the climate crisis and by unearthing the theologies and epistemologies embedded in this literature. She explores and proposes the conceptual architecture required for an earth-centered, de-colonizing, trauma-informed approach for the field. Chapter three, by Un-Hey Kim, draws from ecofeminist theologies and the new materialism for her theo-ethical reflection on the climate catastrophe, re-interpreting humans in terms of the interdependence and inter-relationality of all reality. She explores moves to liberate the human subject from the bondage of human exceptionalism and toward Earth's justice. In the fourth chapter, Mary Hess offers a creative exploratory essay that weaves through multiple narratives from diverse contexts. In her generative narrative weaving, she seeks out "sacred ground within which to root embodied, theologically astute pedagogies" (abstract) for the field. Together, these chapters offer perspectives, resources and approaches to re-imagine the epistemology, theology and methodologies of practical theology.

Theological Reflection on Experiences of Environmental Crisis and Reconceiving Theology

The second cluster of chapters, chapters five through eight, all reflect theologically on lived experiences of climate and environmental crises and seek to reconceive theological concepts through these disruptive experiences. Chapter five, by Christine Tind Johannessen, presents ethnographic theological research on university students' experiences of climate stress. Drawing on her data, and theories from anthropology, psychology and theology, she proposes a model for pastoral care that re-imagines an experiential Trinitarian theological framing for experiencing and perceiving the Divine. In chapter six, Danielle Tumminio Hansen draws on Sallie McFague's body of God metaphor and explores what is at stake theologically when we interpret environmental crises as sexual violation of the Earth. Drawing this metaphor further, she proposes trauma-informed practices for living that shift us away from hierarchical notions of creation. Ryan LaMothe, in chapter seven, interprets environmental crisis theologically as a disruptive revelation of a non-sovereign God. He considers the political, existential and ontological implications of a non-sovereign God and calls readers to reimagine political theologies that frame how we live together. In chapter eight, Tallessyn Zawn Grenfell-Lee draws on a case study from a Swedish experience of crisis to re-interpret experiences of climate disruption in ways that serve resilience and creativity. She concludes with an exploration of hope through a Eucharistic theology of abundance in the face of planetary catastrophe. All these chapters engage either micro- or macro-experiences of climate disruption and explore creative theological constructs and practices to serve life.

Future-Leaning Models for Renewed Eco-integrated Practice, Teaching and Research

The five final chapters, chapters nine to thirteen, all present models or approaches for renewed eco-integrated practice, teaching and research among the different guilds of practical theology. Together, they represent a forward-thinking trajectory that seeks to transform tools of the field toward Earth-centered practices. In chapter nine, Jeane Peracullo and Rosa Bella Quindoza examine how a Catholic Filipino faith-based community addresses multiple environmental crises within their context. They draw forth the wisdom of the community's practices to present a viable model that moves beyond anthropocentrism and builds capacity for ecological social justice. Chapter ten, written by Leah Shade, presents a case study of the author's development and use of a pedagogical tool designed to teach ministry students about ecological interconnectivity and habitat. The tool, called "Who is My Neighbor?", supports students to engage with issues of environmental justice and to integrate these into their ministry practices. In chapter eleven, HyeRan Kim-Cragg draws on Paul Ballard's work to build a practical theological model for preaching that integrates Scripture as a resource and source to engage with the environmental crisis. Not only does she draw out the elements of the model, but she also shares a sermon that utilizes the model in its construction, demonstrating how it can be adapted into homiletical practice. In chapter twelve, Panu Pihkala presents an in-depth review of the pastoral theological literature on eco-anxiety. He itemizes distinct areas of focus for the discipline at present and projects areas for further research. He also identifies helpful conversation partners for the further development of a body of research for the discipline. Chapter thirteen, written by Joyce Ann Mercer, like the chapters in the first section, includes a call to the field as a whole through an ecofeminist practical theological perspective. We chose to place it here because, with its focus on children and change, it leans towards the future by offering a lens for "toward participatory empowerment for change" (abstract). Mercer examines the experiences of children in terms of the distress they carry and the need for a theology of *oikos*—of home, of habitat—to support them toward engagement and justice, even in the face of environmental chaos. The five chapters in this section all provide concrete examples and specific foci for re-imagining ministry and congregational practices to serve ecological and social justice.

Conclusions

We wish to extend our gratitude to all the authors for their committed and creative engagement of the topic. It has been a joy to work with you. We also wish to thank our Associate Editor with MDPI, Ms. Gloria Qi, whose gracious guidance and support has enabled the coming together of this publication. With deep passion and sense of calling we in practical theology are ready to engage with you in the journey of re-imagining our field from outside its anthropocentric roots. This book is an invitation to enter into this difficult conversation with courage, openness and a sense of realistic and grounded hope—a hope inspired by the Earth, our mother, who generously holds and nurtures all creatures, calling forth new life even in the face of overwhelming destruction and death.

Author Contributions: Both authors contributed equally to the paper. All authors have read and agreed to the published version of the manuscript.

Funding: This research received no external funding.

Conflicts of Interest: The authors declare no conflict of interest.

Notes

[1] For example, the recent meeting of the Society for Pastoral Theology included the inaugural gathering of a special interest study group devoted to Pastoral Theology and Climate Change, chaired by Christine Tind Johannessen and Pamela McCarroll; Beginning in December 2022, The Academy of Homiletics will have a new workgroup on climate crisis and creation in preaching, chaired by HyeRan Kim-Cragg and Leah Schade. Jennifer Ayers's recent book, *Inhabitance*, has garnered much attention within the disciplines of religious education, preaching and ministry. In the area of spirituality there appears to be the most publications in relation to climate and environmental crises (Miller-McLemore, forthcoming) though these, again, are distributed across several books and journals.

References

Ayers, Jennifer R. 2019. *Inhabitance: Ecological Religious Education*. Waco: Baylor University Press.
Ayers, Jennifer R. 2021. Recovering Mysteries: Ecological Encounters and Practical Theological Ways of Knowing. *International Journal of Practical Theology* 25: 75–93. [CrossRef]
Clinebell, Howard. 1996. *Ecotherapy: Healing Ourselves, Healing the Earth*. Philadelphia: Haworth Press.
Kim-Cragg, HyeRan. 2018. *Interdependence: A Postcolonial Feminist Practical Theology*. Eugene: Pickwick, pp. 128–49.
LaMothe, Ryan. 2021. A Radical Pastoral Theology for the Anthropocene Era: Thinking and Being Otherwise. *Journal of Pastoral Theology* 31: 54–74. [CrossRef]
Marlow, Hilary. 2022. Creation, Humanity and Hubris in the Hebrew Bible. *Practical Theology*. Available online: https://www.tandfonline.com/doi/full/10.1080/1756073X.2022.2069541 (accessed on 20 June 2022).
McCarroll, Pamela R. 2020. Listening for the Cries of the Earth: Practical Theology in the Anthropocene. *International Journal of Practical Theology* 24: 29–46. [CrossRef]
Miller-McLemore, Bonnie. 2018. The Living Human Web: A Twenty-five Year Retrospective. *Pastoral Psychology* 67: 305–21. [CrossRef]
Miller-McLemore, Bonnie. 2020. Trees and the "Unthought Known": The Wisdom of the Non-Human (or Do Humans have "Shit for Brains"?). *Pastoral Psychology* 69: 423–43. [CrossRef]
Miller-McLemore, Bonnie. forthcoming. Climate Violence and Earth Justice: A Research Report on Practical Theology's Contributions. *International Journal of Practical Theology*.
Moore, Mary Elizabeth. 1998. *Ministering with the Earth*. Nashville: Chalice Press.
Pihkala, Panu. 2018. Death, The Environment and Theology. *Dialog* 57: 287–94. [CrossRef]
Williams, Cate. 2018. Brueggemann, The Land and the Forest: A Forest Church Perspective on the Theology of the Land. *Practical Theology* 11: 462–76. [CrossRef]

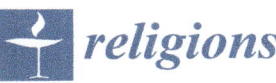

Article

Responding to a Weeping Planet: Practical Theology as a Discipline Called by Crisis

Mary Elizabeth Moore

School of Theology, Boston University, Boston, MA 02215, USA; memoore@bu.edu

Abstract: Practical theology is by nature a discipline of crisis, standing on the edge of reality and potential, what is and what can be. Crises can be gentle turning points, opportunities for radical transformation, or catastrophic moments in time. In the geological age of the Anthropocene, people face devastating planetary effects of human agency, which have created and escalated a climate crisis beyond the boundaries of imagination. Practical theology belongs at the epicenter of ecological crises, which have already produced harsh results, ecological despair, and a time-dated urgency for daring decisions and actions. Change is knocking at global doors—the necessity, foreboding, and hope for change. This article probes practical theology's role in change, giving primary attention to changes in practical wisdom (phronesis) and life practices. Methodologically, the article draws from ecological scholars and activists, philosophers and theologians, indigenous communities, and the earth itself, presenting descriptions and analyses of their shared wisdom across time, culture, and areas of expertise. From these sources, the study identifies challenges, practices, and alternate worldviews that can potentially reshape practical wisdom and climate action. In conclusion, this paper proposes life practices for climate justice: practices of attending, searching, imagining, and communal living and acting.

Keywords: practical theology; crisis; practical wisdom; ecological justice; life practices; climate change

Citation: Moore, Mary Elizabeth. 2022. Responding to a Weeping Planet: Practical Theology as a Discipline Called by Crisis. *Religions* 13: 244. https://doi.org/10.3390/rel13030244

Academic Editors: Pamela R. McCarroll and HyeRan Kim-Cragg

Received: 31 January 2022
Accepted: 3 March 2022
Published: 11 March 2022

Publisher's Note: MDPI stays neutral with regard to jurisdictional claims in published maps and institutional affiliations.

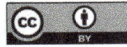

Copyright: © 2022 by the author. Licensee MDPI, Basel, Switzerland. This article is an open access article distributed under the terms and conditions of the Creative Commons Attribution (CC BY) license (https://creativecommons.org/licenses/by/4.0/).

1. Background and Methods

One day in the summer, I walked down the street in my Boston home, where smoke filled the sky and burned my eyes. The smoke had traveled here from Canada and the Western United States, where wildfires were storming across the land. Smoke and fire debris had etched the skies across North America, and the western fires continued to break records in terms of heat produced and land destroyed. A few days later, the Dixie Fire in Northern California was depositing smoke and ash in a continual flow within a 1000 mile radius of its flames. Weeks later, the western fires had further heightened the vulnerability of the atmosphere to extreme weather conditions, including raging rains and floods, and culminating yet again in mud slides and radical damage to soil, clean water, hillsides, forests, habitats for animals, and plants. As fires speed deforestation across the world, rising temperatures increase drought conditions, and dramatic increases of evaporation escalate catastrophic rainfalls, some of which are in the very regions where the heat has risen and forests and foliage have dramatically decreased, and some many miles away. Compound events continue to rise.

We in North America are facing ecological crisis on a massive scale, as are lands and peoples across the world. On our shared continent, we face crises of water and habitats as well as forests aflame, intensifying storms, and dramatic changes in temperatures and rain and snow falls. Consider the rivers that no longer provide habitat for salmon and other fish, the aquifers that have diminished or disappeared, the land that has been stripped of its nutrients in the quest for industrialization and corporate and individual profit, and the habitat networks that have been diminished and separated by industrial or human development so that animals and plants are less and less able to travel between habitats in changing conditions. All these issues are interconnected both physically and socially, and are well documented in international scientific studies (IPCC—Intergovernmental Panel on Climate Change 2021; IPCC—Intergovernmental Panel on Climate Change 2022).

A striking example is the Keystone XL (KXL) Pipeline, an extension of Keystone that was stopped after more than 10 years of struggle; it would have run through five provinces and states and through tribal lands. The southern portion of that pipeline extension had already been completed, running through two new states, as it added to the existing pipeline that already ran through eleven provinces and states, carrying tar sands oil from the borealis forest of Alberta, Canada, for conversion into flowing oil in the United States. The KXL project, if completed, would have dramatically increased the rate of tar sands extraction, destruction of the boreal forest, rate of leakage and spills (higher than for other kinds of oil), destruction of farms and habitable land, and greenhouse gases and carbon released in processes of extraction and refining. In all these escalations, the pipeline threatened to escalate the poisoning of indigenous lands and peoples. These are the same people who have been affected by other industrial development projects that have dammed and diverted rivers, leading to water shortage in some areas and flooding in others. Politically, the people most affected—indigenous communities, farmers, ranchers, and others—are rarely included in decision-making before projects are formulated, or even before projects are set in motion by industries and governments. The dangers and disasters described here represent a complex of crises that date back to the arrival of European settlers, displacement of indigenous peoples, and hundreds of decisions that benefited industry and harmed the people who live on this land, while wreaking havoc on the land itself. Innumerable activists protested the KXL crisis with words and actions and helped stop the extension from becoming a reality (Gilio-Whitaker 2019, pp. 10–24; McKibben 2013, pp. 17–44).

What is the nature of these crises, and how do they relate to practical theology? Methodologically, I will focus on the nature of crisis and then turn to the practical wisdom (phronesis) of ecological scholars and activists, theologians and philosophers, and indigenous communities as they approach earth wisdom and earth caring in their unique ways. By analyzing these sources, I will portray their shared wisdom across time, culture, and areas of expertise. Curiously, their various approaches all include some version of reflection on practices for the sake of future practice, disclosing a resonance with the work of practical theology. On the other hand, indigenous people and many of the activists reflect on practices of the entire natural world, not just human beings, thus challenging the dominant anthropomorphic focus of practical theology. The entire study illumines how diverse scholars and activists contribute to practical wisdom, or phronesis, through reflection on their unique experiences, and how they contribute to human ways of being in and with the world. In particular, the study identifies challenges, practices, and alternate worldviews that can potentially reshape practical wisdom and climate action, and it concludes with proposals for practice toward climate justice.

2. Crises

Crises are turning points or moments when forces meet, facing people and other beings with critical decisions that will shape the future. They are often associated with dramatic or disastrous moments, but the term is also broad. Crises exist in daily lives when people live detached from God's creation and from communion with other people and trees and soil. Crises appear when people face choices whether to continue their customary life patterns or consider alternative ways of relating with the earth, with other creatures, and with themselves. These daily crises (often unrecognized) are connected with catastrophic ones. The catastrophic crisis of climate change was set in motion by countless decisions made in everyday life over countless years to suck life from the planet for human gain and without regard for the life of the planet and all that lives on it. Likewise, the catastrophic plight of indigenous peoples in North America did not emerge in one traumatic moment, but in millions of traumatizing acts of war and murder; kidnapping and enslavement;

colonialization; displacement; broken treaties; and destruction of lands rich with fish, clean water, plants, soil, and game.

Crisis moments often go unnoticed without conscious reflection, especially when they are part of prevailing life patterns and worldviews that are taken for granted; yet people make small and large decisions to act in certain ways, which affect both the immediate and long future. Consider how theories of individual autonomy and individual well-being, taken for granted in most Western Christian cultures, have conflicted with indigenous theories of relationality and communal–ecological well-being, leading to the overtaking of land for individual gain or the economic gain of industrialists. These actions can be cataclysmic over time, creating and reinforcing patterns of injustice that destroy peoples, cultures, and the earth. The actions often appear innocuous at first, but the narratives of European settlements in North America reveal how settler communities, individuals, churches, and state/provincial and federal governments have contributed to the amassing of injustice toward indigenous peoples and toward the earth.

Beneath these actions are theologies or worldviews that generate and reinforce the actions. The interplay of practices and worldviews reveals the dynamic of what Don Browning describes as theory-laden practice and practice-laden theory, as well as "tradition-saturated ideals and practices" (Browning 1991, pp. 5–7, 10–12, 45–49). For him, any ethical or theological question needs to be explored with these complex relationships in mind: theory, practice, and tradition. I add poesis to this list to acknowledge the role of creativity and beauty.

Whether far-reaching or small and local, crises were turning points for European settlers in North America as they made daily judgments and decisions: how best to live in this land; whether and where to clear forests for farming; how to keep their people "safe" from peoples they feared or considered less than themselves; how to establish Christianity in this land; or how to ensure control over land, water, and peoples different from themselves. The decision points took many forms. They were *habitual*, continuing engrained patterns; *anticipatory*, seeking to build or protect a future; and/or *reactive* to immediate situations. All of these together have brought the world to a point of catastrophe.

Practical theology is by nature a discipline of crisis, standing on the edge of reality and potential, what is and what can be. The multiple meanings of crisis are all relevant in this geological age of the Anthropocene in which human agency is the dominant determinant of the fate of the climate and earth. Crisis can be understood as a troubling situation, a moment for decision-making, and/or a moment in which a bad situation is likely to become markedly worse or better. Within macro-crises are also micro-occasions or events described in process-relational theologies in which the objective past and habits of being are met with God's initial aim and the potential of a new decision. An emerging event, through its subjective aim, sets a direction and a new occasion is formed, only to be followed by billions of others. This micro process also takes place in more complex organisms as a fox or forest or human being, as they carry their respective pasts, relationships, and accumulated wisdom into a new moment of time, making a new decision for this moment. The decisions may be repetitive of the immediate and dominant streams of the past, or they may move in novel directions. I propose that we recognize all these decision moments as crises, each representing change (however small or large) and each revealing the necessity, foreboding, and hope for change.

The challenge is for practical theologians to attend even more intentionally to the dynamics of change, building on current movements. For example, practical theologians regularly respond to habituated practices with *proactive responses*, encouraging people to examine their habitual patterns for the sake of comprehending, critiquing, and reshaping or reinforcing them. Consider the work of public practical theologians, cultural analysts, pastoral counselors and caregivers, educators, and homileticians. Climate crisis underscores the need for these same theologians to reflect on engrained habits that have contributed to ecological crises, and the habits that are needed to prevent further destruction in the future. Closely related, practical theologians also engage crises with *anticipatory responses*, analyzing historical and contemporary trajectories of practice (e.g., practices of destructive human relationships or ecological neglect) and anticipating alternative futures. Finally, practical theologians often offer *reactive responses*, addressing threats of disaster, analyzing actions and underlying causes, and posing immediate responses to large-scale threats. In this Anthropocene age, all three responses are needed, as they flow in and out of one another and often take place simultaneously.

Practical theologians have largely focused on crises in the individual and community lives of human beings, but the time has come when that focus needs to be amplified with sustained attention to *all* the natural world and to ecological crises, seeking to protect and regenerate a threatened planet. What is tragically clear in the global climate crisis is that reactive responses are urgent, but the necessity for proactive and anticipatory responses is clear as well. Urgency cannot turn people away from the important work of proactivity and anticipatory action, as it often does. In all this work, practical theologians have an important role to play with their specialized attention to theory-laden practice, practice-laden theory, and tradition-saturated ideals and practices. To play that role requires that we attend to the relationship of practical wisdom and life practices.

3. Practical Wisdom: Reshaping Theology, Worldviews, and Relational Patterns

One of the profound challenges for addressing climate crises is the inadequacy of dominant theologies and world views, intertwined with inadequate relational patterns, as in colonial structures, patterns of dominance of some people over others, emphases on individualism and progress, and the dominance of humans over the land and sea. A prime example is the anthropocentricism of most Christian theologies, focusing on the superiority of humans over all other life forms, the salvation of human beings without reference to other beings, and the accompanying idea that the nonhuman natural world is a resource for humans to use and enjoy, or to tend as an inferior "other." Such views are often intensified in their ecological effects by elitist social structures in which individuals, social groups, and companies with the most economic and political power determine the "uses" of the eco-system and the limits to its protection. In anthropocentric, hierarchical worldviews, the flourishing of the planet is set aside, and the world's complex patterns of mutuality and interdependence go unrecognized. Such views lead to environmental strategies based on what appears best for people (or for people with power) without regard to the value of other beings, like animals, plants, and bodies of water.

What is needed is a deeper engagement with practical wisdom (or *phronesis*), or *deeper understandings of the world as formed in the process of living, relating, and reflecting over time*. Phronesis is a word with a complex of meanings. Different translations of Aristotle's *phronesis* highlight different emphases, most prominently practical wisdom, practical reason, practical virtue, prudence, or moral understanding. Each of these has unique nuances, but each represents a large view of the world. In my effort to capture the full-bodied, guiding force of phronesis, I use the term *practical wisdom*, which is shaped by relationships, practices, worldviews, and moral understandings. It thus includes a capacity to discern common good or ethical futures, and to discern pathways toward goodness. When practical theologians attend to crises of climate change, the turn to practical wisdom is critical—attending to practice and reflection on practice, to moral issues in the practices, and to the potential of alternative futures and actions that contribute to those futures.

The turn to *phronesis* is not new to practical theology. We see it in Don Browning, who emphasizes practical reasoning in the tradition of Aristotle and many later philosophers, recognizing the interpenetrating relationship between philosophies, theologies, and worldviews and the practices of human beings. Bernard Lee and Thomas Groome also accent phronesis, but with emphases on future good and ethical action toward that good. I stand more in the tradition of Lee and Groome, but I also accent the fullness of knowing through all the senses and with all one's being, a view more closely aligned with Jennifer Ayres (Ayres 2013, pp. 37–38). Such holistic knowing is vital as people question and transform theologies and worldviews to reflect more fully on God–world relationships and evoke visions of ecological justice.

My working definition of practical wisdom is the embodied, accumulating knowledge and ethical insight that arise from human and creaturely experience of the world and the numinous. Note that I include the experience of both humans and other creatures, thus recognizing that trees and grasses and animals and people are knowing creatures, albeit in diverse ways, and they have capacities to communicate with one another. Further, all beings have multiple ways of relating with the earth—through senses and sensors, fact-gathering, intuitive or instinctive impulses, esthetic experience, and analysis. Both human and earth knowledge accumulate over time, and values are inherent in the knowing, e.g., the value of preserving life. For humans, practical wisdom is never complete, and it is never without ethical influence. It is a way of knowing and being in the world, and is critically important if we are to understand and respond well to the climate crisis.

3.1. Challenging Practical Wisdom

The dominant forms of practical wisdom neglect much of the world, often justifying social, economic, and ethnic stratifications and human abuses of land and seas for the sake of monetary or techno-industrial progress. Ecologists have long recognized the need to question dominant world views and theologies, seeking to replace individualistic views with communal ones; accents on progress with accents on well-being; anthropocentric views with ecocentric or cosmocentric ones; technological solutions with holistic ecological ones; focus on economic expansion with focus on sustaining and regenerating the ecology; political competition with communal collaboration; and hierarchies of power with deep listening to all beings of creation. I will focus here on the issues and insights posed by some of the most influential ecologists of the past 80 years, recognizing that equally important challenges and alternatives are offered by indigenous peoples, to whom I turn in the next section.

Aldo Leopold was an early pioneer in the modern ecological movement, especially with the posthumous publication of his seminal *A Sand County Almanac* (1949). He was far beyond his time in his understanding of the urgent need for compassion and justice for the whole natural world, including human beings, who were both a beneficiary and a danger to the rest of the natural world. Leopold's land ethic was a guide for human understanding and responsibility, though seriously marred by a lack of racial sensitivity and racist comments. He saw a contrast between conservation and Abrahamic concepts of land, which he identified with commodification. In his foreword, he argued, "We abuse land because we regard it as a commodity belonging to us. When we see land as a community to which we belong, we may begin to use it with love and respect" (Leopold [1949] 2013, pp. 16–17). *Herein lies a major challenge to practical wisdom—to reject worldviews of commodification and to understand the land as community.* An additional challenge has to be addressed to Leopold himself, namely *the challenge to question hierarchies of value, including those that value some peoples over others.*

Rachel Carson carried a different, but complementary, message. She was a marine biologist, ecologist, and science writer, who had a gift for communication in scientifically accurate, poetic prose, thus catching the attention of a broad public. In her earliest book, *Under the Sea Wind*, she told stories of sea animals—birds, fish, turtles, and other creatures—as they lived their daily lives (Carson [1941] 2007). This is a series of narratives that invite readers into the actual worlds of these creatures and their waters. Carson challenges the practical wisdom of viewing the world from human perspectives by narrating an ecology of life among animals related to the sea and one another. In sum, *she challenges dominant forms of practical wisdom by decentering human experience.* Carson ([1962] 2002) offers another challenge in her most famous book, *Silent Spring*, in which she explains the effects of chemicals and pesticides on humans and other living beings, focusing particularly on DDT and its uses in agriculture. Here *her challenge is twofold, revealing the permeability of humans to chemicals, to poisons and contaminants outside themselves, and revealing the enormous damage that can be done to people, plants, and land by chemical pesticides*. This particular work won widespread attention and eventually led to the elimination of DDT and other pesticides from U.S. agricultural use, but sadly not from exports.

Others continued the accents of Leopold and Carson. One of the people who explicitly raised issues of worldviews and practices was the educator Chet Bowers. He sought to connect ecojustice with educational practices in childhood, youth, and higher education (Bowers 1995, 1997, 2001, 2016). From 1974 to 2016, Bowers addressed *worldview challenges, explicitly worldviews grounded in individualism, progress, economic–political power, and human dominance over the earth*. He argued for a "deep cultural" movement, critiquing education for reproducing the very cultures that are destroying the earth by perpetuating the cultural myths that magnify ecological crises. Bowers decried simple answers, even the practice of blaming capitalism; he made a case that *all* assumptions need to be questioned (Edmundson 2017). As a fierce advocate for changes in worldview, he drew especially on indigenous traditions and values to discern and encourage cultural alternatives.

Many other advocates for ecological justice and flourishing have offered ecological alternatives and reshaped worldviews, drawing upon Christianity, Hinduism, Buddhism, Confucianism, indigenous traditions, and others (Grim and Tucker 2014; Tucker 2003; Vaughan-Lee 2016) and upon particular theological traditions such as African American (Baker-Fletcher 1998); Lutheran and ecumenical (Rasmussen 2015; Chicka 2019; Santmire 2020); and process–relational (Cobb 2020; Cobb and Castuera 2015; Birch and Cobb 1981). In all these and more, people have questioned and proposed alternatives for the development of practical wisdom, echoing the challenges named above.

Some ecological authors of the past 40 years have also highlighted the close relationship between environmental destruction and the ideological or physical crushing of women and the poor. Women have frequently raised issues of the mutually reinforcing oppression of the earth, women, and marginalized peoples (Johnson and Wilkinson 2020; Shiva 2015, 2016a, 2016b; Ruether 1995, 1996, 2006; Gebara 1999, 2003; Halkes 1989). Some compilations have brought together voices of women across the world (Ruether 2006) and activist women in diverse cultures and roles (Johnson and Wilkinson 2020). In addition to analyzing gender, gender identities, and environmental perspectives, these women often identify with and speak strongly on behalf of the poor, as do liberation theologians across the world (Boff [1997] 2000). The cries of the earth and the cries of the poor are intertwined. *The challenge is to explore ecological crises from the perspective of multiple religious and cultural traditions and multiple oppressions.*

I have portrayed some of the early work associated with the ecological justice movement to reveal the wide range of concerns and ideas from the 1940s to the present. What is still lacking is the hard work of listening deeply to one another and the earth itself, and the close questioning and reshaping of practical wisdom. What is also lacking is attention by practical theologians to issues of ecological justice and the climate crisis in particular. Pamela McCarroll has diagnosed the situation well, identifying the anthropocentrism of methods and goals in practical theology and in Western theologies more generally, together with the spreading of eco-anxiety that can stimulate defensiveness and thwart action (McCarroll 2020). HyeRan Kim-Cragg's critique is similar, with an emphasis also on the destructive forces of colonialism (Kim-Cragg 2018), as highlighted above by Gilio-Whitaker and others. While practical theologians have made a case for the field's engagement with public theology (Graham 2013; Forrester 2004) and social witness (Ayres 2019b), direct engagement with ecological injustice and crises is limited to fewer works (such as (Ayres 2013, 2019a, 2019b; McCarroll 2020; Kim-Cragg 2018)), even in the face of climate catastrophe. *The challenge now is to study both human and nonhuman practices—practices of trees and rivers and antelope—and to assess and reshape practical wisdom accordingly, so that daily life, community activism, and political action will be transformed.*

3.2. Stretching Practical Wisdom

To live toward a new future, we need to do more than analyze challenges; we need to stretch the largely white Western inheritance of practical wisdom. The previous section offered an arc of ecological concerns from the 1940s to the present, drawing largely on North American ecological leaders, mostly white. By itself, this approach is flawed. Gilio-Whitaker (2019) critiques the crediting of Rachel Carson's *Silent Spring* in 1962 and the first Earth Day in 1970 as the origins of a modern ecological movement, offering a more complex perspective. She especially decries the nineteenth century naturalists, such as John Muir, whose environmental perspectives were grounded in human superiority and colonial views of indigenous people. As much as they contributed, these hierarchy-oriented naturalists left a heritage that continues today in colonial approaches to the earth and to indigenous people. She encourages people to seek a fuller history (pp. 106–110). Thus, I turn primarily to North American indigenous authors in this section as they point to wider wisdom of the earth. In so doing, I acknowledge that other voices also need to be discussed in another work, voices from Africa, Latin America, Asia, Europe, and the Pacific. This too is urgent, as argued by Vanessa Nakate, a young Ugandan activist who decries the dismissal of African voices and points toward a "bigger picture" (Nakate 2021).

Dina Gilio-Whitaker lays much of the ecological crisis at the foot of colonial modes of theorizing and structuring the world, documenting case after case in which the domination of indigenous people and the destruction of ecosystems went hand in hand. She offers a sharp critique, supported by details of cases, laws, history, and activist efforts. She also describes traditions that undergird much indigenous life, including "a philosophical paradigm very different from that of dominant Western society," a paradigm that is often ignored in legal decisions and practices of appropriation (p. 157). She elaborates on the connections that indigenous people have with their homelands—the lack of "separation between people and land, between people and other life forms, or between people and their ancient ancestors whose bones are infused in the land they inhabit" (p. 157.). Others have also accented the profound connections indigenous people have with place and land, such as Vine Deloria, Jr., and George Tinker.

How can people in non-indigenous cultures value and learn from indigenous peoples without abusing and distorting their sacred traditions? The challenges of those traditions to most Western worldviews are so vital that we need to find ways to learn without objectifying and to collaborate without dominating or colonizing. Fortunately, some authors point the way, even as they warn about the dangers noted above. Sherri Mitchell, of the Penobscot people of Maine and the Maritimes, is an advocate of people's learning from one another and seeking harmony, even as she narrates massacres, Indian school tragedies, displacements, destruction of land, and the trauma of her people. She recognizes that the United States "was founded on genocide and slavery" (Mitchell 2013, p. 69), yet she appeals to the potential for healing. Her starting point is to recognize that humanity is at "a teetering point of choice that will determine the future of all life" (p. 22). Mitchell's vision is to weave Penobscot teachings with other views to harmonize and align "with common purpose," a vision of oneness without sameness (p. 23). To that end, she shares the sacred teachings of her people and invites readers to listen to and respect all living things (p. 28). Writing with a sense of urgency, she recognizes that the human family is on "the precipice of an evolutionary leap, one that requires us to transcend our differences and integrate into a more harmonized way of being" (p. 40).

Mitchell's gift is sharing the history and teachings of her people, paired with a vision of a world that can be. Her approach suggests how people might learn from one another and from all living things as they join in stretching practical wisdom. Robin Wall Kimmerer (2013) builds in a similar direction in *Braiding Sweetgrass*. She describes the worldviews of her Potawatomi people, a Native nation originating between Lake Michigan and Lake Huron (later dispersed) and akin to other tribes and first nations of the Great Lakes region in worldview, language, and life practices. Kimmerer herself lives and teaches in upstate New York, where she explores and lives with forests and family. In her writing, she narrates the life of plants and her life among them, drawing from her knowledge as an environmental and forest biologist and the lifeways and traditions of her people. Like Mitchell, she understands her writing as an offering and an invitation for others to learn from the wisdom of her people and the life of plants.

Kimmerer highlights details that I identify as practical wisdom. She describes the wisdom of pecan trees that have airborne communication systems (via pheromones) to warn other trees against pests and connections, which in turn produce defensive chemicals. Pecan trees are also connected underground via fungi and fungal strands that, based on current evidence, gather the excess carbohydrates from some trees to share with others, thus spreading the bounty and enabling the whole pecan grove to bear pecans at the same time, rather than creating a divide between bearing and non-bearing trees. She sees the communication systems as the ways that trees talk with one another as her ancestors taught her to believe (pp. 11–21, esp. 19–21).

Kimmerer also describes the gifts of wild strawberries and black ash, living interdependently with the Potawatomi people, who gratefully receive nourishment from the strawberries and basket makings from the black ash, while other animals also receive from them and while people care for the plants and trees by careful selection and pruning (pp. 22–32, 141–55). Kimmerer further describes what she learns from maple trees and grasses and how they live mutually with other life forms in their habitats (pp. 63–71, 156–166). For the Potawatomi, primal values are grounded in gratitude and the aliveness of creation, which inspire practices of mutuality and reciprocity for the sake of the living whole.

Kimmerer further stretches practical wisdom as she describes the living nature of her native language, learned as an adult. Baffled by the complexity of words and grammatical structures, she experienced an epiphany when her sister sent her a box of word tiles and an Ojibwe dictionary, given the close relationship between her language and that of Ojibwe people. Kimmerer was ready to quit when she discovered an unusual word, "to be a Saturday" (p. 66). How could a noun be expressed in verb form? She reacted: "I grabbed the dictionary and flipped more pages and all kinds of things seemed to be verbs: 'to be a hill,' 'to be red,' 'to be a long sandy stretch of beach,' and then my finger rested on *wiikwegamaa*: 'to be a bay,' 'Ridiculous!'" Then, in a sudden moment of realization, she could smell and see and hear the bay. The moment was an epiphany: "A bay is a noun only if water is *dead*. When *bay* is a noun, it is defined by humans, trapped between its shores and contained by the word. But the verb *wiikwegamaa*—to *be* a bay—releases the water from bondage and lets it live" (p. 66.). The practical wisdom conveyed in these language forms communicates that everything is alive. Kimmerer calls this "the language of animacy," and the animacy extends to rocks and mountains, fire and places, and medicines and songs (p. 67). I have shared Kimmerer's discovery to reveal the nature of practical wisdom, embodied in language and in the relationships of pecans, strawberries, maple trees, and black ash with their habitats and the plants, people, and other animals that dwell therein.

Kimmerer's discoveries are not unique to her or her people. The Hopi language, while different from the Potawatomi, is also marked by relationships and movement, as discovered long ago by linguist Benjamin Lee Whorf (1956). He noted that the Hopi word to describe a wave in the ocean is not an isolated "wave"; rather, it appears in multiple verb forms that indicate a range of movement, such as sloshing, "kicking up a sea," or undulating. The words describe movements of the water in relationship with the sea, rather than isolating the wave from the movement in which it flows (pp. 52–53). Whorf explains that the Hopi preference for verbs contrasts with the English preference for nouns; thus, the Hopi language "perpetually turns our propositions about *things* into propositions about *events*" (p. 63). Space and time are merged, as are subjects and predicates.

Whorf's analysis of the complex Hopi language is more nuanced than my summary, but one can see the movement nature of the language, which echoes Kimmerer's description of movement in Potawatomi and Ojibwe languages. Whorf also observes connections between language and worldviews; "Most metaphysical words in Hopi are verbs, not nouns as in European languages" (p. 61). Language has the power to shape and be shaped by worldviews; thus, people do not experience time and matter in the same ways because their experiences are mediated through diverse languages (p. 158). Language affects what people experience, and their experiences help shape language.

I have shared in some detail the teachings of indigenous peoples, pecan trees and wild strawberries, and diverse languages, all stretching the limits of practical wisdom in North America. If we are to respond well to a weeping planet, we need to face the limitations of the assumed wisdom that modern/postmodern people have inherited within a techno-industrialized, progress-seeking, individual-focused, capital-oriented society. We need to stretch practical wisdom in order to learn from many ancestors (including our own), many living beings, many language worlds, and the spiritual experiences and instructions of peoples living closely with the earth.

3.3. Reshaping Practical Wisdom

Practical wisdom is not sufficient if we hold tightly to dominant views and relational patterns, which keep us inside the confines of prevailing assumptions. What is needed first is *to face the limits of dominant views and patterns, and to stretch our own ways of thinking and relating* by engaging deeply and respectfully with the assumptive realities of diverse peoples, including ourselves. Second, we need *to engage with the traditions, texts, and practices of our own religious communities*, as exemplified by many who have explored questions about God, Christology, creation, and planetary well-being in Christian tradition (Copeland 2020a; Keller 2017; McFague 2008, 2021). These authors and others engage in the process of reshaping practical wisdom in dialogue with the traditions of Christianity. Another approach is generating new work on biblical texts. One representative of that work is Rebecca Copeland, who approaches texts with ecomimetic interpretation in which she invites readers to identify with the nonhuman characters in a text, such as the characters of water, birds, leaves (Copeland 2020b, 2020c, 2021). Such an approach decenters human-centered interpretations, and it also opens fresh questions and insights. Third, we need *to touch–see–listen–taste–smell the living earth*, receiving its wisdom and relating with mutuality. Such engagement contributes to reverence for wisdom itself, for ourselves and others, for the earth, and for the numinous.

These approaches magnify the potential for stretching and reshaping practical wisdom as we engage with ourselves, with the wisdom of diverse peoples and traditions, with the trees and seas, and with the sacred. In the next section we turn to practices that can enhance our human ability to critique and reshape practical wisdom, at the same time reshaping ethical values and relationships so we might respond to a weeping planet.

4. Life Practices

In the face of crisis, practices are critical, intertwined with the practical wisdom that shapes and is reshaped by practice. The significance of practice is clear in Rachel Carson's close observation of sea creatures, and Robin Wall Kimmerer's existential and scientific engagement with wild strawberries and pecan trees, and her study of the Potawatomi language. Here I identify four practices that are important to reshaping and deepening practical wisdom for ecological justice: attending, searching, imagining, and communal living and acting. To ground the proposals, I draw especially on the wisdom of activist scholars and scholar activists.

4.1. Attending

Virtually all writing on ecological justice begins with attending—attending to the gifts of the earth; the lives of plant and animal creatures and water, rocks, and soil; and the tragedies of land and habitat destruction, carbon escalation, heavy burdens on poor and marginalized communities, and global warming. Living in reverent relation with the ecological community is an important starting point for reshaping theologies, worldviews, and practices. Reverence begins with attending: being present to, learning from, and caring with and for creation.

Diana Ventura describes the central method of practical theology as "prayerful attentiveness for human flourishing" (Ventura 2021), a definition rich in possibility. I propose stretching her definition to "prayerful attentiveness for cosmic flourishing." The term "prayerful" suggests a posture of openness to all that the world has to communicate, including the sacred endowment of every being. "Attentiveness" suggests that people open all their senses so they may experience the fullness of the earth in living detail. The aim of cosmic flourishing embraces and cares for the whole of creation. Following this path, practical theologians would attend to shrinking wetlands, communities suffering from food insecurity, and trees and forests. Their attending would not only include the damage and destruction thrust on these communities, but also the lifegiving practices of the wetlands, communities, and trees themselves, practices that reveal their beauty, strength, and potential. Others have already paved this pathway in works such as *The Hidden Life of Trees* (Wohlleben 2016) and *The Songs of Trees* (Haskell 2018). To be attentive is to walk among the trees and wetlands, opening to their wisdom, and to engage in interdisciplinary study so foresters like Wohlleben and biologists like Haskell and Kimmerer can teach us and awaken our senses.

Attending requires that we use all our senses beyond seeing and hearing, which often function as primary in Western societies. I advocate, with Richard Kearney, the practice of touch, which he calls our "most vital sense" (Kearney 2021). If we are to attend to creatures of the natural world, we need to touch and smell and taste as well as see and hear. All the senses reveal uniquely, and each can be employed as appropriate to the subject of our attending. Touching and smelling a leaf or the soil of a farm reveal far more than sight alone.

Attending also requires that we observe communities and systems, as Leopold, Bowers, Boff, Gilio-Whitaker, and Kim-Cragg have done. Separating land from people, one creature from others, a wave from an ocean, a tree from a forest will distort our knowing. Relationality is vital to understand if we are to expand practical wisdom. Climate scientist Katharine Hayhoe has discovered that the best way to communicate climate change with other people is to point out the tangible effects of climate on what matters most to them. She does not try to convince people to elevate the priority of climate change, but to recognize how climate change affects the issues they already hold as top priorities: health, families, jobs, the economy, community well-being, and the well-being of persons on the margins (Hayhoe 2020, pp. 136–37). Hayhoe is doing more here than offering practical advice; she is underscoring the importance of attending to communities and systems—to wholes. Attending to systemic relationships can uncover surprises, as when ecologist Jane Zelikova traces the relationship of ants with the seed dispersal of trees and climate change (Zelikova 2020, pp. 335–36). Attending involves observation and reflection on both details and wholes in the ecosystem.

Practical theologian Jennifer Ayres has offered a good example of attending to details and wholes in her work on food (Ayres 2013), which narrates particular stories and events as well as food systems, attending to them directly and through the work of others. Attending is a pathway to better understanding and action, deepening our practical wisdom and living practices.

4.2. Searching

A second practice arises from the first, namely searching. Knowing and relating with the earth requires an attitude of openness, curiosity, and humility. Just as Kimmerer (2013) was eager to understand the plants in the pond behind her home, so Mitchell (2018) and Gilio-Whitaker (2019) were eager to understand the relationship between colonialism and ecological destruction. So, also, was Carson ([1962] 2002) eager to learn the effects of chemical pesticides on human, animal, and plant life. In all these cases, the authors searched to increase their understanding and guide their action, whether the action was cleaning a pond, political advocacy, or the elimination of pesticides in agriculture. These author-activists shed light on the future work of practical theologians: (1) searching the ecosystems in our home contexts to inspire awe and inform our understanding and action; (2) searching the practices of congregations and people of faith; and (3) searching sacred texts, ritual patterns, and religious structures and practices to reflect on the teachings and values therein, and to critique and reshape them when we find them lacking.

Searching is a familiar theme in practical theology, one that is clearly important to a discipline rich in research and effective in shaping actions for the common good. Wanda Stahl, for example, has engaged in a long-term study of Wild Churches to discover their congregational practices and embedded theologies and values (Stahl 2021). The Wild Churches regularly gather in community in their local habitat (often with pets), and they reshape practical wisdom as they do. Stahl has discovered that their theologies often change over time, moving toward pan*en*theism and an accent on salvation for the whole planet.

Searching is a form of opening ourselves to that which we have only glimpsed, have never encountered, or have been avoiding. It is also a form of seeking reversals or asking hard questions (Moore 2004, chp. 5; 2021). The searching process can fill gaps in a community's knowing, or present major challenges as new discoveries, radical questions, and alternative futures unfold. It is not purely intellectual work, however, but quiet, meditative work as well. In theistic contexts, searching includes spiritual opening and discernment of God's movements, as well as complex deliberations on God and the world, and analysis of climate change and other crises. Searching is an endless practice, but it enriches the lives of searchers and the communities in which they live.

4.3. Imagining

Responding to crises also requires imagination, the capacity to discern opportunities and alternate futures. Imagination is grounded in the world that people know through life encounters and study. At the same time, imagination transcends the "known" world and soars into a world of possibility, offering a potential antidote to human despair and passivity, anger and blame, and life-defying ideas about God and the earth. Consider the ways ecological despair permeates the lives of individuals and communities, perpetuating a sense that no action can ever make a difference. Consider the patterns of blame that block people from considering new information and new possibilities. Consider the sense of hopelessness that is reinforced by theologies centered on original sin or on popular beliefs that humans are autonomous, self-serving beings.

One practice vital to imagination is storytelling. Kendra Pierre-Louis has focused on the problems and possibilities of narratives in telling ecological stories and spinning tales of new possibilities. She argues that some stories create problems for ecological responses, actively "hurting us" (Pierre-Louis 2020, p. 175). She offers an alternate story of the Wakanda, a fictional, roughly historical country in Africa that uses technology to maintain ecological health. She encourages readers to search for and create stories that narrate climate change as an opportunity (p. 179), seeking new and ancient stories; stories in sacred texts and traditions; and stories in our daily lives. The possibilities for stirring imagination through stories are boundless.

4.4. Communal Living and Acting

If we are to respond to the climate crisis with more full-bodied practical wisdom and robust action, we need to begin with community, embracing historical, contemporary, and ecological communities. Individualism is widely credited as a major factor in climate crisis and ecological destruction. The practical wisdom sought in this essay is accessible only through community, particular and global, human and nonhuman. When I wrote *Ministering with the Earth* (Moore 1998), I already knew that hope for the earth depended on an interdependent, intersubjective relationship between the human family and the rest of creation, hence ministering *with* the earth. I have come to see far more complexity in that relationship and the urgency of radically reshaping practical wisdom and relationships if we are to practice "with." Responding to the climate crisis requires far-reaching changes in the ways we relate to and conceptualize the world, ways we live and act in community. Where do we begin?

I propose three paths of practice for communal living and acting. First is to remember the communities from which we come, the peoples and lands that have made us who we are and depend on us for their well-being. The memories may be sweet or harsh or bland, but they are part of the universe with which we are related. Many of the authors in this article share memories of people and lands that have formed them (Mitchell 2018; Kimmerer 2013), recognizing the formative and transformative power of memory. Memory could be included much more actively in practical theological research and action, searching the memories revealed in communities (human and nonhuman), habitats, religious practices, and literature and folklore.

If we are to respond to a weeping planet, a second path is to *draw upon the legacies of people and waters and lands to guide environmental action*. Those legacies will be mixed in their values, but critical awareness of multiple legacies is vital if we are to uncover fresh perspectives on climate protection and regeneration in a time of extreme urgency. Many of the human legacies will be offered by peoples whose ancestries or ways of living in the world are non-dominant. Tara Houska is one who awakened me when she highlighted the difference between life with her people (Zhaabowekwe, Couchiching First Nation) and the practices of environmental protection in corporate boardrooms, in which metrics and campaign outcomes dominate (Houska 2020, pp. 257–59). How might ecological leaders and practical theologians reshape environmental action and climate crisis if we reshaped standard boardroom procedure to account for the legacies of people who live close to the earth? Might board members spend more time walking the land, observing the life patterns of plants and animals, listening to people's stories, observing the geological and climatological patterns, and seeking truly radical approaches to the climate crisis?

Many people have drawn their ecological inspiration from the legacies of human and earth communities. Rachel Carson ([1962] 2002) lived closely with the legacies of oceans and farmlands as she reshaped scientific communication and farming practices. Heather Toney (2020) turned to her African American community and the eco-system to guide her in leading environmental organizations and serving as Mayor of Greenville, Mississippi. Her community legacy fed her, and she laments that communities are usually ignored in facing ecological issues, even though they are "vital for identifying real solutions" (p. 102).

A third path of practice is to *create new experiments and patterns of living in and with communities, local and global.* Practical theologians focus on many areas of life, so the potential actions are many. Leah Penniman (2018) draws upon the wisdom of her African American ancestors to create Soul Fire Farm and to practice farming in a way that is sustainable and life-giving today, guided by their wisdom. Chet Bowers (2001) proposes new approaches to teaching that will reshape cultures and foster community, rather than reinforce individualism and separation from the nonhuman natural world. Networks of women across the world have shared ecological wisdom to change the way human beings conceptualize and live in the world (Johnson and Wilkinson 2020; Gebara 1999, 2003; Ruether 2006; Halkes 1989). Further, many environmental leaders have sought to build coalitions based on common concerns for moms, food justice, water or land protection, justice for communities of color, and so forth. These efforts all focus on community.

I have erred on the side of sharing many narratives because practical theologians need the wisdom of many persons, communities, creatures, and habitats if we are to respond to the weeping planet. We can no longer prevent climate crisis; the crisis is here. We *can* still respond to the crisis with a full range of proactive, anticipatory, and reactive responses. All are needed to prevent further destruction and to help regenerate that which can be regenerated. Can you imagine a community of practical theologians who accept responsibility to act with and for the good of our planetary community? We could become a network of scholars and activists who learn from the wisdom of diverse peoples and forests and deserts, seeking together to halt global warming and heal the earth.

Funding: This project received no external funding.

Institutional Review Board Statement: Not applicable.

Informed Consent Statement: Not applicable.

Conflicts of Interest: The author declares no conflict of interest.

References

Ayres, Jennifer R. 2013. *Good Food: Grounded Practical Theology*. Waco: Baylor University.
Ayres, Jennifer R. 2019a. *Inhabitance: Ecological Religious Education*. Waco: Baylor University.
Ayres, Jennifer R. 2019b. *Waiting for a Glacier to Move: Practicing Social Witness*. Eugene: Wipf & Stock.
Baker-Fletcher, Karen. 1998. *Sisters of Dust, Sisters of Spirit: Womanist Wordings on God and Creation*. Minneapolic: Fortress.
Birch, Charles, and John B. Cobb Jr. 1981. *The Liberation of Life: From the Cell to the Community*. Cambridge: Cambridge University.
Boff, Leonardo. 2000. *Cry of the Earth, Cry of the Poor*. Translated by Phillip Berryman. Maryknoll: Orbis. First published 1997.
Bowers, Chet A. 1995. *Educating for an Ecologically Sustainable Culture*. Albany: SUNY.
Bowers, Chet A. 1997. *The Culture of Denial: Why the Environmental Movement Needs a Strategy for Reforming Universities and Public Schools*. Albany: SUNY.
Bowers, Chet A. 2001. *Educating for Ecojustice and Community*. Athens: University of Georgia.
Bowers, Chet A. 2016. *Reforming Higher Education: In an Era of Ecological Crisis and Growing Digital Insecurity*. Anoka: Process Century Press.
Browning, Don S. 1991. *A Fundamental Practical Theology: Descriptive and Strategic Proposals*. Minneapolis: Fortress.
Carson, Rachel. 2002. *Silent Spring*. 40th Anniversary Edition. New York: Houghton Mifflin Harcourt. First published 1962.
Carson, Rachel. 2007. *Under the Sea Wind*. New York: Penguin. First published 1941.
Chicka, Jessica. 2019. God, Self, Humanity, Earth: Christian Ecological Ethics in Local Contexts. Ph.D. dissertation, Boston University School of Theology, Boston, MA, USA.
Cobb, John B., Jr. 2020. *Salvation: Jesus' Mission and Ours*. Anoka: Process Century Press.
Cobb, John B., Jr., and Ignacio Castuera, eds. 2015. *For Our Common Home: Process-Relational Responses to Laudato Si'*. Anoka: Process Century Press.
Copeland, Rebecca L. 2020a. *Created Being: Expanding Creedal Christology*. Waco: Baylor University.
Copeland, Rebecca L. 2020b. 'Their Leaves Shall Be for Healing': Ecological Trauma and Recovery in Ezekiel 47:1–12. *Biblical Theology Bulletin* 49: 214–22. [CrossRef]
Copeland, Rebecca L. 2020c. Women, Wells, and Springs: Water Rights and Hagar's Tribulations. *Biblical Theology Bulletin* 50: 191–99. [CrossRef]
Copeland, Rebecca L. 2021. Ecomimetic Interpretation: Ascertainment, Identification, and Dialogue in Matthew 6:25–34. *Biblical Interpretation* 29: 67–89. [CrossRef]
Edmundson, Jeff. 2017. In Memoriam: Chet Bowers. *Educational Studies* 53: 671. [CrossRef]
Forrester, Duncan B. 2004. *Christian Justice and Public Policy*. Cambridge: Cambridge University.
Gebara, Ivonne. 1999. *Longing for Running Water: Ecofeminism and Liberation*. Minneapolis: Fortress.
Gebara, Ivonne. 2003. Ecofeminism: An Ethics of Life. In *Ecofeminism and Globalization: Exploring Culture, Context, and Religion*. Edited by Heather Eaton and Lois A. Lorentzen. Lanham: Rowman and Littlefield, pp. 163–76.
Gilio-Whitaker, Dino. 2019. *As Long as Grass Grows: The Indigenous Fight for Environmental Justice from Colonization to Standing Rock*. Boston: Beacon.
Graham, Elaine. 2013. *Between a Rock and a Hard Place: Public Theology in a Post-Secular Age*. London: SCM.
Grim, John, and Mary Evelyn Tucker. 2014. *Ecology and Religion*. Washington, DC: Island Press.
Halkes, Catharina J. M. 1989. *New Creation: Christian Feminism and the Renewal of the Earth*. Louisville: Westminster/John Knox.
Haskell, David George. 2018. *The Songs of Trees: Stories from Nature's Great Connectors*. New York: Penguin.
Hayhoe, Katharine. 2020. How to Talk about Climate Change. In *All We Can Save: Truth, Courage, and Solutions for Climate Crisis*. Edited by Ayana Elizabeth Johnson and Katharine K. Wilkinson. New York: One World, Penguin Random House, pp. 133–40.
Houska, Tara. 2020. Sacred Resistance. In *All We Can Save: Truth, Courage, and Solutions for Climate Crisis*. Edited by Ayana Elizabeth Johnson and Katharine K. Wilkinson. New York: One World, Penguin Random House, pp. 257–64.
IPCC—Intergovernmental Panel on Climate Change. 2021. *Climate Change 2021: The Physical Science Basis. Contribution of Working Group I to the Sixth Assessment Report of the Intergovernmental Panel on Climate Change*. Edited by Valérie Masson-Delmotte, Panmao Zhai, Anna Pirani, Sarah L. Connors, Clotilde Péan, Sophie Berger, Nada Caud, Yang Chen, Leah Goldfarb, Melissa I. Gomis and et al. Cambridge: Cambridge University, *in press*.

IPCC—Intergovernmental Panel on Climate Change. 2022. *Climate Change 2022: Impacts, Adaptation, and Vulnerability. Contribution of Working Group II to the Sixth Assessment Report of the Intergovernmental Panel on Climate Change*. Edited by Hans-O. Pörtner, Debra C. Roberts, Melinda Tignor, Elvira S. Poloczanska, Katja Mintenbeck, Andrés Alegría, Marlies Craig, Stefanie Langsdorf, Sina Löschke, Vincent Möller and et al. Cambridge: Cambridge University Press, in press.

Johnson, Ayana Elizabeth, and Katharine K. Wilkinson, eds. 2020. *All We Can Save: Truth, Courage, and Solutions for the Climate Crisis*. New York: One World, Penguin Random House.

Kearney, Richard. 2021. *Touch: Recovering Our Most Vital Sense*. New York: Columbia University.

Keller, Catherine. 2017. *Intercarnations: Exercises in Theological Possibility*. New York: Fordham University.

Kim-Cragg, HyeRan. 2018. *Interdependence: A Postcolonial Feminist Practical Theology*. Eugene: Pickwick, pp. 128–49.

Kimmerer, Robin Wall. 2013. *Braiding Sweetgrass: Indigenous Wisdom, Scientific Knowledge, and the Teachings of Plants*. Minneapolis: Milkweed Editions.

Leopold, Aldo. 2013. *A Sand County Almanac and Sketches Here and There*. Edited by Curt Meine. New York: Literary Classics of the United States, Inc. First published 1949.

McCarroll, Pamela R. 2020. Listening for the Cries of the Earth: Practical Theology in the Anthropocene. *International Journal of Practical Theology* 24: 29–46. [CrossRef]

McFague, Sallie. 2008. *A New Climate for Theology: God, the World, and Global Warming*. Minneapolis: 1517 Media, Augsburg Fortress.

McFague, Sallie. 2021. *A New Climate for Christology: Kenosis, Climate Change, and Befriending Nature*. Minneapolis: Fortress.

McKibben, Bill. 2013. *Oil and Honey: The Education of an Unlikely Activist*. New York: Henry Holt and Co.

Mitchell, Sherri. 2018. *Sacred Instructions: Indigenous Wisdom for Living Spirit-Based Change*. Berkeley: North Atlantic Books.

Moore, Mary Elizabeth. 1998. *Ministering with the Earth*. St. Louis: Chalice.

Moore, Mary Elizabeth. 2004. *Teaching as a Sacramental Act*. Cleveland: Pilgrim.

Moore, Mary Elizabeth. 2021. The Hidden Force of Gender and Sexuality: A Pedagogy of Truth-Seeking. *Religious Education* 116: 440–53. [CrossRef]

Nakate, Vanessa. 2021. *A Bigger Picture: My Fight to Bring a New African Voice to the Climate Crisis*. New York: Mariner Books, HarperCollins.

Penniman, Leah. 2018. *Farming While Black: Soul Fire Farm's Practical Guide to Liberation on the Land*. White River Junction: Chelsea Green.

Pierre-Louis, Kendra. 2020. Wakanda Doesn't Have Suburbs. In *All We Can Save: Truth, Courage, and Solutions for the Climate Crisis*. Edited by Ayana Elizabeth Johnson and Katharine K. Wilkinson. New York: One World.

Rasmussen, Larry L. 2015. *Earth-Honoring Faith: Religious Ethics in a New Key*. Oxford: Oxford University.

Ruether, Rosemary Radford, ed. 1996. *Women Healing Earth: Third World Women on Ecology, Feminism, and Religion*. Maryknoll: Orbis.

Ruether, Rosemary Radford. 1995. Ecofeminism: Symbolic and Social Connections of the Oppression of Women and the Domination of Nature. *Feminist Theology* 3: 35–50. [CrossRef]

Ruether, Rosemary Radford. 2006. Religious Ecofeminism: Healing the Ecological Crisis. In *The Oxford Handbook of Religion and Ecology*. Edited by Roger S. Gottlieb. Oxford: Oxford University, pp. 1–14.

Santmire, Paul. 2020. *Celebrating Nature by Faith: Studies in Reformation Theology in an Era of Global Emergency*. Eugene: Cascade.

Shiva, Vandana. 2015. *Soil Not Oil: Environmental Justice in an Age of Climate Crisis*. Berkeley: North Atlantic Books.

Shiva, Vandana. 2016a. *Staying Alive: Women, Ecology, and Development*. Berkeley: North Atlantic Books.

Shiva, Vandana. 2016b. *The Violence of the Green Revolution: Third World Agriculture, Ecology, and Politics*. Lexington: University Press of Kentucky.

Stahl, Wanda J. 2021. Healing Our Divide with the Nonhuman World: Theological Foundations and Pedagogical Practices within the Wild Church Network. *Religious Education* 117: 61–73. [CrossRef]

Toney, Heather McTeer. 2020. Collards Are Just as Good as Kale. In *All We Can Save: Truth, Courage, and Solutions for the Climate Crisis*. Edited by Ayana Elizabeth Johnson and Katharine K. Wilkinson. New York: One World, Penguin Random House, pp. 100–9.

Tucker, Mary Evelyn. 2003. *Worldly Wonder: Religions Enter their Ecological Phase*. Chicago: Open Court.

Vaughan-Lee, Llewellyn, ed. 2016. *Spiritual Ecology: The Cry of the Earth*, 2nd ed. Point Reyes: The Golden Sufi Center.

Ventura, Diana. 2021. Prayerful Attentiveness: A Practical Theological Approach Toward Disability and Health. Paper presented at the Center for Practical Theology Annual Lecture, Boston University School of Theology, Boston, MA, USA, November 9.

Whorf, Benjamin Lee. 1956. *Language, Thought and Reality: Selected Writings of Benjamin Lee Whorf*. Edited by John B. Carroll. New York: MIT and John Wiley & Sons, Available online: https://ia802605.us.archive.org/7/items/languagethoughtr00whor/languagethoughtr00whor.pdf (accessed on 10 January 2022).

Wohlleben, Peter. 2016. *The Hidden Life of Trees: What They Feel, How They Communicate-Discoveries from A Secret World*. Translated by Jane Billinghurst. Vancouver: Greystone Books.

Zelikova, Jane. 2020. Solutions Underfoot. In *All We Can Save: Truth, Courage, and Solutions for Climate Crisis*. Edited by Ayana Elizabeth Johnson and Katharine K. Wilkinson. New York: One World, Penguin Random House, pp. 335–41.

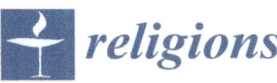

Article

Embodying Theology: Trauma Theory, Climate Change, Pastoral and Practical Theology

Pamela R. McCarroll

Emmanuel College of Victoria University, University of Toronto, Toronto, ON M5S 1K7, Canada; pam.mccarroll@utoronto.ca

Abstract: Since 2009, the amount of literature focused on the psychological and social dimensions of the climate crisis has increased exponentially. This growing interest in the topic is signaled especially in the American Psychological Association (APA)'s multiple reports on the mental health impacts of climate change. More recently, across different disciplines, links have also been made between trauma theory and the climate crisis. These rich discussions include overlapping concerns, areas of potential fruitfulness and theological implications for all the practical theological disciplines, especially for pastoral theology and practices of care. Given the implicitly existential, theological and spiritual dimensions embedded in the realities of both trauma and the climate crisis, there is an important opportunity for pastoral theology in particular, and practical theology more generally, to engage, learn from and contribute to the interdisciplinary conversation. In this paper, I first offer a brief overview of the literature in pastoral theology related to the climate crisis. Second, I present literature specifically on trauma theory and the climate crisis, outlining several of the key themes emerging across the interdisciplinary discussion. Third, I reflect theologically on the presented content, discussing and drawing forward areas of theological, epistemological and practical fruitfulness for practical and pastoral theology.

Keywords: climate trauma; eco-anxiety; climate crisis; ecological emotions; practical theology; pastoral theology; earth-centered; decolonizing; trauma theory; trauma-informed

Citation: McCarroll, Pamela R. 2022. Embodying Theology: Trauma Theory, Climate Change, Pastoral and Practical Theology. *Religions* 13: 294. https://doi.org/10.3390/rel13040294

Academic Editor: John Jillions

Received: 23 February 2022
Accepted: 24 March 2022
Published: 29 March 2022

Publisher's Note: MDPI stays neutral with regard to jurisdictional claims in published maps and institutional affiliations.

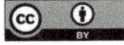

Copyright: © 2022 by the author. Licensee MDPI, Basel, Switzerland. This article is an open access article distributed under the terms and conditions of the Creative Commons Attribution (CC BY) license (https://creativecommons.org/licenses/by/4.0/).

1. Introduction

The literature linking climate change with mental health, psychology and social processes began to proliferate following the American Psychological Association's (APA) first large report on the topic (Swim et al. 2009). Since then, the amount of literature on the topic has increased exponentially. Clayton and Manning identify three primary areas of focus "in somewhat chronological order ... first, ways in which people perceive and come to understand climate change; second, human behavioral responses to climate change; and third, impacts of climate change on human health and well-being." (Clayton and Manning 2018, p. 5). Policy makers and those involved in risk mitigation and adaptation in relation to future modelling for climate change have also shown interest in the individual and collective psychological dynamics anticipated in the face of natural disasters, the destruction of infrastructures of transportation, power and water, food shortages and threats to global security. (Berzonsky and Moser 2017; Moser 2012, 2020). Additionally, researchers beyond the disciplines of pastoral and practical theology have begun to consider this research in relation to cosmological frameworks, spirituality and spiritual practices (see, for example, B. Roszak 1995; Albrecht 2019; Fisher 2013).

Many terms have arisen within and beyond the field of psychology to describe the kinds of emotions and mental health impacts of the climate crisis on individuals and communities. While this paper focuses specifically on the links between trauma and the climate crisis, it is helpful to locate our topic within the larger body of research around climate emotions. Environmental philosopher, Glenn Albrecht has coined several terms to identify specific emotional phenomena experienced in the face of different aspects of the environmental crisis. Most notable is the term *solastalgia* to describe the sense of deep homesickness experienced by humans whose home and habitat have been destroyed by climate disasters (Albrecht 2011, 2019). His recent book, *Earth Emotions* (Albrecht 2019), includes some terms well known in the field and others that are new. In large measure, the growing taxonomy for climate related emotions draws from early sources in the Ecopsychology movement of the 1990s with the work of Betty and Theodore Roszak and our own Howard Clinebell, to name a few. For example, terms such as *biophilia* and *biophobia* (Roszak et al. 1995; Clinebell [1996] 2013) are taken up by Albrecht to refer to the phenomena of love, reverence and awe for the earth, on the one hand, and fear, disgust and rejection of the earth on the other. Similarly, *ecoalienation* and *ecobonding* (Clinebell [1996] 2013) have also found new resonance in more recent research (Fisher 2013). These terms both speak to the extent to which a human individual or community is in 'right relationship' with the earth—alienated from or bonded with the earth. *Ecological grief* (or eco-grief) was an area of focus early in the Ecopsychology movement (Clinebell [1996] 2013; Roszak 1995) and recently has been introduced more widely in the work of Cunsolo and Ellis—"the grief felt in relation to the experienced or anticipated ecological losses, including the loss of species, ecosystems and meaningful landscapes due to acute or chronic environmental change." (Cunsolo and Ellis 2018, p. 275).

Panu Pihkala, a theologian by training and title, has become a foremost researcher on eco-anxiety, often engaging interdisciplinary methodologies, conversations and publications (see Pihkala 2022a, his publication in this *Special Issue*). *Eco-anxiety* describes experiences of "chronic feelings of anxiety, worry and fear" related to the environmental crises (Pihkala 2018a). His recent article (Pihkala 2022b) is a "preliminary exploration of the taxonomy of climate emotions" necessary for future research given the "profound but complex ways emotions shape people's reactions to the climate crisis" (Pihkala 2022b, p. 1). The study is a thoughtful review of the literature relating emotions with the climate crisis.

Particularly since the 2017 report, released by the American Psychological Association (APA) and Eco-America, the amount of literature relating specifically to trauma and the climate crisis has increased across several disciplines. This report found both acute and chronic trauma responses effecting the mental health of an increasing percentage of the population. The acute (or direct) reactions include "increases in trauma and shock, post-traumatic stress disorder (PTSD), compounded stress, anxiety, substance abuse, and depression." The chronic (or indirect) reactions include "higher rates of aggression, violence, more mental health emergencies, an increased sense of helplessness, hopelessness, or fatalism, and intense feelings of loss" (Clayton et al. 2017, p. 7). Beyond psychology, researchers from sociology and the ecological humanities discuss *climate trauma*, making links between trauma theory, the arts and public discourse and the implications for mitigating and managing public anxiety in the face of climate disaster (Kaplan 2016; Zimmerman 2020; Craps 2020). Public policy makers and those concerned with climate adaptation and mitigation are also looking at the psychological, social and political impacts of trauma responses to the climate crisis (Moser 2012, 2020; Berzonsky and Moser 2017).

I share this brief outline to demonstrate how literature in the area is proliferating across several disciplines and to locate the topic of trauma and the climate crisis within some of the larger conversations. All of these discussions include overlapping concerns, areas of potential fruitfulness and theological implications for the practical theological disciplines, especially those of pastoral theology and care. While there is a growing body of literature, sustained focus on the climate crisis has had little traction in the larger field and even less so in the discipline of pastoral theology, the theological discipline most closely connected with psychology and mental health (McCarroll 2020; Miller-McLemore 2020; Swain 2020). In this article, I am particularly interested in examining literature on trauma and the climate crisis as I see much here that is relevant for pastoral and practical theology. Given the implicitly existential, theological and spiritual dimensions embedded in the realities of both trauma and the climate crisis, there is an important opportunity for practical and pastoral theology to engage, learn from and contribute to the interdisciplinary conversation. In this paper, I first offer a brief overview of the literature in pastoral theology related to the climate crisis, including Storm Swain's invitation to build a postcolonial, post-traumatic pastoral theology. Second, I present literature specifically on trauma theory and the climate crisis, outlining several of the key themes emerging across the interdisciplinary discussion. Third, I reflect theologically on the presented content, discussing and drawing forward areas of theological, epistemological and practical fruitfulness for practical and pastoral theology.

2. Pastoral Theology and Climate Crisis

Other than the pioneering work of Howard Clinebell and Larry Graham in the 1990s (Clinebell [1996] 2013; Graham 1992) there has not been much published in pastoral theology on the environmental crises until 2015. Since then, there has been a steady increase in the number of articles and chapters published in the area.[1] The hope is that this *Special Issue* and the conversations it engenders will be an important step in carving out more sustained focus on the climate crisis within the disciplines represented here and in the field of practical theology as a whole. Within the literature so far, there have been calls for a complete re-thinking of the discipline of pastoral theology from the ground up (Lartey and McGarrah Sharp 2016; Lee and Gibson 2021; LaMothe 2021a, 2021b, 2021c; Swain 2020). Some important preliminary work explores dimensions of what a reconceived pastoral theology might look like, including an intersectional, postcolonial, earth-centered reconstruction of the discipline's theological moorings and a critique of the violence of anthropocentric framings (Swain 2020; LaMothe 2021a, 2021b, 2021c; Miller-McLemore, forthcoming; Pihkala 2022a).

Most notable among those publishing in the area of pastoral theology and the climate crisis is Ryan LaMothe, whose recent articles and book begin to reconstruct theological frameworks for pastoral theology (LaMothe 2016, 2018, 2021a, 2021b, 2021c). His work emphasizes the political dimensions of the topic. LaMothe examines categories of care, human suffering and flourishing in relation to the polis. He challenges pastoral theology to reconstruct the theologies that undergird practice (LaMothe 2021b) and offers a pastoral theology for dwelling in these tumultuous times (LaMothe 2021a, 2021c).

In my review, I found several others who had published research on pastoral theology and the environmental crisis. Robert Saler (2015) explores the art of congregational pastoral care in the face of eco-devastation. Andy Calder and Jan Morgan (Calder and Morgan 2016) share their creative and inspiring earth-centered approach to Clinical Pastoral Education. Philip Helsel (2018) considers pastoral practice in terms of place attachment and loving the world. Rowley (2015) calls for intersystemic attentiveness as an approach to pastoral theology. Additionally, Panu Pihkala (2016, 2018b, 2022a) offers interdisciplinary work on eco-anxiety that intersects a good deal with concerns of pastoral theology. In her 2020 article, Bonnie Miller-McLemore challenges the field to acknowledge how the climate crisis changes everything and bemoans the neglect of the field thus far (Miller-McLemore 2020). However, in her more recent research review (Miller-McLemore, forthcoming), she recognizes that while there has not been a sustained conversation in pastoral and practical theological circles regarding the climate crisis, there is a surprisingly large body of literature on the topic.

In a recent publication on theology and climate change, Storm Swain and Elizabeth Tapia offer chapters (the latter a response to the former) on pastoral theology (Swain 2020; Tapia 2020). Swain seeks to carve out space for an ecological pastoral theology that engages postmodern, postcolonial and post-traumatic approaches to "decentre the human species while recentring the ecological body that continues to suffer" (Swain 2020, p. 616). Tapia's response brings Swain's methodological concerns down to earth. Their call for a postcolonial, post-traumatic approach to climate crisis reflects, in part, the motivation for my article here. Their nod to the traumatic, colonizing ethos of the status quo invites response (see also, Lartey and McGarrah Sharp 2016). I now present interdisciplinary literature on trauma and climate change in order to examine opportunities, areas of generativity and theological implications for pastoral and practical theology.

3. Trauma and Climate Crisis

As noted, literature on trauma and the climate crisis is located within larger conversations regarding ecological emotions, public discourse, policy, cultural studies and the arts. In the following section, in an effort to acquaint readers with the basic arguments and to highlight areas of potential interest for pastoral and practice theology, I outline several themes emerging in the interdisciplinary literature.

3.1. Flight, Fright, Fight and Freeze Responses to Climate Crisis

Much of the literature on trauma and climate change makes implicit or explicit links between the fight, flight, fright and freeze trauma responses and various recognizable reactions to the climate crisis in larger publics. In general, the climate crisis is understood as the precipitating stressor that triggers protective trauma responses. Studies identify several psychological reactions that function as "defense mechanisms" (Pihkala 2018b; Woodbury 2019), "protective strategies" (Berzonsky and Moser 2017), "defensive psychic processes" (White 2015) and "psychological coping strategies" (Haltinner et al. 2021). While not all researchers listed here use the language of trauma theory, per se, they point to reactions such as denial, skepticism, indifference, rage, anger, fear, addiction, distraction and so on as unconscious reactions intended to protect persons from rising anxiety, from unacceptable thoughts and a sense of overwhelming threat (Pihkala 2022b; Moser 2020; White 2015; Woodbury 2019).

The fight response is observed in "polarized political discourse" (Woodbury 2019, p. 5); in reactive denial of climate change and anger at those who acknowledge it; in practices of blaming and shaming so common in our increasingly polarized society and in perpetuating cycles of violence the expression of which function as a kind of cathartic release valve (see also, Berzonsky and Moser 2017). The flight response can include a proclivity to intellectualize as a means to flee into mental constructs and ideas (Stanley 2019) as well as addictions of various sorts that distract from the stressor (Woodbury 2019). The fright response can include behaviors such as obsessing over the science of climate change (Woodbury 2019, p. 5) as well as eco-anxiety, which can include sleeplessness, sweating, elevated heart rate and anxious thoughts (see Pihkala 2018b). The freeze response is related to dissociation, when "we simply don't feel or don't allow ourselves to feel . . . ". Dissociation makes sense of the "intrapsychic processes . . . that have allowed climate change to emerge and persist."(White 2015, p. 194)[2]. Climate denial and indifference are seen as dissociative responses, a kind of "psychic numbing" (Lifton) or paralysis. However they are categorized, trauma responses are full-body experiences involving our thoughts, emotions, nervous and limbic systems (Woodbury 2019; Stanley 2019; Fisher 2013). All around us and within us we perceive how climate change can trigger any number of these self-protective mechanisms.

3.2. Distinctives of Climate Trauma

Within the increasingly mainstream work of ecopsychologists, Zhiwa Woodbury tracks the ways *climate trauma* is a distinctive form of trauma in order to develop appropriate psychological frameworks to help individuals, communities and societies (Woodbury 2019). When climate change "is viewed . . . through the lens of traumatology, this deepening existential crisis presents an entirely new, unprecedented, and higher-order category of trauma: Climate Trauma . . . What is unique about this category of trauma is that it is an ever-present, ever-growing threat." (Woodbury 2019, p. 1). Since climate trauma is "superordinate" and ubiquitous, it can compound "past traumas—personal, cultural and intergenerational and will continue to do so until such as time as it is acknowledged" (ibid.). As an existential threat, climate trauma triggers all other traumas and thereby causes widespread dissociation that distracts people from doing anything about the climate crisis.

Kaplan and Craps consider climate trauma a form of "pre-traumatic stress" wherein images of the future, rather than the past, haunt the present. Pre-trauma "describes how people unconsciously suffer from an immobilizing anticipatory anxiety about the future." (Kaplan 2016, p. xix; Craps 2020, p. 279). Craps' work on climate trauma includes "pre-traumatic stress disorder" or "Anthropocene disorder" to distinguish the phenomena from post-traumatic stress, which is commonly understood. Craps' chapter is generative and in line with critiques of anthropocentrism from across many disciplines. It challenges readers to reconceptualise trauma in non-anthropocentric terms and acknowledges the interconnectivity of human and more-than-human forms of trauma. "A traumatized earth begets traumatized people." (Craps 2020, p. 281). The author proposes "geo trauma" (ibid.) as a term that can help us to reconceptualise suffering beyond human exceptionalism from a post-humanist, materialist perspective—"[disrupting] the dominance of human bodies as the only mournable subjects." (Craps 2020, p. 282, quoting Cunsolo and Landman 2017).

Another important distinction of climate trauma is the way shame and guilt can function. Unlike situations of interpersonal violence wherein "victims" experiencing trauma are not its cause, with climate trauma, many who experience it know that they are also a cause of it. Guilt and shame, therefore, are appropriate in climate trauma in a way that they are not in other forms of trauma. The presence of guilt and shame and even self-loathing in relation to climate trauma can compound the trauma reactive response, further entrenching unhelpful defense strategies.

3.3. Collective and Contagious Trauma and Public Narratives

Climate trauma reactions have become collective, socialized such that whole groups and societies experience elements of indirect or direct trauma. "Socially constructed silence" (Pihkala 2018b, quoting Norgaard) and "normalized denial" (Zimmerman 2020, p. 1) perpetuate collective silence about the elephant in the room. Additionally, we see collective trauma responses in expressions of rage, anger, blaming and shaming between groups of people—where polarized discourse sets one group up against another. Trauma is "contagious", creating a "backdrop of culturally reinforced psychosocial defense mechanisms" that manifest in chaotic "cultural and political expressions of group pathology" (Woodbury 2019).

Both actual experiences of extreme climate events as well as discourse about the climate crisis can trigger trauma responses in various publics. How public narratives regarding climate change are framed and expressed have a powerful impact. When narratives highlight the threat, crisis and catastrophic trajectory of the climate crisis, they can function to harden people into defensive postures (Zimmerman 2020), triggering reactions that result in avoidance of the crisis thereby further perpetuating it (Zimmerman 2020; Moser 2020; Pihkala 2018b; Haraway 2016). It is a vicious and messy cycle. Pragmatically and strategically speaking, then, leaders are called to soften the threat discourse. We can recognize here the deeply political dynamics embedded in the realities of climate trauma.

3.4. Grief and Climate Crisis

Public responses to the climate crisis such as denial, anger, anxiety and depression are interpreted also through the lens of grief (rather than trauma) over the painful realization of death[3]—the death of species from habitat destruction and climate disasters and the slow death of modern metanarratives and anthropocentric epistemologies (Moser 2012; Berzonsky and Moser 2017). Effective leadership for today includes acceptance of death from the climate crisis. It is through their own journey to acceptance that leaders may prepare to accompany others through grief and mourning. Mourning is a first step to enable action toward climate justice. Collective opportunities to acknowledge and process the pain of loss through mourning nurture a sense of connectivity, gratitude and love for nature and open up space and energy for action toward climate justice (Moser 2012; Berzonsky and Moser 2017; Cunsolo and Landman 2017).

3.5. Trauma Theory, Climate Crisis and Body Knowing

While the primary focus in literature on climate change and trauma has so far focused on using trauma theory as an assessment lens to interpret what is going on, trauma theory offers much potential for imagining what healing might look and feel like, particularly in relation to the body. The shift to the body has been a central focus in the healing of trauma. "The body keeps the score", as van der Kolk so aptly named his text (van der Kolk 2014), sums up the findings of how intrinsic the body is to the experience of and healing from trauma. In his work on radical ecopsychology, building on the work of Joanna Macy and Gestalt therapy, Andy Fisher focuses on recovering a *felt sense* of the human body as the primary vehicle for knowing. As a kind of resistance to ubiquitous and often unconscious suffering required by the neo-liberal capitalist order, Fisher shares exercises to help us reconnect with our bodies. It is by listening to our bodies, and the many ways they manifest and communicate earth's suffering, that we may discover pathways for earth-bound healing (Fisher 2013). Like Fisher, scholars in other fields critique Western epistemologies that disconnect knowing from being, citing that such epistemologies have contributed to the crisis (Zimmerman 2020; Berzonsky and Moser 2017). Zimmerman comments ironically, "the more we know about the climate crisis, the more we emit greenhouse gases" (Zimmerman 2020, p. 12). Informational "knowledge" does not motivate change. Rather, it is in connecting with our body knowing that epistemologies may emerge that serve rather than hinder the flourishing of the earth.

Robin Wall Kimmerer's exquisite book, *Braiding Sweetgrass*, offers much that is relevant in terms of the deeply embodied ways of being, knowing and loving. As an example, she shares findings of recent research showing "that the smell of humus exerts a physiological effect on humans. Breathing the scent of Mother Earth stimulates the release of the hormone oxytocin, the same chemical that promotes bonding between mother and child, between lovers. Held in loving arms ... " (Kimmerer 2013, p. 236). Our bodies hold a kind of knowing, the reclamation of which leans towards healing.

3.6. Earth's Trauma Is Human Trauma—Ecosystems Thinking

As suggested, there is an important focus on the deep interconnectivity of human mental and physical crises with the earth's crises—human trauma and earth trauma. Ecopsychologists emphasize the intrinsic organic ways human emotions and bodies are part of the earth and expressive of its distress in specifically human form (Fisher 2013; Roszak 1995; Clinebell [1996] 2013). It is a deep systems way of thinking that re-connects human bodies with the ecosystem processes in which we participate and by which we are a sustained. The increase in depression, anxiety, suicide and even pandemics are seen as bodily expressions in the human species of the trauma of the earth with the destruction of the natural healing processes intrinsic to the earth (Fisher 2013, p. 158ff). The argument goes that humans are so deeply entangled in the ecosystems of the earth, they are completely dependent and emotionally and physically regulated as part of the earth; when the earth is in distress, humans are in distress. Our bodies are the ground of our being, the organism through which the earth manifests and communicates. However, in an effort to deny or overcome the suffering of the earth known in our bodies and emotions, we have cut off from our bodies and are no longer in touch with the rhythms and movement of life within and through us. Indeed, the presence of 'coping strategies' reflects the extent to which humans are cut off from our bodies' intrinsic knowing—a situation required by neo-liberal capitalism in order for humans to adapt to an inherently violent socio-political system bound to its own destruction. (Fisher 2013, p. 74). These arguments identify the need for frameworks to interpret human phenomena as participating in the organic systems of entanglements of the earth's processes. Awakening humans to our intrinsic earthiness is essential for a change of perspective. *Falling in love* with the earth—*biophilia, ecophilia*—is a primary starting point toward healing the trauma (Roszak 1995; Clinebell [1996] 2013; Fisher 2013). We cannot save what we do not love. Love reflects our interconnectivity with other beings. It is a generative energy that builds human and more-than-human communities and can nourish and sustain us even when we face the cataclysmic depths of crisis, and the trauma responses overwhelm us.

This brief overview of literature on trauma and climate crisis offers much for pastoral and practical theology to consider and engage, an invitation to which I now turn.

4. Trauma and the Climate Crisis—Pastoral and Practical Theology

4.1. Thinking Theologically about Trauma and the Climate Crisis

Whichever way we look at it, when we bring a theological lens to bear on trauma and the climate crisis, one thing is clear. Trauma responses—whether fight, flight, fright or freeze—reflect a human struggle against existential contingency, our creatureliness. The cataclysmic reality of the climate crisis signifies in real time our ultimate fragility, finitude and earth-bound vulnerability and raises questions of existential and theological import. Using the lens of trauma theory enables us to discern a deep-seated fear[4] that lies beneath all the various reactions in response to the overwhelming threat of the climate crisis. It invites us to perceive the extent to which our own self-protective mechanisms guard and distract us from embracing our humanity and, of course, result in the deepening of the climate crisis.

In her work on trauma, Elizabeth Stanley outlines the many ways our body-minds are wired for trauma responses, having developed this way over millennia to support human survival in hunter–gatherer societies (Stanley 2019). Trauma responses can be triggered when one perceives they are powerless, helpless and lack control over whatever is threatening. "The less agency we perceive we have, the more traumatic the experience will be for our body-mind system." (Stanley 2019, p. 16). As a consequence, the need to control, colonize, manage and/or deny that which threatens can reactively come into play. In fact, she argues convincingly that intellectualizing is a form of trauma response—a practice of colonizing and seeking control when we feel threatened (Stanley 2019).

Of course, this phenomenon of seeking to colonize, control and/or deny that which threatens us is a dynamic many of us can sense in ourselves on a micro level. It is part of the human predicament and identified in various ways from the book of Genesis to the myth of Prometheus, from Augustine to Nietzsche and Freud. What trauma theory helps us notice is that beneath the multivalent ways trauma responses manifest and wreak havoc is a deeper fear from which we are desperate to escape—a fear of our own creatureliness, vulnerability, dependence and finitude. Indeed, it is a spiritual crisis writ large—a failure to discern human purpose and meaning in ways that are life-giving. Trauma theory also helps us recognize that reactive responses are not inevitable. Fight, flight, fright and freeze are not the only options for human responses in the face of threat. However, before we get to that, let us consider some of the ways trauma theory brings a different lens to assessing theology.

We can imagine how certain theologies can both represent and feed the *fight* and *flight* responses through intellectualizing—seeking to colonize, control and avoid that which threatens. Such trauma responses may be discerned in theological infrastructures that privilege human-centered control/power while "protecting" us[5] from seeing things for what they are. Theologians of the cross call such infrastructures "theologies of glory"—theologies that lie about what is obscuring creaturely vulnerability and finitude with promises of glory, power and ultimate victory (McCarroll 2014, 2021; Hall 2012). Indeed, Lynn White's scathing critique of Western Christianity as "the most anthropocentric religion the world has seen", a primary cause of ecological devastation (White 1967), still stands as a challenge for Christian doctrine, witness and practice. When deconstructed through trauma theory, doctrines or theological frameworks that privilege colonizing motifs of human and divine power/control may be perceived as trauma reactive responses—intellectual attempts to deny and overcome the realities of existing. Similarly, when deconstructed through trauma theory, doctrines or theological frameworks that shift our gaze to some far-away god or promise of heavenly bliss and away from the present realities of our earthen material embeddedness may be perceived as trauma responses—attempts to deny and distract from the realities of existing.

An excellent chapter by eco-theologian Heather Eaton argues that the very architecture of Christian theology normalizes denial and indifference as a response to worldly plights and feeds anthropocentrism. Christian theologies that emphasize world-denying ontologies; promise other-worldly salvation and offer doctrines that locate G-d "outside" creation all feed denial and ultimately are a cause of the species extinction and crises at hand (Eaton 2017). "Christianity has developed an extreme opposition to, even refusal of, the conditions of life ... As a result, Christianity supports attempts to escape, resist, or control life's requisites ... because of the refusal to accept the conditions of life, Christianity ... is involved in domination." (Eaton 2017, p. 33). In line with Eaton and others, theologies that image G-d[6] as powerful and in control and those that locate G-d/the Sacred elsewhere in some disconnected realm outside of earth may be interpreted to both reflect and feed trauma reactive responses. By distracting our gaze from life as it is and placing our sense of the sacred in an other-worldly "person" or place, we not only reject the earth as sub-standard, we are also unable to learn from it and perceive its sanctity. So too, with theologies that emphasize human exceptionalism— for example doctrines of *imago dei* (Deifelt 2017)—such theological architecture could well be deconstructed through the lens of trauma theory. By placing human beings at the center of our conceptions of reality, of the divine and of history we are unable to perceive the wisdom of the earth and its processes, to acknowledge our deep dependence and to discover our meaning and purpose as earth-formed creatures.

Eaton goes on to say, "if domination [is] considered to be the result of refusing the conditions of life—meaning vulnerability, mortality and finitude—then a way forward is to embrace them, difficult as that is." (Eaton 2017, p. 34). My argument in many ways follows Eaton's line of argument, though it offers the clarifying lens of trauma theory, which helps us to perceive that, beneath the human opposition and resistance to the conditions of life, lies a deep fear of being human. The difference is slim but significant in terms of contemplating a way forward. With the lens of trauma theory we are able to perceive the powerful role played by spiritual, emotional and psychological fear that quickly co-opts human attempts to "embrace [our] vulnerability, mortality, finitude," throwing us into trauma reactive ways of being. Instead, trauma theory invites us first to acknowledge the fear, to move toward it and be present to it in a spirit of compassion. As we are present to the fear within ourselves and with others the power of the threat can be unhinged and stranglehold of fear released. By perceiving the root problem as fear (rather than resistance and refusal, for example) and tapping into compassion, we can break the cyclical hold of trauma reactivity in our relating and existing.

Interestingly, in my review of the literature on trauma and climate crisis, I found no reference to the *window of tolerance* (or *optimal zone*).[7] I believe it is a helpful concept for considering the options for responding in the face of threat and its relevance for theology and practice. Conceived and mapped out by Daniel Siegel, *the window* offers a helpful phenomenological description of the psycho-spiritual-relational dynamics present when human persons are at our best in a context of threat. It refers to the optimal zone in the face of crisis—a state of equilibrium "beyond" the hyperarousal zone of the fight, fright and flight responses and the hypoarousal zone of the freeze, dissociative response (Siegel 1999). When in this zone, humans are able to recognize the threat but do not seek to escape it. Rather, by moving toward our sense of fear with openness, compassion and curiosity, the power of the fear is loosed. When humans are in this zone, we are able to both think and feel; we are connected with our bodies and to the present moment; we can hold paradox and ambiguity, and we are open, compassionate, curious and present both to ourselves and to others. Mindfulness and somatic-based practices common in trauma care support people to move from trauma reactive states into this state of equilibrium within their window (van der Kolk 2014; Stanley 2019). Long-term goals for trauma care often focus on *widening the window* such that self regulation is enabled through mindfulness and body-based awareness and practices (Stanley 2019). The window of tolerance describes a way of being present in the face of threats and highlights specific practices to support this process. Again, this is not about denying the threat or fighting or overcoming it. Rather, such practices support human people to acknowledge our fear and sense of threat and invite ways to live compassionately and courageously amidst these realities.

How can we, as a discipline and a field, retrieve and develop theological frameworks, practices and epistemologies that do not reinforce the denial of or escape from our earth-entangled human condition? How can we retrieve and develop theological frameworks, practices and epistemologies that support humans to embrace our humanness in all its earth-formed vulnerability? How might theological frameworks, practices and epistemologies enable us to lean into and widen our window—to live courageously as creatures in the here and now within the givens of the earth's claim on us? I turn now to explore some of these questions.

4.2. Toward an Earth-Centered, Decolonizing, Trauma-Informed Approach

From the discussion above, we can discern the centrality of bodies and the focus on the present materiality of existence in terms of theology, practice and epistemology. Of course, practical theology as a whole, more than any other theological field, is concerned with the material realities of life. "Matter matters" (Simone Weil) for practical theology and certainly for pastoral theology. In many ways, practical theology is *the* theological field most equipped to articulate theological constructs, practices and epistemologies grounded in bodies and the present materiality of existence. Our discussion on climate trauma and theology suggests that there is an affective, phenomenological dimension embedded in all discourse and practice that can lean toward trauma reactive responses or toward the equilibrium of our optimal zone, our window of tolerance. In this final sub-section, I propose some questions for de-constructing our theological, practice-based and epistemological priorities and suggest resources for moving forward in these areas. I close in identifying opportunities for further research.

Drawing from the literature on trauma, climate change and theology, I propose here several questions that build on the questions above to help our discipline and field to de-construct theological frameworks, practices and epistemological sources and to move toward more earth-centered, decolonizing, trauma-informed approaches.

In relation to our theological constructs, practice and epistemologies:

1. Do they honour bodily and affective ways of knowing? Or do they reflect an escape into mental constructs that seek to master and colonize that which is "other" including human and other-than-human species and processes? ?
2. Do they take the material realities of existence seriously? Do they flee from the world to uninhabited mental worlds or do they engage the world as it is more deeply? Do they build up and open the theological imagination to recognize the sacred in the midst of creation rather than in some distant time-space?
3. Do they ground us in our bodies and the multiplicity of relationships within and by which we exist? Or do they distract us from our earthen-ness? Do they honour the embodied material integrity of what is, or do they deny and dismiss it?
4. Do they represent colonizing ways of reading and engaging earth and other human and other-than-human persons? Or do they open space to experience what is through the eyes of compassion—in awe and gratitude, in mourning and lament, in actions of care and resistance?
5. How does our research and practice help to widen the window, broaden the optimal zone, within the human species such that humans are freed to embrace our vulnerability with each other and within the community of creation?

In considering theological sources that may serve earth-centered, decolonizing and trauma-informed approaches to pastoral and practical theology, there are several areas to draw from within the larger Christian tradition. Theological frames are important because they provide a hermeneutical landscape for experiencing life with theological imagination. As Eaton notes, of concern is how doctrines and theological sources support humans to embrace, rather than run from, the materiality and exigencies of being. Additionally, it is important to consider how theological frames can support earth-centered, rather than colonizing, approaches to life as these make all the difference to human living and experiencing. In the Christian tradition, helpful sources to draw on are those that enable humans to perceive the sacred in the here and now of existence. Notions of the Divine that include and focus on the earth and its processes help to re-sacralize matter and to expand theological imagination. While some have resistance to *panentheism*—the notion that G-d is in all things and all things are in G-d—it is a rich and abiding theological construct that offers much for an earth-centered, decolonizing, trauma-informed approach. It invites us to perceive the Sacred in the organic interconnectivity, ecosystemic resilience, relational reciprocity and gracious givenness in the earth and its processes.

Similarly, Christology that emphasizes the bodily reality of the G-d in earthen form offers much. Notions of the ubiquity of Christ (Luther), the Logos becoming flesh (John 1) and the incarnation can ignite theological imagination toward earth-centered approaches.[8] Not only do such lenses offer ways of interpreting Christ's presence here and now within the goodness of creation, they also help to broaden notions of the suffering of Christ within the suffering of creation itself. These doctrinal re-imaginings of G-d and Christ can open our theological imaginations to perceive the sacredness in creation, the holy in the ordinary materiality of what is. Indeed, we can feel it in our bodies when theology opens up vistas for experiencing the sacred close-up. We can imagine that such theology may well help us lean into our window of tolerance/optimal zone where openness, curiosity and spaciousness emerge.

In terms of theological anthropology, needless to say, it is important to re-image the place of the human within the creation in a way that honours the distinctive gifts of humans within the organic body of the earth. Indeed, the modern *imago hominis* of the "human as master" of the earth has been replaced by the late-capitalist "human as consumer" of the earth. Arguably, both images reflect colonizing trauma responses that deny and/or resist human vulnerability and finitude and have consequently led to devastation. Traditionally, pastoral theology and some eco-theology have imaged humans as "stewards" of the earth, caring for the earth. However, this image disconnects humans from the earth, as if earth is an object for humans' care. Additionally, it inverts the deeper truth—that humans are actually dependent on and recipients of the earth's stewarding care, not vice versa. As such, *the steward* reflects a soft colonizing motif. Reimaging the role and purpose of humans within the community of creation invites us to consider organic images of reciprocity and systemic interconnectivity as well as images that point to distinctive gifts of the human species within the larger community. By drawing on our capacity for awe and reverence, for mourning and grief, for creative expression, for conscious agency to confront and resist systems of colonizing oppression, pastoral and practical theology have much to offer in reconceiving the *imago hominis*.

In considering practices and epistemologies that serve an earth-centered, decolonizing, trauma-informed approach, this research challenges us to embrace practices and ideas that ground us where we are—as bodies within the multiple organic systems enabling existence. Developing our capacity to listen to and learn from the interconnected systems of the earth, including our bodies, is a steep learning curve in our context where prescriptive mental constructs of reality have colonized our imaginations and narrative frameworks. Central to this journey will be a capacity to honour the intrinsic systemic integrity of what is, being open to learn from it in a spirit of curiosity. For example, when we recognize the phenomenon of eco-anxiety or climate trauma, not only can we acknowledge it and normalize it—a "normal" human response to a sense of overwhelming threat—we can go further to perceive the intrinsic integrity of these phenomena as they arise in human experience. Indeed, rather than pathologies, eco-anxiety and climate trauma reflect how deeply bonded human persons are as part of the systems of the earth, experiencing the earth's own distress in human bodies and emotions. Our epistemologies and practices can acknowledge our deep participation in the earth's systems and process. This relates also to our field's focus on suffering and flourishing. How might we expand our intersectional epistemology to recognize systemic interconnectivities of our earthen-ness? All suffering/flourishing reflects earth's suffering/flourishing. Suffering is experienced in relationships not rightly ordered among and within species and processes. The reciprocity of relationships means that when one suffers and is out of a right relationship, there is a whole interconnected system that also manifests and processes the suffering. So too, with flourishing, it is known when life is ordered in a right relationship within and among species and the earth. Earth-centered intersectional epistemologies and practices tend to the dynamic interconnectivities of being.

Finally, I present here some areas for further research in pastoral and practical theology:

1. Moral Distress/Injury—When we consider the ways trauma theory plays out in terms of the climate crisis, it would be interesting to explore the phenomena of moral distress and moral injury in relation to the climate crisis and to consider the theological resonance (see also Hickman et al. 2021). Notably, the presence of shame and guilt in the phenomenon of climate trauma alerts us to its moral dimensions and the potential for moral injury and distress. Given pastoral theology's research expertise on moral injury and distress, how might we contribute to the interdisciplinary conversation in this area?

2. Leadership—Amid the climate and related political-economic-social upheavals to come in the next decades, it will be wise to develop leaders across all fields and professions who are able to resist the urge toward trauma-reactive polarization or indifference and, instead, to lean into their window of tolerance. Especially for spiritual-religious, public and academic leaders, it will be important for us to develop a wide enough window to support populations to acknowledge and process their trauma, grieve their losses and to constructively facilitate earth-centered communal actions toward life. This kind of leadership presence will require much inner work, self-awareness and communal support (Moser 2012; Berzonsky and Moser 2017). How might theological education and practical/pastoral theological research contribute to the formation of leaders amid the climate crisis?

3. Ritual, spiritual and communal practices that acknowledge the sacredness of material processes and honour body knowing—One of the challenges with the trauma responses in the face of the climate crisis is the extent to which underlying grief, sadness and fear remain unacknowledged and, therefore, powerful. Facilitating spaces and practices that name, normalize and acknowledge the grief invites a cathartic release for and witness of these emotions and opens up space, widening the window and enabling positive actions. How might theological education and practical/pastoral theological research continue to build capacity in this area?

4. Stories of ecological creativity and resilience can feed hope and open up horizons of possibility. Sharing stories of hope is essential for widening the window and enabling us to remain present with the challenges of these times. How might our scholarship, research and teaching provide venues for sharing stories that expand and generate hope in times such as these?

5. Conclusions

In this paper, I have covered some vast terrain. My hope is that, in using trauma theory as a lens to explore human responses to the climate crisis and considering the theological import of this for pastoral and practical theology, this paper can contribute to the ongoing work of re-imagining the discipline and the field from an earth-centered, decolonizing, trauma-informed perspective. As a means to invite more sustained conversation in the discipline and the field, I have presented interdisciplinary research on trauma and the climate crisis acknowledging its theological and spiritual dimensions. I have deconstructed how theological frameworks can manifest trauma reactive responses that reinforce anthropocentric, colonizing control/mastery. I have suggested avenues of potential fruitfulness by identifying theological sources, epistemological orientations and practices that enable us to perceive the sacred in the bodied materiality and interconnectivity of being. May we, as a discipline and a field, contribute to widening the window amidst the threat of climate crisis—being present with courage, compassion and equanimity.

Funding: This research received no external funding.

Acknowledgments: I am grateful to Emmanuel College of Victoria University for supporting my research leave wherein this research was completed.

Conflicts of Interest: The author declares no conflict of interest.

Notes

[1] For this brief review of the pastoral theological literature on the climate crisis, I acknowledge the important work of Bonnie Miller-McLemore in her research review for the *International Journal for Practical Theology* (Miller-McLemore, forthcoming) and that of Panu Pihkala whose extensive review of this literature appears in this *Special Issue* (Pihkala 2022a).

[2] White is quoting trauma researcher Ruth Lanius from a presentation, "Healing the traumatized self" 2014 Unpublished proceedings from the Boulder Institute for Psychotherapy and Research Front Porch Lecture, Boulder CO.

[3] It is helpful to note that behind their discussion of grief is Elizabeth Kubler Ross's cycles of grief model

[4] In *The Courage to Be*, Paul Tillich agrees with other existential thinkers when he distinguishes between fear and anxiety. Fear is considered to be related to an embodied threat, whereas anxiety is considered to be ultimately connected to nonbeing. The goal is to transform anxiety into fear so that the threat can be met with courage. In the face of climate crisis, fear and anxiety coalesce with striking ferocity. I choose the language of "fear" rather than "anxiety" to intimate the possibilities for courage and mindful agency in times such as these.

[5] "Us" is used here to identify those who wield power by colonizing approaches. This manifestation of trauma response—the wielding of power/control over "otherness" and difference perceived as threat—may be seen as the primary *modus operandi* of colonial patriarchy that has functioned to colonize and control minds, hearts, bodies, species, habitats and the earth.

[6] I use "G-d" to point to the reality that the divine source, reality and energy cannot be contained in human words and ideas.

[7] I use this term here as it is a recognized term within trauma theory. It refers to a capacity to tolerate the sense of threat related to a triggering event or situation. I acknowledge of the complexity of experience in relation to "tolerance" as it has been used to colonize and undermine people who have been "othered" by the status quo. As much as possible I will use "optimal zone" or "the window" in this paper to refer to the same phenomenon.

[8] Certainly understandings of incarnation have been an important theological frame for both pastoral and practical theology over the last few decades, particularly since the emergence of theologies of liberation.

References

Albrecht, Glenn. 2011. Chronic Environmental Change: Emerging Psychoterratic Syndromes. In *Climate Change and Human Well-Being: Global Challenges and Opportunities*. Edited by Inka Weissbecker. New York: Springer, pp. 43–56.

Albrecht, Glenn. 2019. *Earth Emotions: New Words for a New World*. Ithaca: Cornell University Press.

Berzonsky, Carol L., and Susanne C. Moser. 2017. Becoming Homo Sapiens: Mapping Psycho-cultural transformation in the Anthropocene. *Anthropocene* 20: 15–23. [CrossRef]

Calder, Andy S., and Jan E. Morgan. 2016. 'Out of the Whirlwind': Clinical Pastoral Education and Climate Change. *Journal of Pastoral Care and Counseling* 70: 16–25. [CrossRef]

Clayton, Susan D., and Christie Manning, eds. 2018. *Psychology and Climate Change: Human Perceptions, Impacts and Responses*. London: Elsevier Academic Press.

Clayton, Susan D., Christie Manning, Kirra Krygsman, and Meighen Speicer. 2017. *Mental Health and Our Changing Climate: Impacts, Implications, and Guidance, March 2017*. APA, Climate for Health, Eco-America. Available online: https://www.apa.org/search?query=climate+change&sort=ContentDateSort+desc&page=5 (accessed on 2 February 2022).

Clinebell, Howard. 2013. *Ecotherapy: Healing Ourselves, Healing the Earth*. Oxford: Routledge. First published 1996.

Craps, Steph. 2020. Climate Trauma. In *The Routledge Companion to Literature and Trauma*. Edited by Colin David and Hanna Meretoja. Oxford: Routledge, pp. 275–83.

Cunsolo, Ashlee, and Karen Landman, eds. 2017. *Mourning Nature: Hope at the Heart of Ecological Loss and Grief*. Montreal: McGill-Queen's University Press.

Cunsolo, Ashlee, and Neville Ellis. 2018. Ecological Grief as a Mental Health Response to Climate-Change related Loss. *Nature Climate Change* 8: 275–81. [CrossRef]

Deifelt, Wanda. 2017. And G*d Saw it Was Good—Imago Dei and Its Challenge to Climate Justice. In *Planetary Solidarity: Global Women's Voices on Christian Doctrine and Climate Justice*. Edited by Grace Ji-Sun Kim and Hilda P. Koster. Minneapolis: Fortress Press, pp. 119–133.
Eaton, Heather. 2017. An Earth-Centric Theological Framing for Planetary Solidarity. In *Planetary Solidarity: Global Women's Voices on Christian Doctrine and Climate Justice*. Edited by Grace Ji-Sun Kim and Hilda P. Koster. Minneapolis: Fortress Press, pp. 19–46.
Fisher, Andy. 2013. *Radical Ecopsychology: Psychology in the Service of Life*, 2nd ed. Albany: SUNY Press.
Graham, Larry. 1992. *Care of Persons, Care of Worlds: A Psychosystems Approach to Pastoral Care and Counseling*. Nashville: Abington Press.
Hall, Douglas John. 2012. *Waiting for Gospel*. Eugene: Cascade Books.
Haltinner, Kristin, Jennifer K. Ladino, and Dilsani Sarathchandra. 2021. Feeling Skeptical: Emotions and Support for Environmental Policy Among Climate Change Skeptics. *Emotion, Space, and Society* 39: 100790. [CrossRef]
Haraway, Donna. 2016. *Staying with the Trouble: Making Kin in the Chthulucene*. Durham: Duke University Press.
Helsel, Philip Browning. 2018. Loving the World: Place Attachment and Environment in Pastoral Theology. *Journal of Pastoral Theology* 28: 22–33. [CrossRef]
Hickman, Caroline, Elizabeth Marks, Panu Pihkala, Susan Clayton, R. Eric Lewandowski, Elouise E. Mayall, Britt Wray, Catriona Mellor, and Lisa van Susteren. 2021. Young People's Voices on Climate Anxiety, Governmental Betrayal and Moral Injury: A Global Phenomenon. Preprints with the Lancet. Available online: https://papers.ssrn.com/sol3/papers.cfm?abstract_id=3918955 (accessed on 2 February 2022).
Kaplan, Ann E. 2016. *Climate Trauma: Foreseeing the Future in Dystopian Film and Fiction*. New Brunswick: Rutgers University Press.
Kimmerer, Robin Wall. 2013. *Braiding Sweetgrass: Indigenous Wisdom, Scientific Knowledge and the Teaching of Plants*. Minneapolis: Milkweed Editions.
LaMothe, Ryan. 2016. This Changes Everything: The Sixth Extinction and Its Implications for Pastoral Theology. *Journal of Pastoral Theology* 26: 178–94. [CrossRef]
LaMothe, Ryan. 2018. *Pastoral Reflections on Global Citizenship*. Lanham: Lexington Books.
LaMothe, Ryan. 2021a. A Pastoral Theology of Dwelling: Political Belonging in the Face of a Pandemic, Racism, and the Anthropocene Age. *Journal of Pastoral Theology* 31: 89–109. [CrossRef]
LaMothe, Ryan. 2021b. A Radical Pastoral Theology for the Anthropocene Era: Thinking and Being Otherwise. *Journal of Pastoral Theology* 31: 54–74. [CrossRef]
LaMothe, Ryan. 2021c. *A Radical Political Theology for the Anthropocene Era: Thinking and Being Otherwise*. Eugene: Cascade Books.
Lartey, Emmanuel Y., and Melinda A. McGarrah Sharp. 2016. Seeking Steadiness in Storms: Pastoral Theology in the Midst of Intercultural, Political and Ecological Trauma. *Journal of Pastoral Care* 26: 149–51. [CrossRef]
Lee, K. Samuel, and Danjuma Gibson. 2021. Caring Over Troubled Waters: Creative and Critical Pastoral Theological Imaginations in the 21st Century. *Journal of Pastoral Theology* 31: 1–3.
McCarroll, Pamela R. 2014. *Waiting at the Foot of the Cross: Toward a Theology of Hope for Today*. Eugene: Pickwick.
McCarroll, Pamela R. 2020. Listening for the Cries of the Earth: Practical Theology in the Anthropocene. *International Journal of Practical Theology* 24: 29–46. [CrossRef]
McCarroll, Pamela R. 2021. What are People For? Re-Imaging Theo-Anthropology in the Anthropocene. In *Christian Theology after Christendom: Engaging the Thought of Douglas John Hall*. Edited by Patricia Kirkpatrick and Pamela R. McCarroll. Lanham: Lexington/Fortress Academic, pp. 85–100.
Miller-McLemore, Bonnie. 2020. Trees and the "Unthought Known": The Wisdom of the Non-Human (or Do Humans have "Shit for Brains"?). *Pastoral Psychology* 69: 423–43. [CrossRef]
Miller-McLemore, Bonnie. forthcoming. Climate Violence and Earth Justice: A Research Report on Practical Theology's Contributions. *International Journal of Practical Theology*.
Moser, Susanne C. 2012. Getting Real about it: Meeting the Psychological and Social Demands of a World in Distress. In *Environmental Leadership: A Reference Handbook*. Edited by Deborah Rigling Gallagher. Thousand Oaks: Sage Pubs.
Moser, Susanne C. 2020. The work after 'It's too late' (to prevent dangerous climate change). *WIREs Clim Change* 11: e606. [CrossRef]
Pihkala, Panu. 2016. The Pastoral Challenge of the Environmental Crisis: Environmental Anxiety and Lutheran Eco-Reformation. *Dialog* 55: 131–40. [CrossRef]
Pihkala, Panu. 2018a. Death, The Environment and Theology. *Dialog* 57: 287–94. [CrossRef]
Pihkala, Panu. 2018b. Eco-Anxiety, Tragedy, and Hope: Psychological and Spiritual Dimensions of Climate Change. *Zygon* 53: 545–69. [CrossRef]
Pihkala, Panu. 2022a. Eco-Anxiety and Pastoral Care: Theoretical Considerations and Practical Suggestions. *Religions* 22: 192. Available online: https://www.mdpi.com/search?authors=pihkala&journal=religions (accessed on 15 February 2022). [CrossRef]
Pihkala, Panu. 2022b. Toward a Taxonomy of Climate Emotions. *Frontiers in Climate* 3: 738154. Available online: https://www.frontiersin.org/articles/10.3389/fclim.2021.738154/full (accessed on 3 February 2022). [CrossRef]
Roszak, Betty. 1995. The Spirit of the Goddess. In *Ecopsychology: Restoring the Earth, Healing the Mind*. Edited by Theodore Roszak, Mary E. Gomes and Allen D. Kanner. New York: Sierra Club, pp. 288–300.
Roszak, Theodore, Mary E. Gomes, and Allen D. Kanner, eds. 1995. *Ecopsychology: Restoring the Earth, Healing the Mind*. New York: Sierra Club.

Rowley, Genny C. 2015. Intersystemic Care: How Religious Environmental Praxis Expands the Pastoral Theological Norm of Justice. *Journal of Pastoral Theology* 25: 107–21. [CrossRef]
Saler, Robert. 2015. Pastoral Care and Ecological Devastation: Un-Interpreting the Silence. *Journal of Lutheran Ethics* 16: 1–6.
Siegel, Daniel. 1999. *The Developing Mind*. New York: Guilford Press.
Stanley, Elizabeth. 2019. *Widen the Window*. New York: Penguin Random House.
Swain, Storm. 2020. Climate Change and Pastoral Theology. In *T & T Clark Handbook of Christian Theology and Climate Change*. Edited by Ernst Conradie and Hilda Koster. London: Bloomsbury Pub., pp. 615–26.
Swim, Janet, Susan Clayton, Thomas Doherty, Robert Gifford, George Howard, Joseph Reiser, Paul Stern, and Elke Weber. 2009. *Psychology and Global Climate Change: Addressing a Multi-faceted Phenomena and Set of Challenges*. APA Task Force. Available online: https://www.apa.org/search?query=climate%20change (accessed on 2 February 2022).
Tapia, Elizabeth. 2020. A Response to Storm Swain from the Philippines. In *T & T Clark Handbook of Christian Theology and Climate Change*. Edited by Ernst Conradie and Hilda Koster. London: Bloomsbury Pub., pp. 627–30.
van der Kolk, Bessel. 2014. *The Body Keeps The Score: Brain, Mind, and Body in the Healing of Trauma*. New York: Penguin.
White, Benjamin. 2015. States of Emergency: Trauma and Climate Change. *Ecopsychology* 7: 192–197. [CrossRef]
White, Lynn. 1967. The Historical Roots of Our Ecological Crisis. *Science* 155: 1203–7. [CrossRef] [PubMed]
Woodbury, Zhiwa. 2019. Climate Trauma: Toward a New Taxonomy of Trauma. *Ecopsychology* 11: 1–8. [CrossRef]
Zimmerman, Lee. 2020. *Trauma and The Discourse of Climate Change: Literature, Psychoanalysis and Denial*. Oxford: Routledge.

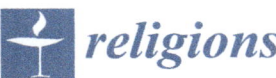

Article

Christian Planetary Humanism in the Age of Climate Crisis

Un-Hey Kim

Presbyterian University and Theological Seminary, Seoul 04965, Korea; uhk@puts.ac.kr

Abstract: This paper attempts to reconstruct the ethics of human response-ability as a theological reflection on the current climate catastrophe, seeing humans as moral actors or a moral actor network. In the meantime, I will argue the relationality and interdependence of matter and discourse, nature and society, and humans and non-humans through crosstalk between ecofeminist theologies and new materialism. In doing so, I reinterpret the human subject as a potential for liberation from modern human exceptionalism, acknowledging the subversive power of the concept of the subject.

Keywords: planetary humanism; climate crisis; deep incarnation; matter and mattering; ethics of responsibility

Citation: Kim, Un-Hey. 2022. Christian Planetary Humanism in the Age of Climate Crisis. *Religions* 13: 224. https://doi.org/10.3390/rel13030224

Academic Editors: Pamela R. McCarroll and HyeRan Kim-Cragg

Received: 1 February 2022
Accepted: 2 March 2022
Published: 7 March 2022

Publisher's Note: MDPI stays neutral with regard to jurisdictional claims in published maps and institutional affiliations.

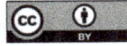

Copyright: © 2022 by the author. Licensee MDPI, Basel, Switzerland. This article is an open access article distributed under the terms and conditions of the Creative Commons Attribution (CC BY) license (https://creativecommons.org/licenses/by/4.0/).

1. Introduction

Mark Jerome Walters suggested that infectious diseases closely linked to ecological changes should be called an "Ecodemic" (Walters 2003). This pandemic urgently requires traditional Western theology to reconsider not only our understanding of nature but also the ways we have dealt with "matter" and to see our material entanglement. However spiritual humans may be, they cannot live without the material environment. They exist in the entanglement of beings, of which there is no outside, despite the fact that human beings are commonly considered to be discrete and independent. Humans have misused this material entanglement in selfish and anthropocentric ways, and this pandemic comes with the dark clouds of climate change, ecological destruction, and the sixth extinction.

It is widely acknowledged that humans are the main cause of today's climate catastrophe. Nevertheless, I believe that humans still have the ability to change the course of the lives of all things on this planet toward "sympoiesis" as well as symbiosis (Haraway 2016, p. 58). This seeming contradiction urges human beings to take responsibility as response-ability (ability to respond) to all forms of beings on this planet. Although humanism is at the center of criticism as far as the cause of these crises is concerned, the uniqueness of being human is still required, if there would be any hope left. To be precise, what needs to be criticized are none other than anthropocentrism and human exceptionalism that have made us ignore human entanglement with nonhuman beings. The idea that humans can take responsibility for what they have done for these crises still seems to be modern and theologically very arrogant.

Therefore, the task of theology today is to construct a new humanism beyond anthropocentrism and human exceptionalism. It is to see humanism through the eyes of deep incarnation, which acknowledges the deep interwovenness of humans, nonhumans, and nonliving beings. This requires a theologically critical dialogue with new materialism. In other words, the theological response to the present crises will not be the abolition of humanism, but it will alternatively re-delineate planetary humanism for the sake of "reworlding". It is to see in humanism "transformative subjects, driven by potential, and subversive face of power" (Braidotti 2022, p. 43). In this context, this paper attempts to reconstruct the ethics of human response-ability by proposing planetary humanism as a theological response to the current climate catastrophe, seeing humans as moral actors or as part of a moral actor network. I argue for the relationality and interdependence of matter and discourse, nature and society, and humans and non-humans through crosstalk between ecofeminist theologies and new materialism. In doing so, I reinterpret the human subject as a potential for liberation from modern human exceptionalism, acknowledging the subversive power of the concept of the subject. Thus, planetary humanism identifies human responsibility in the material environment surrounding humans, non-humans, and objects by pursuing expanded human responsibility through the interpretation of deep incarnation.

2. Criticism of the Modern Humanism: From Reason to Matter

With COVID-19, humanity is facing a new era, in which invisible viruses that exist at the border between abiotic and biotic have broken through the safe zone of human civilization and created threats to the very fabric of its existence. Although countries around the world have done their best to protect civilians from the virus, human societies have been already exposed to the real face of chronic problems such as hidden greed, hatred, inequality, and exclusion over the long period of quarantine policies. As the term, Anthropocene,[1] as a new geological era wherein humans have been the primary determinants of change, already implicates, the exclusive and destructive relationship between humans and the natural environment has led us to this climate catastrophe.

The core spirit of modernity is the expansion of human reason with the myth of progress. Ironically, human supremacy based on rational power has led modernity to this destructive end of humanity. The pandemic challenges us to draw attention to human exceptionalism of modernity and the ecological destruction of the so-called Anthropocene era. The fatal flaw of modern anthropocentrism lies in its lack of attention to the agential power of nonhuman beings and matter. As a matter of fact, these nonhuman beings, including matter, have been very important for modern industrialization, only as instrumental for the progress of human civilization. For this reason, Bruno Latour makes the claim that we have to choose now between modernizing and ecologizing. He uses the modernity as a touchstone, where the relationship between society and nature, that between the world of nonhumans and the world of humans, was beginning (Latour 1998).

By modernization, Latour refers to the ways in which nature has been dominated and controlled through human reason, thereby strictly enforcing the separation of subject and object, politics and science, and humans and non-human beings. On the other hand, ecologization seeks to affirm that human government and 'parliament of things' are intertwined and that human political actor-network as the spokesperson can politically represent for nature and nonhuman beings with the help of democratized science and institution. In fact, ecologization for him means the democratization of science and political power. Along with Latour's eco-friendly democracy, recent theories such as new materialism and ecocriticism also have criticized the modern "assumptions that confine ethical and political considerations to the domain of the Human, while feminism has offered decades of scholarly contestations against the very ethics, epistemologies, and ontologies that have underwritten Human exceptionalism." (Alaimo 2011, p. 282).

Modern humanism has played a central role in this deterioration. In other words, the modern humanist ideology has resulted "in an anthropocentrism that overemphasizes rationality, human autonomy, sovereignty and separateness from the rest of the world. Such a disconnectedness has allowed for the exploitation and abuse of the nonhuman world, which has been denied subjectivity as well as agency in its own right, as only humans are seen as proper subjects" (Signas 2020, p. 111) Humanist ideas such as anthropocentrism, rationality, human autonomy, sovereignty, and so on have contributed to the rendering of what we call nonhuman and matter as passive, mute, and objectified, and thus made them consumable (Signas 2020). Rosi Braidotti argues that the human was never a neutral category, but that it is always linked to power and privilege. Hence, our posthuman task today is to move beyond the old dualities in which Man defined himself beyond the sexualized and racialized others that were excluded from humanity (Braidotti 2022, p. 236). In *Politics of Nature*, Latour proposed a nonmodern constitution because the ideal modern constitution—the absolute separation of nature and culture, human and nonhuman, science and the humanities—never actually reflected the reality in which we live (Latour 1993, pp. 46–48).

The pandemic together with the climate change and ecological disaster discloses the faces of the nonhuman beings to us humans in a very critical way. In this context, it is easy to blame humanism for its implicated anthropocentrism, but what we need today is to construct a new model of human subjectivity that is symbiont with nonhuman others, for we are still humans. Thus, instead of a way towards dehumanization, what we need to seek is a new humanism that refers to a new way of life that should not make humans inhuman, acknowledging our interrelatedness with all beings. After all, the deconstruction of modern liberal humanism would give us a chance for a critical 'reworlding' of all intertwined differences of human and nonhumans as well as reason and matter. It is to overcome anthropocentric humanism in a way that is morally and politically responsible, that is, response-able for human entanglement with other forms of beings, and on the other hand, to find the very meaning of being human under posthuman catastrophes.

The basic orientation of various criticisms of the modern anthropocentric humanisms does not call for a return to old humanism but to planetary humanism that affirms the traversal process of cutting-edge technologies (matter) and various mattering and that shares the "flat ontology" (Morton 2013, p. 14), which argues for the ontological parity of all beings in whatever forms of being would be, including human, nonhuman, matter, nature and society. It is to find a new ethical subject by recognizing in its subjective formation the entangled intra-actions of various agencies of other forms of beings such as bacteria, minerals, ecosystem, climate system, cultural and political environments.

In this context, Latour's suggestions of the politics of nature and the parliament of things provide two critical actions we need today: A rejection of the modern distinction between the subject and object on the one hand, and a rejection of the modern epistemology based upon dualistic understandings of reality by turning to ontology on the other hand. The modern political system has never considered any political agency of nonhumans, even excluding them from any ontological domain. If there was a necessity for the being of nonhumans, it was only as instruments for human beings and societies. The current pandemic, which must be considered alongside the global climate crisis and the failure of ecosystems, provides a witness to how nonhuman beings indeed have their own agencies in the society and nature. Thus, the politics we need during and after the pandemic is a political system that makes the political representation of nonhumans in human institutionalized politics possible. Latour argues that humans in this ecological crisis need to be a "spokesperson" (Latour 2004, p. 64) for the nonhumans in the parliament of things, that is, his politics of nature. Although his idea of human political representation of nonhuman beings still seems to cling to the idea of anthropocentrism, it evidently shows us the urgencies of the political representation of nonhuman beings and things. Given the fact that human impact upon the world and its inhabitants are still immense, there is a great need for 'new forms of ethical thought and practice'(Alaimo 2011, p. 283). This urges a planetary perspective that moves beyond human exceptionalism toward an evolving multi-perspectival and multi-agential reality; hence, Latour's concept of the parliament of things becomes quite relevant. His aim is to acknowledge nonhuman agencies in nature and the environment and the role of human political agency in a way that includes the political powers of objects and hyperobjects beyond human cognition.

I agree in this paper that humanity still has a capability to make important changes in this worlding, that is, reworlding, although it cannot be denied that humans are the biggest cause of the crises we are facing today, including this pandemic. The planetary humanism I suggest here goes even further to see that human beings are the media of the divine calling for the sympoiesis of all beings on the earth. It is to acknowledge "the sense of God-with-all-living-things" (Edwards 2006, p. 60). The divine seeks for meaning with us in Its mattering, and this is what I call deep incarnation.

3. A Planetary Humanism and Materiality: From Epistemology to Ontology

In Christian Tradition, there has long been a separation between humans and the rest of the world. Human salvation has often meant saving human souls from the world and the natural environment. In his writing about ecotheology, Latour criticized both Catholics and Protestants in that they were "abandoning the huge masses of non-humans" (Latour 2009, p. 463). Traditional soteriology has its theological grounds in an anthropocentric understanding with a focus on the soul, not the flesh. The soulful salvation has tended to emphasize the superior or exclusive human uniqueness, having seen nature, the environment, and the material world as instruments for human salvation. In this theological tradition, nonhuman beings, let alone matter, have been silenced. The protestant tradition needs theology to include nonhuman beings, animate and inanimate, in its interpretation of salvation. In this context, I emphasize a planetary humanism that acknowledges the following: (1) humans are part of the entanglement of mattering and meaning, (2) nonhuman beings, including inorganic beings, have their own agencies over their worlds, (3) human responsibility lies in their response-ability to the nonhuman agencies which derives from the divine incarnation. Indeed, unlike doctrinal traditions in Christian theology, the Bible, especially Romans 8, says that it is not just humans but all creatures living with humans that wait anxiously for salvation. Therefore, we should consider the relation of humans with all things gathered, collected, or composed in it.

Proponents of new materialism and ecocriticism as well as those in ecofeminist theology have tried to reconsider the issue of mattering and to envision ourselves "as planetary creature in relation to a multitude of specific others rather than as colonizing agents who can encompass the global from a position outside the planet" (Alaimo 2019, p. 405). A new materialist position in particular supports "a middle ground composed by alliances between human and nonhuman agents" (Braidotti 2022, p. 137). Posthuman Feminist theorist Braidotti, who has described these alliances as heterogeneous assemblages, said that "I am posthuman—all-too-human" since she is "materially embodied and embedded living in fast-changing posthuman times" (Braiotti 2019, p. 12). Feminist theologians are among those who struggle with the difficulty of coming to terms with the weight of material entanglement.

The planetary humanism that I propose stems from a dialogue with the new materialist discourses and their insights and embraces a new materialist account of agency (or subjectivity) that challenges any understanding of materiality to being what is simply given to us or mere effects of human agency. This planetary thinking is expressed as a desire to recognize and reclaim matter and uses 'mattering' to denote this process. This planetary thinking is an expressed desire to recognize and reclaim matter, that is, mattering. According to Barad, matter and meaning are emergent phenomena from the entanglement of reality by our agential cut. In this sense, meaning is our response-ability to matter. In this train of thought, responsibility in this sense is none other than the ability to respond to other forms of being or materialization (Barad 2007). While critically reviewing the destruction of nature and the environment brought about by the modern as well as theological perspectives of the human subject and moral actor, the planetary humanism I theologically propose still seeks to clarify the unique role of human beings as morally responsible (response-ableness) actors. Human uniqueness as a moral agent is based upon the idea of human being as a responsive subject to others on Earth. Indeed, the *earth-bound body* of humans is constantly intertwined with numerous elements of matter, and is at the same time a complex collectivity that uses tools and instruments that are part of materiality. What concerns us in this ecosystem and 'nature society' environment is not the end of the world, but a reworlding of human–nonhuman sympoiesis with powers of material nature and against reductionist analysis of the climate crisis.

Recently new materialists have proposed that we acknowledge the fact that nonhumans make up a large part of our bodies and affect our sympoietic worlding. In this sense, Latour, for example, reads new materialism as a programmatic rejection of epistemology in favor of ontology (Herndl and Graham 2021). It aims to acknowledge the reality of object hidden from human instrumentalist perspective and to move toward an object-oriented ontology. In this pandemic, we are witnessing nonhuman things waiting for us to act upon our response-ability. Here we are reminded of the way in which Barad uses the notion of intra-activity to criticize the traditional human autonomous subject, whether it is in the form of linguistic monism, biological determinism, or classical determinism of Newtonian physics. The separation of epistemology from ontology, caused by the modern dualism of language and matter is a reverberation of metaphysics that assumes a dualism of human and nonhuman, subject and object, mind and body, and matter and discourse. According to Bennett, although human consciousness is the effect of language, this language is "a highly complex material system" (Bennett 2010). Onto-epistem-ology—the study of practices of knowing in being—is probably a better way to think about the kind of understandings that are needed to come to terms with how specific intra-actions matter.

The ethics of planetary humanism and its moral responsibility reformulate the relationship of the human and nonhuman agencies at the center. It is an attempt to reformulate the new materialism with an openness to the possibility of responsible human intervention. A materialist elaboration allows matter its due as an active participant in the world becoming and its "reworlding".Barad has argued that agential realism is morally significant because it is our "responsibility to intervene in the world's becoming, to contest and rework what matters and what is excluded from mattering" (Barad 2003, p. 827). For her, it is our responsibility or our moral-ethical duty of obligation, to intervene, contest, and rework the world's becoming, what she calls the politics of possibility implying the innumerable phenomena made by material-discursive intra-activity. However, these activities are not something we humans can control, simply by taking matters into our own hands and reconfiguring the world to our liking. Rather, on an agential realist account, materiality is an active factor in the materialization process. Nature is neither a passive surface awaiting the mark of culture nor the end product of cultural performances. Indeed, agency[2] entailed in reconfiguring material-discursive apparatuses is quite material, and human subjective moral intervention and ethical action are delegated as insignificant, although not impossible. If any moral intervention would be possible, humans need to form an assemblage with other entangled agencies. Any agential cut, that is, any subjective intervention, discloses an aspect of the entanglement, not all but a part of it. In other words, Barad does not allow human subjects an ability to choose otherwise, acting independently of our material entanglement. Thus, material ecocriticism, including Barad's views included, seems to underestimate human moral intervention, stating that agency is not voluntary decision making, thereby making the achievement of human ethical subject an impossibility (Norris 2016).

In order to take our human responsibility, we need a theory in which human ethical intervention is considered to be significant and possible. In a similar vein, Bridotti insists that humanism should not be easily discarded because of, given the relative success of the historical legacy of humanism in its support of equal rights for all. It needs, instead, to be reviewed, historicized, and assessed critically (Braidotti 2022). It is to talk of humanism "in terms of our planetary others and in terms of biology; conversely, we can talk about the biology of history" (Bauman 2014, p. 152). Thus, understanding human behavior as a complex and sometimes unknown relational behavior, interconnected with the material power of things, expands the scope of human ethical and political responsibility. One way of moving beyond the human exceptionalism is through the recognition that our subjectivities, identities, and agencies are not our own. It is to recognize that we are living with other beings and making a life together with them. No matter how much Jesus wanted to convey his love, for example, it was not possible without water and buckets to wash his disciples' feet and towels to wipe their feet. Furthermore, it would have been impossible to have a precious dinner without desks, chairs, bread, wine, and bowls at a dinner with the twelve disciples. Human subjective actions are always—already—accompanied by the agencies of things that are material, natural, and artificial. This can be said a deep incarnation, deep into the matter beyond flesh.

In the idea of "deep incarnation"—the view that the divine incarnation in Jesus presupposes a radical embodiment that reaches into the roots of material and biological existence, as well as into the darker sides of creation—one can see the importance of human agency, as Latour speaks of human political agency as the "spokesperson" for nonhumans(Latour 2004, p. 64). Such a wide-scope view of incarnation allows Christology to be meaningful when responding to the challenges of scientific cosmology (Greg 2015). Nature can live without humans, but humans cannot live without nature. Therefore, planetary humanism does not renounce hope for human possibility as the only species that aims to be, and values being, an ethical being resembling the image of God. In this sense, humanism connected to its tradition is still important in the eco-theological discourses, although it needs to move ahead and beyond it. Only humans can dream and imagine another world, the not-yet not based upon the genetic algorithm. The possibilityies and imagination of another world can only be done by humans. Despite its many problems, humanism is indeed very difficult to discard.

4. Encounter with Deep Incarnation and Matter—Moving toward a Planetary Humanism

The essential elements of Incarnation are body and matter. The body is a form of matter with which all environmental elements are entangled. In order to overcome the epistemological limitations of the modern theology constructed upon the ideas of reason and spirit, ecofeminist theology has persistently highlighted the importance of body and flesh. Traditional ethical theories were based upon an anthropocentric thinking which believed only humans were moral beings with intrinsic values and that animals, creatures, and matter had only instrumental values for human survival and well-being. In this theology, humans enjoyed absolute privilege over all other nonhuman beings. However, given that humanity is, without a doubt, the biggest cause of the climate crisis, violence against animals, and environmental destructions, this anthropocentric theology has reached its end.

In this context, one needs to be reminded that incarnation is "a question of Christ being here and being there at the deepest levels of the material world of flesh as the Incarnate One who both shares and transcends the conditions of materiality" (Greg 2015, p. 251). Thus, to be incarnate is to be immersed within this web of relationships, and the core of incarnation is to give the so-called physical world its orientation and sense. In other words, the incarnate human can think of the not-yet, introducing the inexistent time to the world we live in. In this way, humans live "at the depths" of the whole through the flows of energy and meaning (Mazi 2002). Instead of "passing time", humans become *capable of being time* in their response-ability to the not-yet. The human experience of things "com[ing] together" and "fall[ing] into place" is none other than the experience of having "timed" ourselves with others and with things. Maybe the not-yet is the voice of "the insistence of God" (Caputo 2013, p. 1). As J.D. Caputo argues, the presence of God is experienced with the divine insistence of our being here rather than the existence of God.

The destructive relations between human and nonhuman beings are currently the most serious challenge for humanity. Therefore, the significant aim of theological reflection on the climate crisis is to seek a symbiotic way in which all living beings and things live and make a life together on earth. As we seek an alternative humanism, I propose planetary humanism, seeking humans as that understand human to be moral actors and ethical subjects with response-ability. Theologically, planetary humanism is grounded in the idea of deep incarnation which is made evident in the compassion and radical self-deprecation (kenosis) in Jesus' life and death, whereby incarnation does not represent any deficiency in the divine but rather the full realization of divinity in the material entanglement. Thus, divine transcendence is none other than the ascendence of God into this world. For the planetary humanism, incarnation first means God's eternal commitment to the natural world, and secondly, it is understood as a promise of God's specificity (Edwards 2014). From this point of view, the depth of incarnation is understood as the amazing implications of God himself being with the body and matter forever. Moreover, through the deep incarnation, God is understood as the personal dimension of the not-yet, who desires matter and body. Such a depth of the divine incarnation may help us understand the very meaning of the scripture that says, "the word became flesh and made his dwelling among us."[3] Thus, deep incarnation is a theology of flesh and matter as well as a symbolic interpretation of all creatures, the planet earth and cosmos which is where I position the planetary humanism.

This new interpretation of the deep incarnation supports the Christian ethics of becoming, which does not refer to a qualitative difference between God and humans but rather to a process of self-transcendence of human existence toward others that is possible because of the relationship of deep entanglement between God and all things. The discovery of the divine possibility inherent in humanity is the most radical experience of transcendence and the most specific instantiation of material entanglement. Nevertheless, the planetary humanism proposed in this paper recognizes a qualitative difference between the becoming of relational subjectivity as a process and the completed apocalyptic existence. This planetary humanism differs from the Western individualism, which assumes the atomic and separate individuality of human being from others. Instead, it believes in human flourishing that is possible in a planetary community created with other beings, both animate and inanimate. Catherine Keller suggests "intercarnation" for such a possibility (Keller 2017a). Jurgen Moltmann in a similar gesture has emphasized that faith in a cosmic Christ can help us recover the reconciliation between heaven and all things on earth and accepts all creatures as precious beings that Christ has paid for through his death (Moltmann 2012, p. 252).

Human life is not just social and political but also biological and material. Through the deep incarnation, we are living in 'mattering', through the intra-acting in the entanglement of beings and things. Indeed, life is materialistic in the sense that our living is based upon collaboration with material beings. In the course of salvation, there is nothing a human can do alone. Therefore, the planetary humanism recognizes that the Bible understands salvation to be cosmic in nature to be achieved in the interdependence between humans and nonhuman animals within the planetary community of the kingdom of God. The concept of the new heaven and earth declared by Jesus includes and embraces the whole world, encompassing all things including nonhuman beings and humans. One of the important theological themes of incarnation in the planetary humanism is that God the Holy Spirit came to the place where humanity lived and became a member of the bio-historical community. In Christ, the world as a material reality, that is, the earth, can be a place for the ministry of the Holy Spirit to bless the whole planetary community. For example, the church uses wine, fire, and bread at that moment when expressing the most transcendental experience. Indeed, Catherine Keller explained that everything in the world has been entangled in the universe, "No Christianity could quite throw off the narrative weight of fleshly incarnation, material justice, and bodily resurrection" (Keller 2017b, pp. 111–12). Jane Bennett said that human consciousness is the effect of language, and language is 'a highly complex material system' (Bennett 2010, p. 11). Nevertheless, we easily subject nonhuman beings and matter to the below of humans. The history of salvation does not consist only of words. It should not be forgotten that the Word was proclaimed in the created world and physical environment to which the language refers.

The human condition is always already earthbound as we live together and thus stand in relation to others in our common home-planet Earth (Mazi 2002, pp. 220–21). In this created Earth containing nonhuman beings, our ethics of responsibility should not be an ethics that only speaks about responsibility, but Christian ethics that brings about practical change by actively participating in all material processes, realizing values oriented towards relational entanglement. This planetary humanism seeks responsibility that serves the multiplicity of species.

Therefore, our deep incarnation is not about transcending, but rather about the radical immanence of divinity into our planetary community of becoming, and it is none other than our worlding or reworlding in the divine creation. This incarnational humanism extends its relationality over the nonhuman and all matter, and, in this way, it is a planetary humanism. To a great extent, our species, like our subjective experiences, does not live only on our own terms. Our present experience indeed contains the evolutionary history, which refers to the millions of other species, plants, animals, minerals, and other organisms that have contributed to produce this very moment (Bauman 2014, p. 147). Jesus asks us, 'who is your neighbor?' As we can widen our relational imagination over nonhumans, animals, plants, vegetables, and minerals, they are none other than our 'kins,' as Haraway argues. As a matter of fact, "[m]any religions have jolted us out of the habits of love based upon ego, family, kin, and even nation" (Bauman 2014, p. 166). When Jesus asks us who is our neighbor is, he was issuing an ethical commandment to make a new family based upon love. This commandment to leave one's family and create a new family is not based on kinship, race, or even sex. Family is none other than the one who participates in the saving of one another, instead of seeking one's own interests. It is none other than a compassionate yearning for humans, animals, and the earth that are under the yoke of oppression. By feeling another's pain as one's own, we can become a divine family, and the current pandemic asks us to think of the pain and oppression of nonhumans on the earth. In other words, it is time for us to think about a planetary family.

Imagining a possibility of another world is possible only for humans Thus, human beings still retain their unique presence in the world despite many problems derived from anthropocentric ways of thinking. Therefore, our planetary assemblage that this planetary humanism seeks, especially during the pandemic, must find a sympoietic way to live with nonhuman forms of beings, animate and inanimate, and it will have to find a way to orient all kinds of living on the earth to the divine will. God created humans and other beings as fellow. At the same time, they are all companions for salvation. In Psalm 119, God says, "All things have been built by words", and declares, "All things have become servants of God" (Psalm 119: 89–91). Not just humans but all things are called to be God's servants. It means that human beings are companions of God and other nonhuman beings to fulfill God's will. Why does humanism still matter? It is simply because I am still a human. It is to acknowledge the limitation of the human position and, at the same time, human responsibility as an ethical subject. In this sense, humanism still has to be discussed in our eco-theological discourses of the creative tension between ontological collectivity and ethical responsibility, if we see the whole world as a collective as argued by Latour. This theological reflection will remind us that humanism is still significant for human responsibility, especially in human entanglement with other (human and nonhuman) beings on "Earth Planet". Thus, symbiotic humanism calls for rethinking this issue of responsibility as "response-ability".

5. Conclusions

Humans are the only species that can think of a living ecosystem. However, as the soteriological perspective in the Christian tradition is anthropocentric and other-worldly in orientation and emphasizes only individual repentance, therein lies a theological limitation that prevents Christians from actively contemplating human responsibility for nature and matter. The theological perspective of deep incarnation standing from the dialogue with new materialists emphasizes that we must have a firm response-ability for the entire planet because of our unique response-ability to this world. We must begin to think of the ethics of the planet, recognizing that its agents are members of a collective solidarity for the sake of a planetary community, which is constantly in flux. It requires that we form solidarity with nonhuman beings in order to embody the possibility of the "reworlding" of planetary humanism. This will lead to a symbiotic response-ability more deeply rooted in the biblical-theological ground. In this sense, Christians must immediately stop reckless anthropocentric practices such as development for development, factory-style livestock, and the way of life of mass production and consumption. In addition, human-centered ways of living that treat nonhuman beings simply as means for the progress of human civilization should be changed. The pollution of the air, water, and soil that kills other living beings is in fact driving us to death, as well as this Anthropocene civilization. It means that our world must immediately undergo 're-worlding' from our earthen foundations. Such a 're-worlding' could mean ecological salvation.

Therefore, if earth bodies are affirmed in their myriad forms of entanglement in the planet, sensitively utilizing their capacity for mutual interdependence, our homeostatic balance of well-being can resonate with other forms of beings on the earth. This asks us to change the meaning of responsibility a human individual subject must take into response-ability, which allows us to empathize with each other. As many thinkers have expressed recently, there would be no final solutions but only the ongoing practice of being open to each other, and taking the risk of being vulnerable, so that we might use our ability to respond, our responsibility, to help awaken and breathe life into our new possibilities for living justly. We only remember that God created human beings with the divine image but forget that the earth is co-creating plants and vegetables. That is, God has the earth as a co-creator of living beings on the earth. The co-creativity that is also endowed to humans with the divine image is not only for humans but for the sake of all beings. This is the reason we need to consider the way we live with animals, plants, vegetables, and things, natural and artificial. Humanism is still significant for human responsibility, given that human beings are always already intertwined with everything on "Earth Planet". I still wish to emphasize human responsibility as an ability to respond to all beings, for only humans can imagine the not-yet in order to change the world.

Funding: This research is supported by the Research Fund of the Presbyterian University and Theological Seminary, Seoul, 2022.

Institutional Review Board Statement: Not applicable.

Informed Consent Statement: Not applicable.

Data Availability Statement: Not applicable.

Conflicts of Interest: The authors declare no conflict of interest.

Notes

[1] The term 'Anthropocene', coined in 2002 by Nobel Prize winner Paul Crutzen, describes the current geological era as dominated by the measurable negative human impact on the Earth, through technological interventions and consumerism. It was discussed at the International Geological Congress in August 2016, but was rejected in July 2018 by the International Commission on Stratigraphy, in favour of the 'Meghalayan' era (Braiotti 2019, pp. 12–13).

[2] Agency is not an attribute whatsoever—it is "doing"/"being" in its intra-activity. Agency is the enactment of iterative changes to practices through the dynamics of intra-activity. Agency is about the possibilities and accountability entailed in reconfiguring material-discursive apparatuses of bodily production, including the boundary articulations and exclusions that are marked by those practices in the enactment of a causal structure" (Barad 2003, p. 827).

[3] John 1: 14: The Word became flesh and made his dwelling among us. We have seen his glory, the glory of the one and only Son, who came from the Father, full of grace and truth.

References

Alaimo, Stacy. 2011. New Materialisms, Old Humanisms, or, Following the Submersible. *NORA—Nordic Journal of Feminist and Gender Research* 19: 280–84. [CrossRef]
Alaimo, Stacy. 2019. Wanting All the Specoies to Be: Extinction, Environmental Vision, and Intimate Aesthetics. *Australian Feminist Studies* 34: 102. [CrossRef]
Barad, Karen. 2003. Posthumanist Performativity: Toward an Understanding of How Matter Comes to Matter. *Sign* 28: 801–31. [CrossRef]
Barad, Karen. 2007. *Meeting the Universe Halfway: Quantum Physics and the Entanglement of Matter and Meaning*. Durham: Duke University Press.
Bauman, Whitney A. 2014. *Religion and Ecology: Developing a Planetary Ethic*. New York: Columbia University Press.
Bennett, Jane. 2010. *Vibrant Matter: A Political Ecology of Things*. Durham: Duke University Press.
Braidotti, Rosi. 2022. *Posthuman Feminism*. Cambridge: Polity.
Braiotti, Rosi. 2019. *Posthuman Knowledge*. Princeton: Polity Press.

Caputo, John D. 2013. *The Insistence of God: A Theology of Perhaps*. Bloomington: Indiana University Press.
Edwards, Dennis. 2006. *Ecology at the Heart of Faith*. Maryknoll: Orbis.
Edwards, Dennis. 2014. *Partaking of God: Trinity, Evolution, and Ecology*. Collegeville: Liturgical Press.
Greg, N. H. 2015. The Extended Body of Christ: Three Dimensions of Deep Incarnation. *Incarnation on the Scope and Depth of Christology* 2015: 225–51.
Haraway, Donna J. 2016. *Staying with the Trouble: Making Kin in the Chthulucene*. Durham: Duke University Press.
Herndl, Carl, and Scott Graham. 2021. Getting Over Incommensurability: Latour, New Materialisms, and the Rhetoric of Diplomacy. In *Thinking with Bruno Latour in Rhetoric and Composition*. Edited by Paul Lynch and Nathaniel Rivers. Carbondale: Southern Illinois University Press.
Keller, Catherine. 2017a. *Intercarnations: Exercises in Theological Possibility*. New York: Fordham University Press.
Keller, Catherine. 2017b. Tangles of Matter, Tangles of Theology. *Entangled Worlds* 2017: 111–12.
Latour, Bruno. 1993. *We Have Never Been Modern*. Translated by Catherine Porter. Cambridge: Harvard University Press.
Latour, Bruno. 1998. To modernise or ecologise? That is the question. In *Remaking Reality: Nature at the Millennium*. Edited by Bruce Braun and Noel Castree. London: Routledge, pp. 221–42.
Latour, Bruno. 2004. *Politics of Nature: How to Bring the Sciences into Democracy*. Translated by Catherine Porter. Cambridge: Harvard University Press.
Latour, Bruno. 2009. Will Non-humans be saved? An argument in ecotheology. *Journal of the Royal Anthropological Institute* 15: 459–75. [CrossRef]
Mazi, Glen. 2002. *Earthbodies Rediscovering Our Planetary Senses*. Albany: State University of New York Press.
Moltmann, Jurgen. 2012. *Ethics of Hope*. Minneapolis: Fortress Press.
Morton, Timothy. 2013. *Philosophy and Ecology after the End of the World*. Minneapolis: University of Minnesota Press.
Norris, Marcos. 2016. Ecocriticism and Moral responsibility: The Question pf agency in Karen Barad's Performativity Theory. *Fugitive Environmentalism* 49: 180–1. [CrossRef]
Signas, Jakob. 2020. Who is thy neighbour? On Posthumanism, responsibility and interconnected solidarity. *Approaching Religion* 10: 111. [CrossRef]
Walters, Mark Jerome. 2003. *Six Modern Plagues: And How We Are Causing Them*. Washington, DC: Island Press.

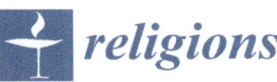

Essay

Shifting Epistemologies, Shifting Our Stories—Where Might We Find Hope for a World on the Brink of Climate Catastrophe?

Mary E. Hess

Luther Seminary, Saint Paul, MI 55108, USA; mhess@religioused.org

Abstract: In the early 1990s, David Orr wrote about the epistemological myths of North American culture, and offered ecological literacy as a form of resistance. In the same decade, Parker Palmer confronted dominant epistemologies in religious institutions, and retrieved early Christian frames by way of resistance. One was writing through the lens of environmental science, and one through the lens of the desert mothers and fathers of Christian history. Neither acknowledged the First Nations, Metis and Inuit epistemologies which offered similarly contesting frames. It may be too late, yet even in a moment of climate catastrophe there is hope that shifting our forms of knowing can invite pedagogical practices that transform our communities. This essay will articulate the congruence between these disparate and diverse stances as sacred ground within which to root embodied, theologically astute pedagogies for the 21st century. Several pragmatic exercises that have emerged as fruitful for learners seeking to embody compelling counter narratives are also offered.

Keywords: environmental education; religious education; indigenous epistemologies; storytelling exercises; story categories; adult development

Citation: Hess, Mary E.. 2022. Shifting Epistemologies, Shifting Our Stories—Where Might We Find Hope for a World on the Brink of Climate Catastrophe?. *Religions* 13: 625. https://doi.org/10.3390/rel13070625

Academic Editors: Pamela R. McCarroll, HyeRan Kim-Cragg and Antonio Muñoz-García

Received: 2 February 2022
Accepted: 1 July 2022
Published: 6 July 2022

Publisher's Note: MDPI stays neutral with regard to jurisdictional claims in published maps and institutional affiliations.

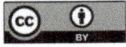

Copyright: © 2022 by the author. Licensee MDPI, Basel, Switzerland. This article is an open access article distributed under the terms and conditions of the Creative Commons Attribution (CC BY) license (https://creativecommons.org/licenses/by/4.0/).

1. Introduction

Story matters. Story offers context and connects to larger contexts. Story helps us to make sense of ourselves and each other. We live embedded in a cacophony of stories, most of which are digitally mediated in some fashion (Hess 2011, 2016, 2018, 2019a, 2020, 2021). In 2022, as the world faces climate devastation, how we tell the story of transcendence, of relationship with God, with the earth, and with each other is impossibly urgent. Yet we must try to find ways to discern how to untangle the knots of destructive stories, and braid those of hope and resilience together.

Let me begin this essay by noting that I grew up near the shores of Lake Winnebago, in Oshkosh, Wisconsin, in the United States. For the last two decades, I have lived a ten-minute walk from the Mississippi River in Saint Paul, Minnesota. Both of these settings are places where people are encouraged to be outside. I grew up bicycling, skating (both roller and ice), canoeing, sailing, even rappelling off state park cliffs. When we moved to Minnesota, we were immediately told that there is no such thing as bad weather only the wrong clothing, and invited into multiple forms of outdoor recreation.

The "outdoors", then, has always been a big part of my life and the contexts in which I have lived. But note the ways in which I was invited to experience the outdoors: always as a place to play, as a form of "recreation", as something to be enjoyed. Yet both of these places—Oshkosh, Wisconsin and Saint Paul, Minnesota—hold haunting histories in their very grounds. "Oshkosh" was the name of a Menominee Indian chieftain, yet I grew up with little or no knowledge of the anguish, injustice, and deep loss endured by the Ho-Chunk (Winnebago) people at the hands of settlers, a history that continues in so many ways. One of my favorite walking paths takes me past the confluence of the Mississippi and Minnesota rivers, a place deeply sacred to the Dakota peoples, the ground of their creation, and also the place of their internment and much death following the US-Dakota war in 1862 (Carley 1961; Westerman and White 2012).

How is it that the "story of the outdoors"—a story that led me to work for a conservation organization shortly after college—has never been shared with me with deep enough memory and care to include these elements of the land's story? At least one response to that question lies at the heart of what it means to do environmental education, and thus the challenges we must face if we as a whole community of creation are to care for our deeply ailing world.

Stories come in multiple forms, some of which are transformative and many of which are "de-formative" and deeply destructive. A story which invites you into more complex meaning, which shares ways to resist oppression, or even simply draws you into deeper empathy, can be profoundly transformative. Stories which constrain imagination, limit connection, dehumanize and polarize, on the other hand, can be deeply destructive.

Who tells stories, the context in which the stories are engaged, and the process by which we share them is an essential element of the meaning we construct with them. The competition over what it means to know, over who is a knower, over who determines what is authoritative, indeed, what it even means "to know" is the challenge we must face if we are to be attentive to the sacred stories at the heart of religious community. The conflict over our central epistemological assertions is clearly visible at the heart of environmental catastrophes. Was the world created in seven 24 h days, or is evolutionary theory a more adequately descriptive frame for seeing each other and the earth? Are human actions implicated in the changes we are detecting in glacial ice, or are such changes predestined and unchangeable manifestations of a deity's transcendent agency?

The challenges here are not about making choices between one reality and another, but rather about understanding with humility and complexity how we can embody stories which frame our world through scientific lenses *and* theological ones. I believe we must draw on the ancient—and still present—meaning-making frames our indigenous siblings offer us if we are to engage deeply both the despair and the hope that resides amidst this catastrophe. Indigenous epistemologies move beyond an either/or framing and more deeply into depicting and embody what it means to know through complex and resilient story-making and storytelling (Antoine et al. 2018; Garod et al. 2017; Reyhner 2015; Cajete 2015; Kirkness 2013).

In the early 1990s, David Orr, arguably one of the most influential of environmental educators, wrote about the epistemological myths of North American culture, and offered ecological literacy as a form of resistance to them (Orr 1994). In the same decade, Parker Palmer confronted the dominant epistemologies of North American religious institutions, and retrieved early Christian frames by way of resistance (Palmer 1983, 1998). The former was writing through the lens of environmental science, and the latter through the lens of the desert mothers and fathers of Christian history. Neither acknowledged the First Nations, Metis and Inuit epistemologies which offered similarly contesting frames. Perhaps they were unaware of these ways of knowing the world, or perhaps they avoided what could have been cultural appropriation? Regardless of why there was no such acknowledgement, much of what they wrote is congruent with indigenous meaning-making, and can be even more deeply transformative for religious communities. One clear way to avoid cultural mis-appropriation is to develop thorough relational accountability, to learn with and from indigenous communities while respecting their complexity and commitment. It may be too late, yet even in a moment of climate catastrophe there is hope that shifting our forms of knowing can invite pedagogical practices that transform our communities.

I need to share one more part of my own story, so as to contextualize clearly from whence this argument arises. I write from a very specific space in ways that might be evocative for others but cannot be prescriptive for people beyond my location. I am a faculty member at an ELCA Lutheran seminary in Minnesota. I have been there for more than two decades as their professor of educational leadership. I am also a Roman Catholic layperson and a white, cis-gendered woman with two adult children and a spouse of more than three decades, all three of whom are male and cis-gendered. That is a very narrow stance from which to observe, and I want to write primarily to people who inhabit that kind of social location, because far too often we are the producers and enforcers of dominant cultural streams. I hope that in doing so I may reach such producer/enforcers, and open up some room for change.

2. Stories and Storying

2.1. A Story of Wolves

There is an ancient story attributed to the Cherokee people[1] which tells us that we are each made up of two wolves, one which is evil and feeds on our anger and other base emotions, and one which is good and feeds on our joys and compassion. The one we feed the most will be the one who lives. This is but one way to speak about the competing and often conflicting impulses and desires that make up what it can mean to be human. Note where human agency resides in this story: in making choices about what to feed, how to nurture, a particular dynamic.

I grew up with Christians in churches who tell a story of conflicting emotions and actions in terms of the Fall in the book of Genesis, and so draw on a theology of original sin to describe the ways in which we as humans must constantly seek forgiveness from a judgmental God who rules in omnipotence. Even the overflowing grace of a God who chooses Incarnation, who chooses to pour Godself out in a kenosis beyond imagining in the body of Jesus the Christ gets interpreted as seeing God's action as a "sacrifice" for our sins, rather than as an exercise in "at-one-ment." For me, at least, this story has been profoundly destructive, leading to shame and a temptation to view myself as "saved" while others are "damned." There are, however, many other ways to tell the stories of Genesis. I have been gifted with biblical colleagues who have helped me to follow the Christ into a sacramental imagination that leads to these other interpretations, each of which tends to "feed the wolf" in differing ways, and several of which invite us into compassion, justice, and clear engagement in global interdependence.[2]

My point here is that we are story people. We tell stories to make sense of ourselves, of our relationships with others, with God, indeed with all of creation. The challenge for religious educators in the uncertainty, constant change, and turmoil of the worlds we inhabit is to ignite curiosity about the stories we hold most dear, to curate versions of them that are life-giving, and to help people develop the practices and capacities necessary for a thriving religious imagination.

2.2. Three Curricula

Educators have long observed, as did Elliott Eisner in 1985, that learning is embodied in three curricula: the explicit, the implicit, and the null (Eisner 1985; Kim-Cragg 2019). The explicit curriculum being that which we intentionally seek to teach, the implicit being those elements, that information, which we pick up unintentionally or around the edges of any explicit curriculum. The null curriculum, perhaps the most powerful of all, is that which we learn through silences, through taboos.

I grew up with an explicit curriculum about the outdoors being a place in which to play, a resource for my enjoyment, a source of beauty and peace. The implicit curriculum of those spaces carried as well the sense that I as a human being had both the right and the ability to plumb those spaces to their depths for my enjoyment. The null curriculum, the silence at its heart, taught me to ignore the histories behind the names of these places I loved, to not listen for the anguish emerging there. It also taught me, a white person growing up in a middle-class space, not to ask where everyone else was. Why were there not people of many other races enjoying these spaces? The native peoples who had tended that land for centuries were simply an ancient stereotype. The enslaved peoples, and the people who had been brought to build the railroad from Asian lands, these people were nowhere to be found in the spaces I inhabited, and that was typical, that was what I learned was the norm, how it was supposed to be. Never mind that Wisconsin as a state in the 1970s and 1980s as I grew up had many communities of people in it from many vastly differing lands and contexts. I learned not to ask certain questions, and I learned not to see, not to feel, certain kinds of pain (Brookfield and Hess 2021).

It is this combination of the three curricula that we need to break open. As renowned scholar of leadership Brené Brown has written: "... numbing vulnerability is especially debilitating because it doesn't just deaden the pain of our difficult experiences; numbing vulnerability also dulls our experiences of love, joy, belonging, creativity, and empathy. We can't selectively numb emotion. Numb the dark and you numb the light". (Brown 2012, p. 137). Refusing to acknowledge the pain and the anguish of these places also means I, like so many others who grew up in these "curricula", have been cut off from the deep joy and love to which our God invites us. Far from feeding only one of the wolves, we are essentially starving ourselves all together (Ayres 2021).

2.3. A Global Pandemic in the 2020s

It is 2022 as I write this piece, and there are diametrically opposed stories vying for our attention and embodiment. We are currently in the third year of a global pandemic due to the SARS-CoV2 virus. The stories swirling around compete constantly for our attention. Is this a mild bug, a mild flu? Is this a devastating virus which has killed more than 1,000,000 people in the US alone? Is this a viral vector deliberately created by sinister entities seeking to implant nanochips in people? Are basic measures like physical distancing and masking social goods to be embraced by all? Or are vaccines and face coverings deceptive and hidden attempts to erase personal freedoms?

Notice, though, how few of these stories lift up the possible origins of this virus in the devastation of our global home, and the climatic changes that are ruining biomes. There is actually a lot of scientific evidence that this virus, and others sure to follow it, are being born and finding pools in which to grow and mutate, because of the profoundly altering impact humans are having on our earth, on our shared home.[3] Here again there is a null curriculum that is preventing us from perceiving deeply that to which our God (at least in Christian settings, the ones from which I speak) is calling us.[4]

What might we observe about this discontinuity, this disconnect between the ubiquitous stories that heighten our fears and anxieties in terms of individual responsibility, and any others that might articulate shared and communal forms of knowing?

The story of the two wolves has been embedded in so much popular culture that it has lost much of its original context.[5] If we could retrieve and reclaim some of that context, we could learn that the native communities telling this story (and so many others) begin within a shared space of collective knowing. Their epistemological standpoint, if you will, is thoroughly communal, deeply relational, and explicitly story-driven. It is not simply that each individual person "feeds" their wolves, but also that the very notion of having within oneself a "wolf" is connected with a way of viewing oneself and creation as deeply entwined. I would caution here against the cultural mis-appropriation of notions of a "spirit animal" that have become so dangerously popular,[6] and emphasize instead that this story arises within an epistemological stance which honors all of creation, and views human persons as but one participant in that creation (Garod et al. 2017; Reyhner 2015; Cajete 2015; Kirkness 2013).

2.4. Genesis Stories and beyond

Christians who inhabit the kind of social location in which I find myself need to be asking profound questions about the Genesis stories, and whether there might be a different standpoint, a different form of knowing, from which to hear and embrace that story (Dahill and Martin-Schramm 2016; Johnson 2014; Rasmussen 2013). For instance, Parker Palmer describes in his book *To Know As We Are Known*, an interpretation of that story which suggests that Adam and Eve

> ... were driven from the Garden because of the kind of knowledge they reached for—a knowledge that distrusted and excluded God. Their drive to know arose not from love but from curiosity and control, from the desire to possess powers

belonging to God alone. They failed to honor the fact that God knew them first, knew them in their limits as well as their potentials. In their refusal to know as they were known, they reached for a kind of knowledge that always leads to death. (Palmer 1983, p. 151)

This is an interpretation of the story which highlights our need to stand in humility and awe, rather than reaching for power. There is a story in Genesis that is far more often told when thinking about creation and the environment, and that is the story of God giving Adam "dominion" over creation. Rather than interpreting that word in its sense of "domain" and "tending to the domain"—an epistemological stance that would be congruent with seeing humanity as part of creation—that text has far too often been understood as granting humans power over creation, and as a license for domination (Chamberlain 2000, p. 137).

3. Teaching with Story

3.1. Four Kinds of Stories

How might we engage these iconic stories in ways that draw people into deeper and more grounded versions, that emphasize the love of which Palmer writes, and the humility of being part of, not owner or controller, of creation? Seeking to understand how to shift interpretation means seeking to understand engaging story, storying, storytelling. It demands that we understand the stance, the epistemologies, we wish to honor. Bell and her team, while working in the field of anti-racism education, have identified four categories of stories that help to illuminate this task of transformative interpretation and learning. They write of "dominant or stock", "concealed", "resistance", and "counter" stories (Bell et al 2008).

"Dominant or stock" stories are those which are "the most public and ubiquitous in dominant, mainstream institutions". They are told by those who hold control in various discursive terrains, and who are able to embed their stories in public rituals, monuments, school curricula, and many other institutional and structural forms. They "tell us a lot about what a society considers important and meaningful".

"Concealed" stories, in contrast, while existing in the same spaces as so-called stock stories, "most often remain in the shadows, hidden from public view". These stories might be "told and retold by people in the margins whose experiences and aspirations they express and honor". Yet there is a seductive element to such stories because only "insiders" know them and in our current information ecology they can be drawn into conspiracy frameworks all too easily.

The third kind of story, "resistance" stories, are "both historical and contemporary, that tell about how people have resisted forms of oppression such as racism, challenged the stock stories that support it, and fought for more equal and inclusive social arrangements". Such stories can teach us about perspectives and practices that have existed throughout our history up to the present time, thus expanding our vision of what is possible in our own work for the kin-dom of God. Note that even a small shift—from "kingdom of God" to "kin-dom of "God"—invites resistance to dominance.

The final category of which they write, "counter stories", contains stories which "are new stories that are deliberately constructed to challenge the stock stories. They build on and amplify resistance stories, they offer ways to interrupt the status quo and work for change. These stories enact continuing critique and resistance to the stock stories and enable new possibilities for inclusive human community" (Bell et al. 2008, p. 19 and following).

3.2. When Counter Stories Get Co-Opted into Stock Stories

It is critical to grasp that indigenous epistemologies are counter stories within hegemonic cultural spaces. They may well offer resistance stories, and to some extent have been concealed from dominant view, but at their heart they are "new" stories, in the sense that they are from an entirely different frame than that which structures the stories of dominance within which I grew up (DeMars and Tait 2019).

Yet at the same time, it is also possible to perceive the ways in which a story that arose in a very specific context, within a very specific epistemology, can be drawn into one of these four categories (Ng 2020). We both know and understand how important context is, and yet need to begin to grasp that context collapse is all around us. Context collapse is part of what occurs when stories from one specific people, told in a specific context and with a specific set of practices, get lifted up and floated on the global digital sea, losing most of that context (Hess 2019b, p. 215). This happens all too often with stories that arise from within indigenous communities. A very famous example might be the teary-eyed Indian commercial/PSA from the 1970s (https://youtu.be/8Suu84khNGY, accessed on 1 February 2022). In that commercial an Indian paddling his canoe down a highly polluted stream evokes a commitment to the land that is now almost past retrieving. His single tear, highlighted by the camera, has an accompanying narration in an ominously deep male voice saying "people start pollution, people can stop it". The "solution"? Write for a pamphlet on how to "Keep America Beautiful".

Here a thoroughly relational element between a person and the land which is characteristic of many indigenous epistemologies is being used to attempt to catalyze opposition to littering. Never mind that genocide and centuries of settler colonialism have erased these peoples from the very land they were connected to, here the native person is constructed wholly as a stereotype and used instrumentally in the service of the dominant story. To be blunt, individual litter was never the real environmental problem (a reality to which the smoke stacks belching smog in the background of the commercial make subtle allusion).

In 2022, a commercial aired selling a package of streaming media (Hulu, Disney+, and ESPN) starring the actor Dave Bautista as he paddled a canoe (https://youtu.be/Cc6QxlXjvWU, accessed on 1 February 2022) down a quiet stream. The version airing within mobile games includes him trailing his hand in the water while saying "I love you, stream". Fifty years of advertising have developed from a native person at the heart of a PSA bemoaning littering, to an ad for streaming media with a person whose physical characteristics subliminally evoke native stereotypes (olive-toned skin, long hair pulled back in a single ponytail, actions which clearly relish the "outdoors") and which seeks to sell digital media streams.

Here a comprehensive connection to the land and its resources, understood within many native epistemologies as a relative, is trivialized and narrowed down to an excuse for staying hooked to a computer screen even while outdoors "in nature". This is an example of how counter stories arising from indigenous epistemologies have been drawn into dominant stories, perhaps identified as somewhat "concealed" or "minoritized"—but nonetheless understood only in relation to a dominant story.

3.3. A Counter Story of Ecological Literacy

In practical theological terms, the challenge is not simply to offer better interpretations of biblical stories, but also to deconstruct the racism and other oppressive dynamics structured into all of our stock representations through their underlying epistemological framing, through what is understood to be "knowledge" and what constitutes "knowing". Hearlson calls this "unmasking of idols" (Hearlson 2021, p. 138).

Scholars and teachers within the movement for environmental education have been seeking for decades to push back against dominant stories. Consider the basic assertions that David Orr (1994), a key figure in environmental education in the US, offered by identifying what he termed "key myths" of US culture.

3.3.1. Myths Which Prevent Ecological Literacy

- Ignorance is a solvable problem
- With enough knowledge and technology we can manage planet Earth
- Knowledge is increasing and by implication human goodness
- We can adequately restore that which we have dismantled

- The purpose of education is that of giving you the means for upward mobility and success
- Our culture represents the pinnacle of human achievement (Orr 1994, p. 8 and following)

The "US culture" he is writing of here is clearly a dominant story that encapsulates white supremacy, and in doing so removes human beings, at least those characterized as white, from connection to the land in deeply relational ways. He asserts, by way of contrast, that learning should be focused as follows.

3.3.2. Ecological Literacy Contrasts

- All education is environmental education (null, implicit, explicit)
- The goal of education is not mastery of subject material but of one's person
- Knowledge carries with it the responsibility to see that it is well used in the world
- We cannot say that we know something until we understand the effects of this knowledge on real people and their communities
- The importance of "minute particulars" and the power of examples over words
- The way learning occurs is as important as the content of particular courses (Orr 1994, p. 8 and following)

3.4. A Counter Story from Christianity

In the same decade that Orr was writing, Parker Palmer published *The Courage to Teach* (Palmer 1998), a book which has become a key text throughout the country in courses focused on helping people learn to teach. Indeed, it has been reprinted so often that it has both a 10th and a 20th anniversary edition. Even prior that book, however, a full decade earlier, Palmer published *To Know As We Are Known* (Palmer 1983). In his books, Palmer sought to retrieve what he identified as an ancient form of knowing rooted in the lives of the desert mothers and fathers. The writings of these people, generally understood to be Christians who lived in first few centuries following Jesus and who fled into the desert regions of what is now Egypt to form monastic communities, have become central to a retrieval of contemplative and communal forms of Christian knowing. Palmer has sought to help contemporary teachers shift their practices to embody this form of knowing he has termed "the community of truth".

Much like Orr, Palmer's arguments sought to dethrone what he labeled an "objectivist myth". His diagrams make his ideas clear, but they cannot be reprinted in this article due to copyright constraints.[7] Palmer's "community of truth" is a profoundly relational, as contrasted with relativist, way to conceptualize what it means to know. In his description, every entity knows, and even that which is known has agency: the topic or subject at the heart of our knowing impacts what we know. How we see shapes what we see, and what we see shapes how we see. To teach within this conception, within this frame of knowing, is to design spaces in which this "community of truth" can be genuinely embodied.

Palmer writes in a later book, with Arthur Zajonc, that physicist Henry Stapp believes that: "it is no longer possible even to think of the atom as a discrete entity . . . an elementary particle is not an independently existing, unanalyzable entity. It is, in essence, a set of relationships that reach outward to other things" (Palmer and Zajonc 2010, p. 26). Further, they draw on the work of philosopher of science, Ian Barbour, to suggest that: "Nature is understood now to be relational, ecological, and interdependent. Reality is constituted by events and relationships rather than separate substances or separate particles. We are now compelled to see nature as "a historical community of interdependent beings (Palmer and Zajonc 2010, p. 26)".

This profoundly interconnected, interdependent conception of reality can be linked, as Palmer suggests, to the ancient work of the desert mothers and fathers (Palmer 1983, p. 207 and following). I often offer students the "sound bite" version of Palmer's assertions by noting that "the more diverse the knowers, the more robust the knowing". This is a story about knowing, an epistemological argument, that is deeply congruent with the contrasting epistemologies shaped by First Nations, Metis, and Inuit peoples in North America. Indeed, some scholars believe that this conception of knowing as thoroughly relational (not relativist), and profoundly embodied in story is a key similarity across indigenous epistemologies the world over.[8]

3.5. Mediated Stories as Entry Points into the Trauma Found in Stock Stories

What could it mean, for those of us embedded in the dominant stories of North America, to find ways to move to a more grounded—and I use that metaphor deliberately—conception of knowing? Knowing through story requires learning a series of embodied practices. Herein lies hope: hope for transformation (James and Brookfield 2014), hope for renewing relationship (Brookfield and Holst 2011), hope for leaning into the sacramentality of creation (Johnson 2014), the embodied and multi-sensory forms of knowing that can be understood as being at the very heart of Christianity (Smith 2004).

Consider the story of the two wolves with which I began this essay. Where did it come from? Who told it? In what context did I encounter it? What elements of my own already existing sense of story did it hook into? A story invites imagination, it invites "feeling with", it casts a vision for how to perceive that which is around and within you. It also narrows focus, and spotlights elements to the exclusion of other elements upon which it casts shadows.

In this third year of the COVID pandemic, Adam McKay wrote and produced a film entitled *Don't Look up* which was then sold to stream online through Netflix. This satirical comedy imagined a giant comet streaking towards the earth, certain to destroy the earth all together.[9] The film highlights the commercial success of misdirected and even patently false information, and the extent to which vast numbers of people with the structural capacity to respond to an existential threat instead are drawn into petty and self-serving dynamics. The president of the US in the film, the military advisors, the mass stream "news" anchors: all of them are in thrall to immediate polling numbers, the latest celebrity scandal, and their own personal anxieties.

As is often stated, if you cannot imagine it, it is difficult to work towards transformation. Further, if you cannot feel it, how are you to desire transformation? Stock stories numb our emotions, they hide and deny anguish, they seek to teach us that helping each other somehow harms us by creating "dependence" (Stone 2008). We have to reclaim our ability to sense and feel pain, and then to heal and grow with it. Just as the two wolves story suggests we must "feed the wolf" of joy and love, we can engage the Christian story of Jesus as one in which Jesus engages in relationship with everyone, no matter how marginalized, and as a story in which "being baptized into death" yet brings forth life.

Resmaa Menakem has described two different kinds of pain that attend trauma. He describes a traumatic event as "an incident that causes physical, emotional, spiritual, or psychological harm. The person experiencing the distressing event may feel threatened, anxious, or frightened as a result. In some cases, they may not know how to respond, or may be in denial about the effect such an event has had". In 2022, we are surrounded by traumatic events, events that are entwined with environmental injustice, with deeply oppressive relationships with creation (or the lack thereof). But Menakem describes trauma not as an endpoint, but rather as the starting point for asking how we are to heal. In doing so he suggests that there are at least two kinds of pain: "clean" pain and "dirty" pain. Clean pain is "pain that mends and can build your capacity for growth. It's the pain you feel when you know what to say or do; when you really, really don't want to say or do it; and when you do it anyway, responding from the best parts of yourself". While dirty pain is the "pain of avoidance, blame, or denial—when you respond from your most wounded parts" (Menakem 2018, p. 26).

Do dominant or stock stories help us to distinguish between clean and dirty pain? Or instead, do they seek to numb us to the pain, hide its origins, and deflect engagement with it? Might they in fact be supporting precisely the kind of "numbing" of which Brown warned? In the film *Don't Look Up*, the only hints of a different way to view reality come in brief glimpses of animals amidst the beauty of nature. In contrast, we see many examples of attempts to ignore, deny, and numb what Menakem would label "dirty" pain in the actions of the main characters. Perhaps one of the clearest examples of dirty pain in that film, of someone who numbs themselves to reality, comes from a scientist who gets drawn into an adulterous relationship with a media celebrity rather than deal with the pain in his family.

The film concludes with a small group of people who sought unsuccessfully to intervene in the disaster, eating one final meal together and sharing their sense of the peace that can come from deep relationality, even as the comet obliterates them. It is a bleak ending, and once again reinforces the notion that it is up to individual human beings ensconced in particular structures of power to change things. It concludes that ordinary, everyday human beings have little or nothing to contribute in transformation. Yet even in that bleakness there is also a glimpse of the hope and joy that can come in sharing a simple meal, in being with loved ones. Indeed, the only depiction of religion in the whole film comes in this final scene when a millennial who has left a conservative evangelical upbringing behind offers a profound prayer. There is hope to be found here, even if it is a bleak hope, in acknowledging that we are all part of one another—indeed of all of creation.

3.6. Digital Stories as Entry Points into Resistance and Counter Stories

There are a nearly infinite number of examples of short pieces available through Youtube that offer an imagination for such hope that is deeper and vividly depicted. There are four that are particularly pertinent here.

The first is a film produced by the Bioneers,[10] with Robin Kimmerer narrating, entitled "the Honorable Harvest". In this piece, Kimmerer offers the insight of a counter story that the honorable harvest is a "covenant of reciprocity between humans and the living world". This covenant demands an understanding that the lives we are taking, when we pick plants, are the "lives of sovereign beings . . . . And in order to accept their gift we owe them at least our attention". She goes on to describe how she has been taught "never to take the first plant that you see . . . If you are going to take a life, you have to be personally accountable for it". This is a way of seeing the world, a way of knowing, that is very much part of the epistemological frames I noted earlier, within native communities. Robin Kimmerer herself is an enrolled member of the Potowatomi Nation. Her description of the "honorable harvest" also has clear resonance with the "community of truth" of which Palmer writes.

A second piece produced by The Intercept, and narrated by Alexandria Ocasio Cortez, is entitled "A Message from the Future".[11] In this short animation, Cortez imagines herself twenty years in the future, looking back on both the climate devastation wrought by humans, and also the hopeful interventions and shifts made possible when human beings organize collectively to offer universal health care, universal income, universal access to work. Hers is a profoundly political message, but one which is shaped by ideas about collective action and collective accountability. She is narrating a resistance story, one which invites an imagination that could develop into a counter story.

A third piece is an excerpt from a much longer film which is an interview with Joanna Macy.[12] In this short excerpt, she describes what it means to "befriend our despair," and in doing so talks about how we as a "planet people" are "sick in our soul". She suggests that we "need pain to alert us to what needs attention". Rather than treating pain as an "enemy to our cheerfulness", we need to understand (as does the first noble truth of Buddhism) that "there is suffering". She remembers her early childhood in the Christian church to draw out a belief that recognizing the pain of our suffering world is essential. "Pain opens the heart and the eyes so you can see the beauty." Here she is offering an example of Menakem's "clean" pain, and inviting us to see—as does Brown—how refusing to numb our emotions is crucial.

Finally, a fourth piece is a short music video by the group Birdtalker, entitled "One."[13] This song uses a poem by Rumi to narrate a string of images which ignite imagination for the heartbeat of creation, a heartbeat in which we all participate. A line from the song, "underneath what's detectable with eyes, every particle's vibrating with the one life", makes clear the interdependent, entwined nature of reality. This is my briefest but perhaps most compelling example of a counter story rooted in this alternate epistemology, this connected and relational and accountable form of knowing.

I offer these four examples because they are diverse, grounded in wildly different spaces, and yet all four offer a narrative, a story, a vision of an inter-connected, interdependent world that is in sharp contrast to dominant narratives. They are available via digital media, they invite curiosity about our deep relationality, they draw on multiple senses—visual, aural—to embody their story, and they each refuse to succumb to despair.

4. Developmental Psychology for Transformation

How are we to engage stories, then, how can we help people to see "through" the satirical lens of dominant media, and to seek out and embrace resistance stories in ways that might move us into the "community of truth" of which Palmer writes, the "ecological literacy" of Orr; indeed, the contrasting epistemological frames offered by long minoritized indigenous communities that provide profound counter narratives?

To return to the biblical stories we first read in Genesis, for those of us working within Christian contexts at least, we have a set of stories that have come to be understood within a fairly narrow range of interpretations. Before we can even begin to articulate alternatives, resistance stories that might help us move to counter stories, we have to understand where people are, how they have understood what it means to be Christian, particularly as part of or in relation to Creation. This is urgent work that demands that we understand working at the level of heart knowledge, not simply cognitive ideas. This is work that demands transformation in the ways we know.

Robert Kegan, a constructive developmental psychologist, is eloquent about how transformation of meaning-making unfolds in adult life. He has demonstrated that adult learning and development proceeds in a spiral fashion that can be identified as "confirmation, contradiction, continuity" (Kegan 1982, p. 123 and following). He and his colleagues have documented different forms of meaning-making that can develop in adulthood. Of specific interest here are the shifts they have observed when people move from what they have labelled a "socialized mind with cross-categorical meanings" to a "self-authoring mind capable of complex systemic" meaning-making. At least for people who carry one or more of the identity markers that confer privilege in our systems of dominance (gender, race, age, ability, economic status, education, and so on), it is a "self-authoring mind" that needs to be cultivated to be able both to see these systems and begin to construct ways beyond them.[14] It is a "self-authoring" mind that invites relational accountability, and offers the capacity to embody such.

As an example, if you are watching the 2022 commercial for streaming services I described earlier, could you differentiate between the experience of joy and curiosity you might experience in engaging stories in such digital streams while at the same time acknowledging the tenuous relationship with the outdoors that is being depicted? If connection to the outdoors truly is to bring connection and joy, how might you be fully present to it? Holding awareness of both at the same time is a deeply challenging stance that emerges within a self-authoring mind.[15] In a similar dynamic, is it possible to engage the stories of Genesis—particularly of the Garden of Eden, of the Fall, of the expulsion from the Garden—as deep truths and at the same time enter into the awe and wonder evoked by scientific explanations of the Big Bang, and the ever expanding and evolving Cosmos?

In the worlds in which the biblical stories first arose as compelling truths, in the social spaces of oral culture, all that we can glean at this many centuries of distance from their first telling suggests that a deep relationship with Creation was the center and heartbeat of that imagination (Johnson 2014; Jennings 2010). When Palmer writes of a "community of truth" that centers on learning a topic, a subject such that that topic, that subject, has real subjectivity and agency itself, he is echoing in the language of rationalist western culture, something that appears to me, at least, to be deeply rooted in the epistemological frames, the stories and practices, of so many indigenous peoples.

Robin Kimmerer (trained in the western practices of environmental and forest biology, and also an enrolled member of the Citizen Potawatomi Nation) is one of the few teacher/scholars I have encountered who is able to speak in these disparate languages (Kimmerer 2013). Her description of the "honorable harvest" I noted above in the short video, offers the two frames side by side, or perhaps intermingled, in a way that bridges some of the distance that might be perceived between them, while at the same time lifting up the essential moral convictions embedded in indigenous epistemologies.[15] Palmer is seeking a similar moral conviction, when he urges readers to recognize that "we know as we are known" by a God who is relational within God's very self, in the social Trinity. So, too, Pope Francis when he urges "care for our common home" (Pope Francis 2015).

Why does this matter to environmental education in religious settings?

Joanna Macy is quoted by ter Kuile (2020) as noting four metaphors for describing our relationship with creation:

> The first is to think of the world as a battlefield in which the forces of good fight the forces of evil. In this frame of mind, the earth is a resource to be mined and shaped to meet our human desires . . . .

> Macy identifies the second paradigm as viewing the world as a trap.

> Instead, argues Macy, we might think of the world as our lover. "When you see the world as lover, every being, every phenomenon, can become an expression of that ongoing, erotic impulse . . .

> The fourth and final paradigm Macy invites us into is seeing the world as self. No longer is nature something outside of us, a landscape for us to admire or even to love—instead, we are nature. (quote in ter Kuile 2020, pp. 142–46)

This is a description that, at a minimum, comes from a "self-authoring mind", perhaps it even stretches into what Kegan calls a "self-transforming mind".[17]

Do those psychological labels matter? Only if we can use them as a way to deepen our empathy for the learning challenges we are facing in doing environmental education entwined with religious education. As Kegan notes, transformative learning proceeds from confirmation through contradiction and beyond **only if and when sufficient continuity is present**. What can offer such continuity? What are the resources, the stories, we can use that will hold us in such a way that we can perceive the contradictions we face without descending into despair? Can we find our way into these forms of knowing that offer hope in the midst of climate catastrophe? Is there a way to be present to our pain, to refuse to ignore or deny what is going on all around us, and instead to live into deep relational accountability?

In this third year of the global pandemic, I want to recall the early months, the summer of 2020, when most of the world was enduring some form of stark lockdown. The enforced physical separation led many of us to mourn what we were losing when our relational patterns were so sharply disrupted. There was a short video spreading wildly, circulating "like a virus" in March of 2020 entitled "#ASCOLTATE #LISTEN—a letter from the virus". Since then, many, many different versions of a "communication from the virus" have been created and shared. One I particularly like is by a group called Sustainable Humans and is entitled "What might we learn from COVID".[18] These pieces which ignited imagination and drew global attention (as evidenced by their wide sharing),[19] imagined the virus as having subjectivity, as acting with intent, the intent being to force humans to slow down, to pause, to quiet ourselves, and to listen to all that we are doing that is harming the earth and its inhabitants. These videos urge us to see human beings intimately bound up with all of creation; to see, as Macy suggests, that "we are nature".

That same summer, in May of 2020, George Floyd was murdered by a police officer near my hometown in Minneapolis, Minnesota. As the urgent uprising following that murder unfolded, and as the funerals and memorials began, many people remarked on how the video that 17-year-old Darnella Frazier filmed as the murder unfolded captured the attention of a nation in lockdown. There was surprise that people were able to focus, to listen, to sense their own anguish and outrage at what was happening, and recognition that that awareness was possible precisely because so many people were bereft of their usual entertainment distractions. The Rev. Al Sharpton, in offering words at George Floyd's memorial in Minneapolis that June of 2020, noted that we are "in a different time, a different season".[20] He was doing a riff on the Ecclesiastes 3 text, and urging people in the midst of a time of COVID disruption, to use the space created by not having popular entertainment to distract us, to use that space to focus a spotlight on the brutality and systemic racism embedded in our systems of policing.

This season—of COVID, of global uprising in relation to racial injustice—has perhaps disrupted our dominant stories just enough for us to long for a different way to view the world, to long for a different form of knowing.

Confirmation, Contradiction, Continuity

In helping us to understand how to support transformative learning with adults, Kegan writes of confirmation, contradiction, continuity. The pandemic brought huge disruptions and exposed deep contradictions in our meaning-making. In some ways, it has created room by stopping us in our tracks, and alerting us to what can happen when we care for each other. Yes, there has been tremendous injustice, hatred, fear, and outrage provoked by this virus. But there has also been renewed awareness of our connections to the natural world. There was already attention being brought to the power of "forest bathing," of "spending time in nature," of rebuilding broken connections prior to the pandemic (Hari 2020), a process which the enforced physical isolation of the pandemic only accelerated.

The pandemic has renewed awareness of the joy of simply being outside, of short walks in a neighborhood, of creating things by hand, and of course, of the deep joy that can come from re-connecting after a time of loss and isolation. It has also, at the same time, brought attention to the plight of those who do not have the privilege of spending joy-filled time outdoors, people who are isolated by their health, by their socioeconomic status, by the conditions of their employment or lack thereof. And perhaps most of all, it has brought attention to those who are unhoused, those who are outside because they have no choice but to be outside.

Such complex storytelling is not only joy-filled storytelling about the outdoors, but rather storying that recognizes the dangerous, anxiety-provoking, anguished lives of those on the margins of our economies. I suspect that some of those stories were told, at least in dominant media streams, because there was finally a recognition of how inter-connected we are, of how much public health is shaped not by the most secure but by the most vulnerable among us. Religious educators need to pick up on and highlight the interconnected relationality evoked here, rather than the fear-mongering and shame of telling these stories as "stock" or dominant stories.

The many and diverse realities of living within a global pandemic offer us elements of what it means to be human that we can "confirm," to use Kegan's language, and in doing so expose the "contradictions" (again, Kegan's language) that are visible when racial injustice is filmed and shared widely, when a pandemic reaches into all corners of the globe and makes clear the inequities and injustice that are pervasive. Our task is now to provide the "continuity" that can nourish transformation. This is the work of so many communities, and an increasing number of authors who are calling us back into relationship, who are demanding that we see our interdependence and the intimate connections we share, as necessary (Ayres 2020). They are offering us "continuity" in Kegan's frame. We are coming to recognize that religious education, that environmental education, must embed us in alternative epistemological frames. The continuity we need to face these contradictions, the ways of knowing the world that can help us to embody deep relationality, have been here all along if only we listen deeply enough.

We must find and share resistance stories, and begin to build up counter stories that draw us into deep empathy, into collective action, into hope even in the midst of climate catastrophe and the despair it can provoke. These are stories that we can draw from deep within our religious traditions, they are stories we can glean, interpretations we can invite, from deep within the history of our tradition, offering continuity and hope (Fleischer and DeMoor 2015). In order to do so, we must bring the "null" curriculum into the light, into focus. We need to ensure that our "explicit" and our "implicit" curricula are aligned with each other, and that the forms of knowing we are nurturing are deeply connected to these relational and profoundly grounded frames.

The power of these widely shared stories—the "letter from the virus" and Darnella Frazier's recording—is clear in what has since unfolded. The challenge to us, in religious communities in particular, is to offer the continuity that can sustain that transformation, that can connect these stories to our traditions, to what we might want to retrieve from the past, to the hope and the faith that creates room for these transformations. That continuity cannot come from dominant frames of knowing, but demands that we retrieve—and learn from other communities—forms of knowing that are thoroughly relational, rooted in a "community of truth," and deeply interdependent.

Having ignited curiosity about alternative frames for seeing, and curating good resources for deepening and sustaining those perceptions, it is crucial to share practices that embody these frames, that strengthen and root and ground them. The first step is in the basic process of "confirmation," following beyond that into "contradiction" and "continuity."

In the rest of this essay, I want to share some of what we are doing in my own contexts, again, not as prescriptive but as evocative examples that I hope will ignite your imagination, offer ways to find and curate good resources, and that can shape practices of storying.

5. Practices That Support Shifting Meaning Frames, That Invite Transformation

5.1. Story Exercises That Begin in Confirmation

Far too many of us are socialized primarily by the stock or dominant stories of white supremacy, of neoliberal capitalism, of narrow forms of rationality taught in higher education. Shifting the underlying epistemologies to meaning-making frames that emphasize, interdependence, and accountability begins in offering respect and care for the persons whose storying we are trying to shift. It is often remarked upon that one of the most sacred practices we can engage in is deep listening. Or, as community organizers note: people do not care what you know, until they know that you care. Yet we are not often taught how to embody such a practice, and certainly the stock/dominant story processes that surround us emphasize disbelief and criticism, rather than careful listening. The first set of exercises I offer here are exercises that invite practices of attention, practices that are multi-sensory, practices that can lead to deeper relationship.

5.1.1. Learning to Breathe

The global pandemic, and renewed attention to police brutality have heightened our attention to our breath. "I can't breathe" are often the last words of people held under the knees of police brutality. "I can't breathe" is also all too often a symptom of the oxygen depletion caused by the SARS-CoV2 virus and its many mutations.

Learning to breathe deeply, learning to recognize when our breath has become shallow—perhaps due to anger, or fear, or outrage—is a very first step. We know, deep in our core, that we can live for days without food, for perhaps a day without water, but not even ten minutes without breath. Breath is the gift of oxygen synthesized by the plant and algae life all around us, the gift scientists have labelled "photosynthesis." Doing something as simple as paying attention one's breath is a first place to begin to embody forms of knowing that are open to our interdependence with all of creation, and Menakem offers multiple ways to practice such attention in the midst of our pain. He shares ways to refuse to numb our emotions but rather to learn with and from them (2018).

5.1.2. Chanting to Sing

Anyone who has learned to sing knows how important breath is to singing. A simple way to invite attention to breath beyond the practices already mentioned, is to draw people into a chant. I am fond of the Julian of Norwich phrase "all will be well, all will be well, and all manner of things will be well." When you chant it in a two-tone phrase it can become a round, and is easily picked up and shared by people. An experience of shared song, in this simple and connected process, invites wonder and eagerness to keep learning. It "confirms" a simple reality of connection.

5.1.3. Acknowledging the Land upon Which You Learn

Land acknowledgements are a tiny, a very small, first step in inviting awareness of the ground upon which we stand in learning. Worked out in concert with members of local native communities, a land acknowledgement can be a good practice in beginning, in grounding people for whatever learning event is to unfold.[21] Such a practice confirms a given context, a shared place, with openness to the painful histories that are inscribed there.

5.1.4. Mindful Walking

There are many, many invitations spread across multiple religious communities to practice "mindful walking." Perhaps one of the more frequently shared comes from the work of Thich Nhat Hanh, he of blessed memory, who wrote a piece in the Buddhist magazine *Tricycle* describing this practice.[22] This practice, like the others named above, is focused being present to one's immediate space. It builds capacity for feeling with, not simply "thinking about."

5.1.5. Digging in Dirt

One of the exercises that was shared with me, years ago when I first ventured into the rural environs of Minnesota, came from the Rev. Dr. Mark Yackel-Juleen (2021), who put down a hula hoop on the ground of the "prairie pothole" in which we were standing at the time, and helped us to see more than 100 species (grasses, insects, small animals) present in that small space. Learning that dirt, that the earthen soil in which our food is grown, is itself a widely varied ecology, is itself a profoundly powerful counter story. Far from the "dirt" which I learned as a child must be swept away, cleaned off, hosed down, not tracked into the house, "soil" is a living organism upon which all of our lives depend. This is actually an example of a practice that begins in "confirmation," by inviting people to be present to the land upon which they stand, but then builds into "contradiction" by asking participants to wonder about our living relationship with this dirt/soil.

5.1.6. Attentive Seeing

Another exercise I frequently use with students is to send them out on a walk through the neighborhood, wherever we are located (whether in a church, a seminary, a campsite) with their phone cameras, and then to ask them to take pictures of anything they see that catches their attention. Next I ask them to walk the same path again, looking for things that do not do so. That is, I ask them first to take photos of beauty, and then to go back and take pictures of things they see that they think are ugly, or at least that their eyes skipped over on the first walk. We bring these photos back into a shared setting, put them up on a screen, and meditate on them together. Where can we see God in these photos? What is in the frame of the camera, and what was left out? Many people think they are taking a picture of something only to look at the photo itself and realize how much was left out, or is not visible. Bringing context to these images invites stories of the walk around, which in turn invites a deeper awareness of what it means to "see" in new ways. Many educators have written about "place-based learning" which clearly has roots in indigenous epistemologies, whether acknowledged as such or not (Sobel 1996, 2004; Leslie et al. 1999; Sterling 2001; Litchfield 2019).

5.1.7. Tracing Water Pathways

The Capitol Region Watershed, a local government entity here where I live, has worked with local churches to develop a curriculum called "Wade in the Water" that helps young people to trace the ways water moves in their community, and to see what feeds that water and what is fed into it that is destructive.[23] Water holds such a powerful place in religious imagination, across multiple traditions, and is an easily accessible entry point into awareness of interdependence.

5.1.8. Listening to Sound (an Exercise in Sonic Environments)

"Create/share/believe" is a circle I often describe as an instantiation of the social Trinity, and when drawn upon for religious education it is a recognition and embrace of our creative "maker" cultures (Hess 2014). The following three exercises become environmentally aware when the prompts used invite stories about relationship with creation.

So many of us have grown accustomed to creating the sonic spaces in which we live by curating music on our phones and keeping that music on all around us, such that it becomes a background for existence and we find it increasingly difficult to be quiet, to inhabit stillness. This exercise is described at length in *Engaging Technology in Theological Education* (Hess 2005, pp. 136–39). The learning goal is to invite people to attend to the ways in which music shapes their emotional senses, and to begin to learn how to listen more deeply. Once people have done the sonic exercise, it can invite conversation about stillness, about quiet, and about what the sounds all around us might be inviting us to hear: whether they are city sounds drowning out any other sounds, or they are the whisper of wind, the creak of insects, and the calls of birds.

5.1.9. Story Listening in Circle

This is an exercise (described at length in *Becoming a White Antiracist*, Brookfield and Hess 2021, pp. 66–83), in which people are invited to sit in groups of four and take turns telling a brief story based on a shared prompt. Each, in turn, then reflects on the story through attending to the feelings, the actions, and the values evoked. It is a way to slow people down to listen to themselves through the ears of others.

5.1.10. Story Listening through Titling

This is another exercise (described at length in *Becoming a White Antiracist*) that invites short story sharing in a circle, where the listening results in proposing various titles for the story. Again, it creates an opportunity to listen closely and build capacity through a process that is in itself enjoyable.

5.2. Story Paths for Confronting and Contradicting Stock Stories and Igniting Resistance

Having developed some basic practices of story listening and sharing, demonstrating respect in a circle, "confirming" if you will, the reality of the people with whom you are learning, it is necessary to move to widen and deepen awareness through contradicting the more narrow and oppressive dominant/stock stories in which we find ourselves (Schroeter 2019).

It is in listening to, engaging, learning from the stories of indigenous communities that those of us who are thoroughly shaped by stock stories can begin to hear what has been concealed from us in ways that nurture resistance. There are so many opportunities to learn from leaders in First Nations, Metis, and Inuit communities, to learn from the indigenous peoples who have long tended this earth, and from many other minoritized communities.

The field of religious education has focused more recently on this kind of storytelling, and there are numerous scholars working in this area. I would highlight in particular the work of Kim-Cragg (2015, 2019); Tran (2017); Parker (2003); Smith (2004); Baker (2010); and Kaunda and Sang-man (2021).

Here in Minnesota the project "Healing Minnesota Stories" (https://healingmnstories.wordpress.com accessed on 1 February 2022) invites people to participate in sacred site pilgrimages led by native guides. These experiential learning events draw people into direct contact with the ground upon which they stand, and then share the stories deeply held by the native communities who have tended that ground.

Film and video streaming have also begun to offer many and varied ways to hear stories that have been concealed by stock/dominant voices, and to begin to learn the stories of resistance without unduly burdening or triggering trauma by constantly asking persons who have been minoritized to share their stories. These are projects that have been created precisely to share stories. Here are just a handful that we use regularly here in Minnesota, but I would encourage you to be in contact with the indigenous communities in your own lands for ideas and resources.

- "Dakota38", a film (full film made available online: https://youtu.be/1pX6FBSUyQI, accessed on 1 February 2022)
- "Say Your Name", a short music video about boarding schools sung by Keith Secola (https://youtu.be/1UftaoCvMxc, accessed on 1 February 2022)
- "Proud to be", a PSA created by the National Congress of American Indians to fight some of the NFL mascot battles. It remains a powerful resistance story (https://youtu.be/mR-tbOxlhvE, accessed on 1 February 2022)
- "We Shall Remain", a short film by the Stylehorse Collective in collaboration with tribal youth programs in Idaho (https://youtu.be/1pX6FBSUyQI, accessed on 1 February 2022)
- "Grace", a poem written and read by poet laureate Joy Harjo (https://youtu.be/dualpWSuT3I, accessed on 1 February 2022)
- More than a single story website (https://morethanasinglestory.com, accessed on 1 February 2022)
- The National Native American Boarding Schools Coalition (https://boardingschoolhealing.org, accessed on 1 February 2022)
- ROCO films (a documentary film production company) (https://rocofilms.com, accessed on 1 February 2022)
- The Hartley Media Impact Initiative (https://auburnseminary.org/hartley/, accessed on 1 February 2022)
- Adam Mazo and Mishy Lesser at the Upstander Project (https://upstanderproject.org/dawnland, accessed on 1 February 2022)

5.3. Creating Counter Stories for Building Self in Deep Relation to the Earth (Continuity)

As noted earlier in this essay, the goal of shifting our storying, the learning frame necessary for coming into deep relationality, for coming to "see ourselves as nature" (Macy), for coming into a "reciprocal covenant" (Kimmerer), requires offering continuity that supports people as they move through the contradictions, many of which are deeply painful and guilt producing, that arise when opening up to wider awareness.

I am reluctant to offer too many examples in this category because I know I am myself so deeply embedded in dominant/stock stories that I find it most helpful to stand with humility and listen to my native siblings as they offer their stories. I have been deeply impacted by authors such as Louise Erdrich, Robin Kimmerer, Peter Razor, Drew Haden Taylor, Diane Wilson, and so on.

I do want to point, however, to contemplative traditions in Christianity, which have in many ways kept alive a respect for and engagement with forms of knowing that are not narrowly rationalist (Smith and Higginbotham 2019). These are the streams which Parker Palmer has drawn on. Maggie Ross in her book *Silence: A User's Guide*, writes of a form of knowing, of knowledge, that arises in "drinking from the well of silence" (Ross 2014). Willie James Jennings (2010), in narrating the many paths Christianity took to create and enforce racialization, notes that there are other paths, roads less traveled, that are evident in the glimpses we still have of Christians who did not perceive such a stark separation between humans and animals, between Creation and ourselves.

I am often struck by how many of my students are deeply connected to yoga, or find certain kinds of Buddhist meditation powerful, but have no idea that similar embodied practices of prayer exist within Christian traditions as well. Often the best way I know to help young adults begin to imagine how Christianity might be a resource for them, is to introduce them to the embodied practices, the rituals, pilgrimages, shrines, and other elements I can draw on within my Roman Catholic community.

6. Concluding Notes

I want to conclude by reiterating that we are storying people. To transform our practices in the midst of climate catastrophe, we must transform our stories. And to do that we must transform the very ways in which we come to know. That process, at least for those of us who have been thoroughly socialized into dominant stories, requires a spiral process of "confirmation, contradiction, and continuity", drawing us ever more deeply into a mutual covenant of relationality and reciprocity. Such a covenant has been embodied and embraced for millennia by indigenous communities, from whom all of us have so very much to learn. Stepping into such deep and accountable relationality is a process that demands that we open ourselves up to a full range of emotions, and that we not numb ourselves to the pain that arises when we are honest about the climate catastrophe we face. First Nations, Metis and Inuit peoples lead the way here, helping us to see that we are all part of one another.

Funding: This research received no external funding.

Conflicts of Interest: The author declares no conflict of interest.

Notes

[1] Like many stories from oral cultures, it is difficult to cite the "first" evidence of this story. The Wikipedia article on the story is regularly updated: https://en.wikipedia.org/wiki/Two_Wolves, accessed on 1 February 2022.

[2] One of the more profound articulations of this other way of interpreting Christianity, with a particularly pertinent congruence to the issues discussed in this essay, is Pope Francis'2015 encyclical *Laudato 'Si: On Care for Our Common Home*.

[3] A good collection of the growing research on this issue can be found at Harvard's T. H. Chan School of Public Health (https://www.hsph.harvard.edu/c-change/subtopics/coronavirus-and-climate-change/, accessed on 1 February 2022).

[4] Please note that I am thoroughly aware that other religious traditions have powerful ways to speak to these realities as well. I am simply seeking to stay specific to my social location.

[5] Here again the Wikipedia article is useful as it points off to multiple popular culture "takes" on this story.

[6] See for instance, Erin Magner, https://www.wellandgood.com/spirit-animal-native-american/ (accessed on 1 February 2022).

[7] On a side note, the reality that certain elements of his argument cannot be reproduced due to copyright restrictions is a small, but powerful, element of the larger argument in which his work is embedded.

[8] A particularly powerful and useful guide to such work on indigenous forms of knowing has been made available in an open textbook format: *Pulling Together: A Guide for Curriculum Developers* by Asma-na-hi Antoine; Rachel Mason; Roberta Mason; Sophia Palahicky; and Carmen Rodriguez de France is licensed under a Creative Commons Attribution-NonCommercial 4.0 International License, except where otherwise noted.

[9] More credits for the film are available online: https://en.wikipedia.org/wiki/Don%27t_Look_Up (accessed on 1 February 2022).

[10] https://bioneers.org/about/purpose/ (accessed on 1 February 2022), and then the link to the video: https://youtu.be/cEm7gbIax0o (accessed on 1 February 2022).

[11] The Intercept (https://theintercept.com/about/, accessed on 1 February 2022), https://youtu.be/cEm7gbIax0o (accessed on 1 February 2022).

[12] You can access the interview with Macy here: https://youtu.be/7fnEUhZIirw (accessed on 1 February 2022).

[13] Birdtalker: https://youtu.be/Odlw8WdsZS8 (accessed on 1 February 2022).

[14] I am writing in this article from a very specific location, but I would note here that Walker and Cariaga (2021) offer an important corrective to this theory by lifting up ways in which hybrid cultural identities must be recognized and engaged.

[15] Kegan and associates have also identified a fifth space of meaning-making, something they term a "self-transforming mind". That frame could be even more conducive to managing the contradictory stories here, but few adults ever get that far in the spiral of adult development.

[16] For a lengthier treatment of these ideas, her book *Braiding Sweetgrass* is a wonderful read.

[17] In a different discursive terrain Hanchin and Hearlson (2020) suggest that what we need is an "ecological and psychic conversion" (p. 258 and following).

[18] Originally created in March of 2020 (https://youtu.be/UEgl_TUYOZo accessed on 1 February 2022), many, many versions of the same idea have been created and shared since then. One I particularly like comes from the Sustainable Humans group: https://youtu.be/XELczQ3JWQY (accessed on 1 February 2022).

[19] Note Jenkins et al. (2013) and their work on "spreadable media" as contrasted with the slang of "viral" media.

[20] Visible here at about the 1:46 mark: https://youtu.be/3egsimHziWg (accessed on 1 February 2022).

[21] There is much wisdom available as to how to craft such an acknowledgement, beginning with connecting with local native communities. Basic information can be found here: https://usdac.us/nativeland (accessed on 1 February 2022).

[22] Available here: https://tricycle.org/magazine/walk-buddha/ (accessed on 1 February 2022).

[23] The curriculum is free to download and available here: http://growinggreenhearts.com/stories/wade-in-the-water-curriculum-for-community/ (accessed on 1 February 2022).

References

Antoine, Asma-na-hi, Rachel Mason, Roberta Mason, Sophia Palahicky, and Carmen Rodriguez de France. 2018. Pulling Together: A Guide for Curriculum Developers by Is Licensed under a Creative Commons Attribution-NonCommercial 4.0 International License, Except Where Otherwise Noted. BC Campus. Available online: https://opentextbc.ca/indigenizationcurriculumdevelopers/ (accessed on 1 February 2022).

Ayres, Jennifer. 2020. Embracing vulnerability: Religious education, embodiment, and the ecological affections. *Religious Education* 115: 15–26. [CrossRef]

Ayres, Jennifer. 2021. A pedagogy for precarious times: Religious education and vulnerability. *Religious Education* 116: 327–40. [CrossRef]

Baker, Dori. 2010. *Greenhouses of Hope: Congregations Growing Young Leaders Who Will Change the World*. Herndon: Alban Institute.

Bell, Lee Anne, Rosemarie Roberts, Kayhan Irani, and Brett Murphy. 2008. The Storytelling Curriculum Project: Learning about Race and Racism through Storytelling and the Arts. Storytelling Project, Barnard College. Available online: http://www.columbia.edu/itc/barnard/education/stp/stp_curriculum.pdf (accessed on 4 August 2019).

Brookfield, Stephen, and John Holst. 2011. *Radicalizing Learning: Adult Education for a Just World*. San Francisco: Jossey-Bass.

Brookfield, Stephen, and Mary Hess. 2021. *Becoming a White Antiracist: A Practical Guide for Educators, Leaders and Activists*. Sterling: Stylus Publishing.

Brown, Brené. 2012. *Daring Greatly: How the Courage to be Vulnerable Transforms the Way We Live, Love, Parent, and Lead*. New York: Gotham Books.

Cajete, Greg. 2015. *Indigenous Community: Rekindling the Teachings of the Seventh Fire*. St. Paul: Living Justice Press.

Carley, Kenneth. 1961. *The Dakota War of 1862: Minnesota's Other Civil War*. St. Paul: Minnesota Historical Society.

Chamberlain, Gary L. 2000. Ecology and religious education. *Religious Education* 95: 134–50. [CrossRef]

Dahill, Lisa, and James Martin-Schramm, eds. 2016. *Eco-Reformation: Grace and Hope for a Planet in Peril*. Eugene: Cascade Books.

DeMars, Tony R., and Gabriel B. Tait. 2019. *Narratives of Storytelling across Cultures: The Complexities of Intercultural Communication*. New York: Lexington Books.

Eisner, Elliot. 1985. *The Educational Imagination: On the Design and Evaluation of School Programs*. New York: Macmillan.

Fleischer, Barbara J., and Emily DeMoor. 2015. Hope for environmental action. *Religious Education* 110: 274–88. [CrossRef]

Francis, Pope. 2015. Laudato 'Si: On Care for Our Common Home. Available online: https://www.vatican.va/content/dam/francesco/pdf/encyclicals/documents/papa-francesco_20150524_enciclica-laudato-si_en.pdf (accessed on 1 February 2022).

Garod, Andrew, Robert Kilkenny, and Melanie Benson Taylor. 2017. *I Am Where I Come From: Native American College Students and Graduates Tell Their Life Stories*. Ithaca: Cornell University.

Hanchin, Timothy, and Christy Lang Hearlson. 2020. Educating for ecological conversion: An ecstatic pedagogy for Christian higher education amid climate crisis. *Religious Education* 115: 255–68. [CrossRef]

Hari, Johann. 2020. *Lost Connections: Why You're Depressed and How to Find Hope*. London: Bloomsbury Publishing.

Hearlson, Christiane Lang. 2021. Converting the imagination through visual images in ecological religious education. *Religious Education* 116: 129–41. [CrossRef]

Hess, Mary. 2005. *Engaging Technology in Theological Education: All That We Can't Leave Behind*. New York: Rowman and Littlefield Publishers.

Hess, Mary. 2011. Learning the Bible in the 21st century: Lessons from Harry Potter and vampires. In *Teaching the Bible in the Parish (and Beyond)*. Edited by Laurie Jungling. Minneapolis: Lutheran University Press, pp. 79–99.

Hess, Mary. 2014. And the Word went viral: Finding God at the intersection of scripture and popular media. *America: The National Jesuit Review*, 21–28.

Hess, Mary. 2016. Teaching and learning comparative theology with millennial students. In *Comparative Theology in the Millennial Classroom*. Edited by Mara Brecht and Reid B. Locklin. London: Routledge, pp. 50–60.

Hess, Mary. 2018. Using digital media and storytelling to unearth racism and galvanize action. In *Teaching Race: How to Help Students Unmask and Challenge Racism*. Edited by Stephen D. Brookfield. San Francisco: Jossey-Bass, pp. 253–72.

Hess, Mary. 2019a. Storying faith: The promises and contradictions of new media in Catholic religious education. In *Global Perspectives on Catholic Religious Education in Schools: Volume II Leading in a Pluralist World*. Edited by M. T. Buchanan and A. M. Gellel. Berlin/Heidelberg: Springer, pp. 357–68.

Hess, Mary. 2019b. Theme-centered interaction: Intersections with reflective practice in North American religious contexts. In *Theme-Centered Interaction in Higher Education: A Didactic Approach for Sustainable and Living Learning*. Edited by Sylke Meyerhuber, Helmut Reiser and Matthias Scharer. Berlin/Heidelberg: Springer, pp. 209–20.

Hess, Mary. 2020. Finding a way into empathy through story exercises in a religious studies classroom. *Religious Studies News*. January 7. Available online: https://rsn.aarweb.org/spotlight-on/teaching/empathy/story-exercises-religious-studies-classroom (accessed on 1 February 2022).

Hess, Mary. 2021. Finding learning amidst the maelstrom: Storytelling, trauma and hope. *Teaching Theology and Religion* 23: 218–30. [CrossRef]

James, Alison, and Stephen Brookfield. 2014. *Engaging Imagination: Helping Students Become Creative and Reflective Teachers*. San Francisco: Jossey-Bass.

Jenkins, Henry, Sam Ford, and Joshua Green. 2013. *Spreadable Media: Creating Value and Meaning in a Networked Culture*. New York: New York University Press.

Jennings, Willie James. 2010. *The Christian Imagination: Theology and the Origins of Race*. New Haven: Yale University Press.

Johnson, Elizabeth. 2014. *Ask the Beasts: Darwin and the God of Love*. London: Bloomsbury.

Kaunda, Chammah J., and Kim Sang-man. 2021. 'Samae Spirit' Assist toward 'Ubuntu Spirit' Model for Rural Adult Christian Education in Zambia. *Religious Education*. [CrossRef]

Kegan, Robert. 1982. *The Evolving Self: Problem and Process in Human Development*. Cambridge: Harvard University Press.

Kim-Cragg, HyeRan. 2015. Theology of resistance in conversation with religious education in unmaking violence. *Religious Education* 110: 420–34. [CrossRef]

Kim-Cragg, HyeRan. 2019. The emperor has no clothes!: Exposing whiteness as explicit, implicit, and null curricula. *Religious Education* 114: 239–51. [CrossRef]

Kimmerer, Robin. 2013. *Braiding Sweetgrass*. Minneapolis: Milkweed Editions.

Kirkness, Verna. 2013. *Creating Space: My Life and Word in Indigenous Education*. Winnipeg: University of Manitoba Press.

Leslie, Clare Walker, John Tallmadge, and Tom Wessels. 1999. *Into the Field: A Guide to Locally Focussed Teaching*. Great Barrington: The Orion Society.

Litchfield, Randy. 2019. *Roots & Routes: Calling, Ministry, and the Power of Place*. Nashville: Abingdon Press.

Menakem, Resmaa. 2018. *My Grandmother's Hands: Racialized Trauma and the Path to Mending Our Hearts and Bodies*. Las Vegas: Central Recovery Press.

Ng, Greer Anne Wenh-In. 2020. Complexities in religious education with Asian/Asian Canadians and indigenous realities: The Truth and Reconciliation Commission Report on Residential Schools. *Religious Education* 115: 315–22. [CrossRef]

Orr, David. 1994. *Earth in Mind: On Education, Environment, and the Human Prospect*. Washington, DC: Island Press.

Palmer, Parker, and Arthur Zajonc. 2010. *The Heart of Higher Education: A Call to Renewal*. San Francisco: Jossey-Bass.

Palmer, Parker. 1983. *To Know As We Are Known*. San Francisco: HarperCollins.

Palmer, Parker. 1998. *The Courage to Teach: Exploring the Inner Landscape of a Teacher's Life*. San Francisco: Jossey-Bass.

Parker, Evelyn. 2003. *Trouble Don't Always Last. Emancipatory Hope Among African American Adolescents*. Cleveland: Pilgrim Press.

Rasmussen, Larry. 2013. *Earth-Honoring Faith: Religious Ethics in a New Key*. New York: Oxford University Press.

Reyhner, Jon, ed. 2015. *Teaching Indigenous Students: Honoring Place, Community, and Culture*. Norman: University of Oklahoma Press.

Ross, Maggie. 2014. *Silence: A User's Guide*. Eugene: Cascade Books.

Schroeter, Sara. 2019. A case for anti-racist and decolonizing approaches to multiliteracies. *Studies in Social Justice* 13: 142–58.

Smith, Jessica, and Stuart Higginbotham, eds. 2019. *Contemplation and Community: A Gather of Fresh Voices for a Living Tradition*. New York: Crossroad Publishing.

Smith, Yolanda. 2004. *Reclaiming the Spirituals: New Possibilities for African American Christian Education*. Cleveland: Pilgrim Press.

Sobel, David. 1996. *Beyond Ecophobia: Reclaiming the Heart in Nature Education*. Great Barrington: The Orion Society.

Sobel, David. 2004. *Place-Based Education: Connecting Classrooms and Communities*. Great Barrington: The Orion Society.

Sterling, Stephen. 2001. *Sustainable Education: Re-Visioning Learning and Change*. Totnes: The Schumacher Society.

Stone, Deborah. 2008. *The Samaritan's Dilemma: Should Government Help Your Neighbor?* New York: Nation Books.

ter Kuile, Casper. 2020. *The Power of Ritual: Turning Everyday Actions into Soulful Practices*. New York: HarperOne.

Tran, Mai-Anh Le. 2017. *Reset the Heart: Unlearning Violence, Relearning Hope*. Nashville: Abingdon Press.

Walker, Anne Carter, and Peter H. Cariaga. 2021. Mixed (up) and messy: Culturally hybrid proposals for vocational exploration. *Religious Education* 116: 493–505. [CrossRef]

Westerman, Gwen, and Bruce White. 2012. *Mni Sota Makoce: The Land of the Dakota*. St. Paul: Minnesota Historical Society.

Yackel-Juleen, Mark. 2021. *Everyone Must Eat: Food, Sustainability, and Ministry*. Minneapolis: Fortress Press.

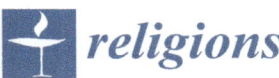

Article

Belonging to the World through Body, Trust, and Trinity: Climate Change and Pastoral Care with University Students

Christine Tind Johannessen [1,2]

[1] Centre for Pastoral Education and Research, Church of Denmark, 8230 Aarhus, Denmark; ctj@km.dk
[2] Faculty of Theology, University of Copenhagen, 1463 Copenhagen, Denmark

Abstract: This article explores how pastoral care is performed in an age of climate change. University students suffer from a wide range of stresses, reducing their well-being. Climate change compounds these stress reactions, even where students are not directly affected. As climate change affects concrete, material matters, human reactions to it may no longer be viewed and treated as purely inner psychic states. Thus, climate change disrupts usual divisions of material, social, and mental features as separate categories, underscoring instead the close-knit relations between them. Given the far-reaching ways climate change affects mental health, the article presents an ethnographical-theologically-driven model for basic conversation in pastoral care with students in the midst of escalating climate events. Making use of theories from anthropology, psychology, and theology, this article builds on in-depth interviews with Danish university chaplains about their pastoral care with students. The model extrapolates from these theories how pastoral care may support students in the era of climate change through a triad of organizing themes that come to the fore in the interviews: "Mothering the Content", "Loving Vital Force", and "Befriending the Environment".

Keywords: pastoral care; climate change; sustainability; psychological stress; university students; ethnography; in-depth interview; feminist theology; trinity; mentalizing; the new climatic regime

Citation: Johannessen, Christine Tind. 2022. Belonging to the World through Body, Trust, and Trinity: Climate Change and Pastoral Care with University Students. *Religions* 13: 527. https://doi.org/10.3390/rel13060527

Academic Editors: Pamela R. McCarroll and HyeRan Kim-Cragg

Received: 9 March 2022
Accepted: 16 May 2022
Published: 8 June 2022

Publisher's Note: MDPI stays neutral with regard to jurisdictional claims in published maps and institutional affiliations.

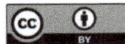

Copyright: © 2022 by the author. Licensee MDPI, Basel, Switzerland. This article is an open access article distributed under the terms and conditions of the Creative Commons Attribution (CC BY) license (https:// creativecommons.org/licenses/by/ 4.0/).

1. Background

"Only rarely do students seek pastoral care specifically expressing a need for help because of stress arising from climate change. However, the whole preoccupation with the climate . . . it is a part of the students' scenario for the future. It enters the pastoral care room through statements like: 'I'm now going to live vegan' or 'What do we do about the globe?' or 'I wonder if we have a future at all?'. The utterances are placed in the periphery. Yet, climate change remains an underlying concern in the foreground conversations. Remarks about food and second-hand clothes, open questions about the acceleration . . . how difficult it is to stop on your own, like: 'Can I change it myself?'"

Student Chaplain H

Pastoral care at university has to work with a multiplicity of stress states in students. Students suffer from different kinds of stress, such as anxiety, depression, bereavement, discrimination, suicidal ideation, failed studies, loneliness, abuse, breakups, troubled relationships, family, and interpersonal functioning (Smith and Khawaja 2011; Field et al. 2011; Haldorsen et al. 2014; Appiah-Brempong et al. 2014; Sharp and Theiler 2018; Ribeiro et al. 2018; January et al. 2018; Thai and Moore 2018; Russell et al. 2019; Klein and Martin 2021). Psychological stress is classically defined as "a particular relationship between the person and the environment that is appraised by the person as taxing or exceeding his or her resources and endangering his or her well-being" (Lazarus and Folkman 1984, p. 19). Studies have shown that high levels of stress reduce students' well-being, and this negatively impacts their performance outcomes (Keech et al. 2018). Even though stress is experienced and often treated individually, it can also be viewed as a collective form of societal reaction (Kirkegaard and Brinkmann 2015).

Studies on students' mental health have shown positive effects of psychological treatment and prevention and social support (Regehr et al. 2013; Rith-Najarian et al. 2019; Maymon and Hall 2021). Further, there is a growing awareness that spiritual well-being and religiousness have a beneficial impact on students suffering from stress (Krägeloh et al. 2015; Fabbris et al. 2016; Hai et al. 2018; Leung and Pong 2021). Hence, the literature indicates that pastoral care may also help youth and students in crisis (Cardoso et al. 2012; Murphy and Holste 2016). Addressing different types of stress and distress in the context of pastoral care, the American pastoral theologian Robert C. Dykstra (1997), in his book *Counseling Troubled Youth*, addressed how young people are overwhelmed by forsaken hopes for a meaningful future. Dykstra drew attention to the importance of pastoral caregivers having "theoretical knowledge and practical wisdom" to offer youth and students on their way to finding their "self".

Following this, recent literature also shows that climate change concerns can lead to different kinds of psychological distress and stress—a phenomenon often called "climate anxiety" (McBride et al. 2021; Pihkala 2020). Young people experience a wide range of emotions related to climate change, including anxiety, anger, grief, fear, powerlessness, and hopelessness, even though they may not directly be affected by the climate changes (Wachholz et al. 2014; van Nieuwenhuizen et al. 2021; Burke et al. 2018; Lancet 2021). Studies indicate that higher pro-environmental behavior among students may be associated with greater well-being, possibly because it satisfies basic psychological needs like autonomy, competence, and relatedness (Senbel et al. 2014; van Nieuwenhuizen et al. 2021). However, while activism may prevent feelings of helplessness and increase young people's sense of empowerment, meaning, and purpose, it may also lead to decreased health due to increasing the stress states (van Nieuwenhuizen et al. 2021).

Studies also suggest that different kinds of psychotherapy may have a positive impact on stress from climate change (Budziszewska and Jonsson 2021). However, climate stress relief may be viewed from other perspectives and disciplines beyond psychotherapy. Climate change stresses are not just feelings to be got rid of but indicate lessons to be learned; climate change stress should not be seen just as a problem to be solved or a condition to be medicated but rather an important encounter with our awareness of our impact on the world (Pihkala 2020). We are dealing with a widespread—and often unconscious—environmental anxiety which posits a pastoral challenge (see, for example, Campbell-Reed and Lartey 2015; Pihkala 2016; Calder and Morgan 2016; LaMothe 2016; Miller-McLemore 2020).

Given the far-reaching ways in which climate change affects psychological well-being among students and the youth, pastoral theology and care may have an important role to play. In developing alternative dialogues, supportive social networks, and a living relationship with the Earth, pastoral theology and care may "think and be otherwise" (LaMothe 2021). Here, some basic questions arise: How might pastoral care conversations with students respond to states of stress under the further pressure of climate change? How might these conversations create a basis for the release of stress whilst simultaneously nourishing opportunities for positive changes in the action and thinking of the students in their relationship with the Earth?

2. Aim, Empirical Research, and Methodology

2.1. Aim, Argument, and Outline

This article explores the basic contact in pastoral care between chaplains and university students, addressing the context of climate change. By scrutinizing empirical practices in pastoral care grounded in theological and psychological theory, the aim is to unfold "a sustainable pastoral care practice" in the midst of escalating climate events.

The argument is that pastoral care, as it is often intuitively done through social and material enactments, may hold an emerging climate pastoral care. Such pastoral care would contain practices concerned with alleviating stress but would also be given through communication and a spacious image of God that is related to the single individual through social-material manifoldness and communality. I aim to show how pastoral care contains a trust-building and embodied practice as a basis for change as it unfolds a doctrine of the Trinity which breaks open traditional images of God. Attaching theory to practice may open new insights and possibilities for pastoral care addressing climate change. Thus, this article establishes a constructive pastoral theological perspective, not with the purpose of being in agreement with one particular theology, but for the purpose of outlining a grasp in pastoral care practice which is consistent with students' contemporary understanding of reality.

As a part of my ethnographical-theological research project "Sustainable pastoral care and stress release", this article builds on my in-depth interviews with Danish university chaplains about their student pastoral care. Seeking some kind of order in the chaplains' many narratives, descriptions of their practices, observations, and interpretations, my analysis takes a point of departure in the chaplains' reflections on how stressors from climate change come to the fore as viewed through the prism of a philosophical-anthropological-inspired repertoire on climate change (Bruno Latour). Using a theological repertoire, making reference to a feminist interpretation of Trinity as "Mother, Lover and Friend" (Sallie McFague), and a psychological repertoire, making use of concepts of "epistemic trust" and "mentalizing" (Peter Fonagy and colleagues), I develop a pastoral care model extrapolated through a triad of organizing themes, as they come to the fore in the interviews: "Mothering the content", "Loving vital force", and "Befriending the environment". The leading idea is that pastoral care conversations transcend differences between everyday language and Christian theological language. In fact, the three themes cannot be separated in pastoral care conversations, rather they unfold together as a network of connections, which transcends the understanding of them individually. These connections create a network of entanglements that tie together the psychological, the pastoral, the theological, and climate-related issues.

2.2. Empirical Material and Method

The empirical data derive from recordings and notes from semi-structured, in-depth interviews with participant observation carried out among eight Danish university chaplains from the Danish Lutheran Church. The inclusion of chaplains intended a wide sociodemographic distribution. The ethnographical method used is in line with ethnographical principles in anthropology and pastoral theology (Spradley 1979; Moschella 2008). The duration of the interviews varied between 75 and 150 min. Audio records were transcribed. The chaplains were asked to describe their practice of pastoral care in detail in relation to different kinds of students' stress.

Ethical guidelines were followed accurately in relation to The European Code of Conduct for Research Integrity (ALLEA 2017) and The Danish Data Protection Agency (Datatilsynet.dk n.d.). The chaplains were provided with information about the research before the interview and informed that they had the right to withdraw from the study. Chaplains gave their written consent. All the names mentioned were converted into random letters to secure anonymity for the persons who participated in the research project.

2.3. Methodology

This article's use of the term "pastoral care" starts from a broad meaning of the concept, as it addresses diversity in gender, age, race, sexuality, social class, and religious and non-religious/secular convictions and values in order to include everyone who seeks pastoral care. Thus, the concept of pastoral care operates in line with Rodney J. Hunter's broad intercultural definition, here cited in a slightly moderated version:

> "Pastoral care is considered to be any form of personal ministry to individuals and to family and community relations by representative religious persons (ordained or lay) and by their community of faith, who understand and guide their caring

efforts out of a theological perspective rooted in the tradition of faith." (Hunter and Ramsay 2005, p. x)

In order to form a useful clinical resource for the pastoral care of that particular emotional dilemma that our ecological crisis creates, I draw on three grounds of theories—from anthropology, theology, and psychology—that inform the practices of pastoral care, as each of them in different ways corresponds through different kinds of perspectives that operate and relate—with their similarities and differences—in constructive ways.

The eco-anthropological theory presented draws on the constructivist Bruno Latour's (1993, 2017) "empirical philosophy". It holds critiques against a modern worldview and argues that humans and nature—instead of separating them from one another—become more and more interconnected as entangled hybrids. As a co-architect of *Actor Network Theory*, Latour is preoccupied with tracing "the enactment of materially and discursively heterogeneous relations that produce and reshuffle all kinds of actors including objects, subjects, human beings, machines, animals, 'nature', ideas, organizations, inequalities, scale and sizes, and geographical arrangements" (Law 2009, p. 141). Thus, Latour claims that religion holds the language and passion for the force of the world in which everything is entangled. In this sense, this amodern approach to science and religion can lead us through our crisis in order to care for the Earth.

In the context of pastoral care practice, a theological "translation" of Latour's anthropological view is necessary in order to address and interpret beliefs, faith, and trust with further regard to the cultural (and confessional) context in Danish society. Turning to theological theory, I present a protestant, constructive, and postmodern perspective by the eco-feminist theologian Sallie McFague (1987, 2008). McFague argues that God is not a distant supernatural force but incarnated in the world as "the body of God"—a God who will hold us "close through our greatest fears" (McFague 2008, p. 172). By use of McFague's theology correlated to anthropology, Latour, in turn, presents a theo-anthropological ground, which unfolds the relation of nature-culture, that shows complementary to McFague's framework. However, McFague's systematic theology and Latour's empirical philosophy raise the question of how theology and anthropology are clinically applicable in pastoral care in order to work as a stress releasing mental health practice related to the individual—as it is simultaneously not only related to self and others but directly connected with communality, the collective, society, and world.

In addressing this clinical need in pastoral care, I turn to psychological theory. The concept "mentalization", developed by Fonagy and colleagues, has strong roots in psychoanalysis. I suggest this therapeutic framework for mental health as a stress releasing and "Earth healing" practice in pastoral care, as mentalizing builds up ("epistemic") trust in care practice through its work with relating self to others and the world. Mentalizing is related to everyday concepts, such as thoughtfulness, empathy, and self-knowledge, and integrates elements from, e.g., psychoanalytical theory, evolution theory, developmental psychology, affect theory, neurobiology, theory of mind, social cognition, meta-cognition, and attachment theory. Mentalization-based therapy (MBT) has proven to be useful in the treatment of mental disorders and has further expanded the knowledge on mentalization in relation to mental health in general.

Emphasizing in this context that pastoral care practice is not MBT in its classical clinical form and that pastoral care does not indicate psychological treatment as such, I suggest that pastoral care may be inspired by the ways that mentalizing, among others, highlights the role of imagination in the intersubjectivity between self, others, and the world. I suggest that this imaging may come near to both Latour's anthropological understanding and McFague's theological interpretation of our connectedness to Earth, indicating a kind of openness towards the spiritual—an openness which is further supported by scholars in mentalization, who point to the fact that clients, in general, are more inclined to talk about religious and spiritual matters than psychotherapists (Allen 2013).

Altogether, I relate these three theories to the empirical material from the University chaplains—as they unfold and crisscross through similarities and differences—and suggest that they create a room of conversation in pastoral care practice, which has the opportunity to use theological and pastoral knowledge and religious beliefs to solve environmental issues. Hence, as I draw on implicit ideas of pastoral care imagined as a "web" (Miller-McLemore 1996) or "network" (Johannessen-Henry 2012, 2013, 2017), I leave the suggested model open as actualizations of unprejudiced, anti-hierarchical, and devotional spaces.

3. "Down to Earth": A Point of Departure for an Ethnographical-Theologically-Driven Pastoral Care Model

"The condition of living with climate change lies as foil on everything in the conversations. They [the students] get in contact with basic anxiety, the anxiety of vanishing. The situation of climate changes appears in one way or the other—intensified by the fact that we seemingly are much, much closer to disaster than we have earlier believed. This triggers conflicts between the generations; it is my boomer-generation who prompted the climate changes and placed the whole responsibility on the youth. So, when we present explanations of meaning (of life), they do not listen at all, saying: 'You have really no idea what you have done. You have created a situation that leads to the Twilight of the Gods'. I feel it through their anxiety: 'What is the meaning of life, if we are not here anymore in a few generations?'. The students raise climate issues directly by saying: 'Well, then there is all that with the climate ... '. It is like blind spots appearing in the conversations that you cannot deal with rationally. It's about gaining more knowledge about it, more, more, more, how to prevent it and what we can do, where is the worst happening, and what is the best to do. It runs constantly on other levels during the pastoral care conversations."

Student Chaplain C

The quotes from Chaplain H and Chaplain C both illustrate how a deep intensity pervades the pastoral care as it takes place. The content of pastoral care concerning stress from climate change is difficult to represent in all its many different and indirect shapes. As a starting point, the direct expressions regarding climate changes are characterized by being sporadically spread out through a diversity of situations, feelings, states, and beliefs. The expressions come to the fore directly almost only through short statements or quick words and questions which fall into the conversation. Because of this, the climate content is impossible to just mark with a label or distil as "pure" climate change stress separate from the rest of the content. Quite the contrary, it seems like we are dealing with invisible connections and lines, which somehow inseparably cling to the students' state of mind as "foil"—or even as something penetrating the things that go on in the lives of the students. Student Chaplain Z phrases the impact of climate change like this:

"It is like all over. Like anxiety of the future. Like their future is in liquidation. I can tell the students that it is not an individual problem. Talk with them about it. In itself that is no comfort. That something outside us sets an agenda, that we do not have the power over."

In many ways, the interviews bear witness to content that takes shape as something intangible and global. At the same time, the narratives are also characterized by being rooted in something local to them—in things that are concrete, bodily, and fleshy, which also "messes" things around in connection to the feelings, thoughts, and beliefs as they flow out during the pastoral care conversations. Continuing with Student Chaplain Z:

"A student said that she had been used to hearing a particular bird coming back to the same place year after year. Suddenly the bird wasn't there anymore. So, the student googled it and found out that it was endanger of total extermination. She became so devastated and sad that life around us is destroyed. Young people are supposed to expand, while biodiversity and climate are about to crash."

As exemplified by this quote (which some term: "ecological grief", Comtesse et al. 2021), the interviews testify that the climate's state is related dynamically to the students' states of mind as both global and local. It is experienced as materially connected to feelings of sadness, despair, loneliness, etc. In other words, we are dealing with some kind of entanglement. Rather than trying to divide or split climate change stress in pastoral care from the rest of the content, the interviews show that the global and local, entities and parts, humans and non-humans are inseparably interwoven.

In this respect, the chaplains' narratives seem to be captured, in different ways, by the thoughts of the philosopher, anthropologist, and sociologist Bruno Latour (2017), not least presented in his book *Facing Gaia*. The pastoral care experiences, at first glance, seem to match his opening image drawn from "The Angel of Geostory" by Stéphanie Ganachaud:

> "A dancer is rushing backwards to get away from something she must have found frightening; as she runs, she keeps glancing back more and more anxiously, as if her flight is accumulating obstacles behind her that increasingly impede her movements, until she is forced to turn around. And there she stands, suspended, frozen, her arms hanging loosely, looking at something coming towards her, something even more terrifying than what she was first seeking to escape—until she is forced to recoil. Fleeing from one horror, she has met another, partly created by her flight." (Latour 2017, p. 1)

Illustrating the force coming at us in this harrowing form—the "emergence of an enigmatic figure, the source of a horror that was now in front rather than behind" (ibid., p. 2)—Latour seeks to draw the contours of the *New Climatic Regime*. In this new regime, the physical framework, which has earlier been taken for granted in the modern way of thinking of the world and reality—the ground on which history had always played out—has become unstable. Contradicting the modern view, Earth seems to react to our actions.

In our climate change situation, Latour argues, this force of the Earth may be captured by the metaphor of Gaia. In the ancient Greek poet Hesiod's narrative, Gaia plays the role of a primordial and ancestral force. Gaia ('Ge' from the ancient Greek root for 'earth') is not a goddess, properly speaking, but a force from the time before the gods (ibid., p. 81). Hence, she is not a figure of harmony. There is nothing maternal about her—in the traditional understanding of "Mother", anyway; her performances are "multiple, contradictory, hopelessly confused" (ibid., p. 82). In Hesiod's telling, she animates her children to castrate their father, her husband Uranus. In that, she is an active prophetess and advisor. Gaia makes others act.

Latour calls attention to Gaia because she is presented as the occasion for a return to Earth that allows for a differentiated vision reduced to more modest, that is, "earthbound" views of reality (ibid., p. 4). Gaia reacts to us, calls us. This way, Latour describes Gaia as a force, which indicates the need for humble, situated actions that can break down or make up the blindness and blind-ended Anthropocene—calling attention to the "terrestrial" (terra) forces to become less anthropocentric, as we interact with birds, foods, seas, air (cf. the quote from Student Chaplain Z), and in our scientific approach of things, including the discipline of theology. Latour holds that when we seek to grasp what is coming at us with climate change, we need to "come back down to Earth" (ibid., p. 87).

Relating Latour's thoughts to the interviews on students' pastoral care, the point is that it matters how each of us thinks and does—coming from a view of our interaction with Earth. In this sense, supporting the students is not about serving "perspectives" on the world, distancing us from it, but about enacting the world (cf. Mol 2002). This means that pastoral care, which seeks to take this new climatic regime into conscious account, is, in the words of Latour, "to discover *a course of treatment*—but without the illusion that a cure will come quickly" (Latour 2017, p. 13). Connecting this point to the above quotes from the chaplains on the lack of any possibility of a traditional "safe comfort" through a modern view of ensuring Earth as a stable object, Latour suggests:

> "There is no cure for the condition of belonging to the world. But, by taking care, we can cure ourselves of believing that we do not belong to it, that the essential question lies elsewhere, that what happens to the world does not concern us.

(...) In these matters, hope is a bad counsellor, since we are not in a crisis. We can no longer say 'this, too, will pass.' We're going to have to get used to it. *It's definitive*." (Ibid., p. 13)

What I suggest here is that in the practice of pastoral care, the local and basic enactments of things, bodily expressions, feelings, and views which drive (and hinder) our being as belonging to the world are not separated from the issue of climate change, but they are interconnected. Climate change is not just something passive "out there" in itself that humans then relate to. Hence, Latour's alternative narrative is that instead of separating the world into a nature/culture binary, as passiveness and activeness, respectively, (which modern thinking has usually done), we ought to realize that our planet is full of 'agents'—things—which have the power to act according to their own intention, will, force, desire, need, or function. Our environments are anything but passive. Humans and things are inextricably connected. As Latour puts it:

"Don't try to define nature alone, for you'll have to define the term 'culture' as well (the human is what escapes nature: a little, a lot, passionately); don't try to define 'culture' alone, either, for you'll immediately have to define the term 'nature' (the human is what cannot 'totally escape' the constraints of nature). Which means that we are not dealing with *domains* but rather with one and the same *concept* divided into two parts, which turn out to be bound together, as it were, by a sturdy rubber band. (...) They were born together, as inseparable as Siamese twins who hug or hit each other without ceasing to belong to the same body." (Ibid., p. 15)

My interviews show precisely that climate change discourse and changes in the environment are not distant issues separated from moods, feelings, beliefs, anger, joy, faith, etc., but are entangled in social activities, disciplines of science being studied, and the imagination of every single student seeking pastoral care. In this sense, climate change is socialized and incorporated into pastoral care practice. "As soon as we abandon the borders between the outside and the inside of an agent, by following these waves of action we begin to *modify the scale* of the phenomena considered" (ibid., p. 104). Latour speaks of a "multiplicity of modes of action that are capable of intermingling (...) human and nonhuman actors" (ibid., p. 50). The Earth is lively, vital, and active, though certainly not as a single agent or a unified subjectivity. Humans and nature are connected as complex, heterogenic entities, as intensely interwoven hybrids (Latour 1993, 2017). They are not distant but entangled in the same multiple bodies of the world (cf. Latour-quotation above).

From this opening analysis, leading into an earthbound approach in pastoral care, we now turn to a theological view that might further unfold the new climatic regime leading to a more specific model for pastoral care practice. For this purpose, we need a form of God-talk which does not address a God of distance, but a present and participating God—a theology approaching exactly our belonging to the world—the Earth—as the body of God.

4. Climate Theology

"I usually inquire into the students' projects as crisis may also grow out from them. To most students who write about sustainability, it is seen as a societal task. They can do something for the environment. But some are confused about how slowly science is moving forward—the stress is related to this, even though it is difficult for them to put it directly into words. Ambitions and career, the character of working stress, contributes to channel that anxiety they feel about what is going to happen in the future. Thus, they do something, going out to look at the trees and birds, prefer to bike instead of driving a car, protest against nuclear power. Much merges exactly there. It is a kind of a monk's understanding of the world, go out and do good. They live by it. Become vegans. Charity. The matter of the climate is such a charity. Sincerely magnanimous motives."

Student Chaplain X

It clearly emerges from Student Chaplain X's quote that, in the "repertoire" of everyday experiences, the awareness of climate change is embodied and material. "Events are necessarily local. Somewhere. Situated" (Mol 2002, p. 180). For that reason, pastoral care practice needs a broad image of God or *imago dei*—a metaphor that is able to hold life's multiplicity, that is, diversity, difference, connectedness, and the entanglement of humanity and nature—addressed by Latour as the new climatic regime. Such pastoral practice requires theological images and models which are able to express the claims of Christianity in contemporary and vigorous language, which contains embodiment, commonality, imagination, and vision.

In connecting Latour's thoughts on climate change to God-talk, associations arise to a range of climate theologies that have advanced through decades, not least those related to thinking of Gaia (Ruether 1992; Primavesi 2009). However, in search of a model of God that can develop an empirically-driven grasp for pastoral care communication, I turn to the American theologian Sallie McFague. McFague (2008) was experimenting with alternative, new languages of God and ourselves, later insisting on the need to find a language that addresses the planetary agenda—"with the hope that different action may follow" (p. 3). According to McFague, we become ourselves by acknowledging our radical dependence on God and on our planet. What McFague presents is exactly a theology, which brings the church—in the words of both Latour (cit. above) and McFague—"back down to Earth" (ibid., p. 32). She proposes a God-talk where God is not supernatural, distant from humans, but in which God and humans are entangled and connected. "Because God is always incarnational, always embodied, we can see God's transcendence *immanently*" (ibid., p. 76). "In the world as God's body, God is the source, the centre, the spring, the spirit of all that lives and loves" (ibid., p. 76). This way God is permanently and "bodily" present to us, in all places and times of our world (McFague 1987, p. 60). Humans are not to "rule" but to be responsible for the world (cf. Gen 1:27). McFague writes:

> "The significance of the truth that the transcendent God is with us cannot be overestimated as we struggle to care for the Earth. It means that we are not alone as we face the despair that creeps over us when at last, we acknowledge our responsibility for climate change. We do not face this overwhelming problem on our own: God is with us as the source and power of all our efforts to live differently". (McFague 2008, p. 77)

Thus, according to McFague (1987, p. xii), theology must try out images which can lead the reality of God's love into the imagination of today's people. Working with ideas of "the body of God", McFague (1987) proposes a metaphor for the Trinity in her book *Models of God*. For the purpose of a pastoral care model, the Christian dogma of the Trinitarian God—traditionally interpreted as Father, Son, and Holy Spirit—offers a symbol or image of God that is fluid, multiple, and relational (Cooper-White 2007). The relations in the Trinity show a true network, a web, an image of God, who is not simple, but rather a multiple One (Keller 2008, p. 64). The image of God as Trinity operates in web structures in the sense that the single parts cannot be separated but hang together as they weave into and out of each other. This web of relations opens for lived and bodily experiences. Through such images, God is experienced physically (Moltmann and Moltmann-Wendel 2003): God *is* body, not released from the body (Moltmann-Wendel 1995). In this sense, faith in God is organic.

As a corrective to a traditional imperialistic image of God, which typically runs through the patriarchal expositions, McFague proposes an image of the Trinity of God as "Mother", "Lover", and "Friend". She understands the metaphors of God as a parent, lover, and friend of the Earth, which is precisely expressive of God's very self (McFague 1987, p. 62). As corrective, she argues, these more concisely call attention to heterogeneity, diversity, and difference, and thereby open us for change. As *imago dei,* humans are called to be Mother, Lover, and Friend to the world, other humans, and non-humans; these specific metaphors originate from the deepest levels of life (ibid., pp. 86–87). To practice the presence of God means to embrace what God embraces: life and love (McFague 2008, p. 172). God is what keeps us from giving up (ibid., p. 173).

In what follows, I make an attempt to organize the chaplains' numerous practices, experiences, considerations, and intentions about pastoral care with students by letting these reflections cross with McFague's metaphoric expression of God's love and rescuing presence. At the same time, I let the interviews and McFague's model be escorted by a "psychological repertoire" on stress-regulating communication by use of the concepts "mentalizing" and "epistemic trust", which are to serve the social understanding. Herein, trust is viewed as crucial in order to be able to open up to and interact with the world.

5. "Mentalizing" and "Epistemic Trust"

"As a chaplain, you let burdens be burdens. The climate problem cannot be fixed. But God makes the whole difference in how the pastoral care conversation turns out, and in exactly that belief lies the relief: The experience of truly speaking about our condition of life here and now. To have trust in life itself, in God, that things are moving, by taking one step at a time."

Student Chaplain L

To have trust, to have trust in life, to have trust in God. "Trust" is a word that recurs again and again in the reflections of the student chaplains, as the interview quote from Student Chaplain L illustrates. This points towards what we might call "down-to-Earth" social and material enactments that go on outside the pastoral care room. Trust is here intimately related to feelings of connectedness—to others, life, the world, and God. Trust and connectedness seem to be central in the related psychology, too.

"To mentalize" (Fonagy 1991) is about attending to mental states in the self and others; it is about "holding mind in mind"—"seeing yourself from the outside and others from the inside" (Allen et al. 2008, p. 3). To be able to mentalize is to be able to imagine what is behind the other's behavior and, at the same time, imagine how one is affecting the other. The point of highlighting the concept of mentalizing in pastoral care is that mentalizing, in its ideal form, provides intimacy. That is, mentalizing can nourish a loving feeling of connectedness with the reality of another person (Allen and Fonagy 2006). In pastoral care, it is necessary that chaplains are able to draw on imagination and ideas, and this is what mentalizing is referring to.

The psychologist Peter Fonagy and his colleagues have argued that mentalizing plays a part in the process of change as a "common language" in the therapeutic process regardless of the details, nuances, or particulars present in the conversation and regardless of the way the professional shapes the conversations (Fonagy and Allison 2014). Drawing on newer research in the area of communication and learning processes concerning "common factors" in psychotherapy, Fonagy and colleagues argue that limitations in clients' capacity to learn from their experiences—that is, where the client is difficult for the professional to reach—can be generally overcome by letting the clients feel understood. To feel understood serves to reconstruct/restore a capacity for social understanding, that is, mentalizing (ibid.).

However, newer developments in the concept of mentalizing have further developed this argument and call attention to the development of "trust" (Fonagy and Campbell 2015). To feel understood does not only restore social understanding but also creates the trust needed to learn from social experience. The prerequisite for being able to open oneself to good advice, guidance, notions, and contact is the willingness of the individual to regard new knowledge as trustworthy and relevant—and thereby as worth integrating (Campbell et al. 2021). "Epistemic trust" is defined as "openness to the reception of social communication that is personally relevant and of generalizable relevance" (Bateman and Fonagy 2019, p. 15). In short, Fonagy and colleagues suggest that a rise in epistemic trust is the potent driving force in therapeutic change and that restoring epistemic trust may be at the core of all effective therapeutic work (Fonagy and Campbell 2015).

Taken together, social understanding (mentalizing) and increased epistemic trust build some basis for life outside the therapy room upon which new information about oneself and the world may be acquired and internalized. Ultimately, this may imply that the changes happening in therapy (or pastoral care) are not just due to new skills or insights which are acquired in the professional room. Rather these are due to the capacity that is implied in the therapeutic (or pastoral care) relationship, which creates a potential for learning about oneself, others, and the world outside the therapy room (ibid.).

Fonagy et al. (2017) describe the therapeutic change in terms of three processes that facilitate the development of epistemic trust and the capacity to mentalize: Communication System 1: "The teaching and learning of content that lowers epistemic vigilance"; Communication System 2: "The re-emergence of robust mentalizing"; and Communication System 3: "The re-emergence of social learning". The following analysis is inspired by these three processes and weaves them together with McFague's Models of God (Mother, Lover, and Friend) and also with the chaplains' efforts in pastoral care based on the interviews. The aim is to show how trust-building activities and movements in Trinity traverse the pastoral conversations taking care of the "blind spots" of stress arising from climate change (cf. Student Chaplain C).

6. A Down-to-Earth Pastoral Care Model: "Mothering the Content", "Loving Vital force", and "Befriending the Environment"

6.1. Mothering the Content

> "The awareness of the climate's changes is experienced by some students as a place of powerlessness. Here, faith becomes involved—in the community together. A student comes and sees me. And then she sobs her heart out. I go round to her and hold her. She is blessed with a nice boyfriend, the right study, a good family. We talk about her sense that she is in some state of powerlessness. She is to discover the things she has got . . . The Mother-Child-feeling appears thinking: 'Oh, you little biscuit'. The care. The young ones are to take responsibility for their lives. Evidently, of course, it is a shock, suddenly to become and be grown up. Feelings storm within them. They have to take a position on so many things—achieve endlessly, love affairs. It is a bit like Ecclesiastes. It is new experience. Then we try to break it down together into many small winds, instead of one big storm. . . . In the gospels we find plenty of love and pain and suffering . . . "
>
> Student Chaplain Z

The quote from Student Chaplain Z illustrates the chaplains' wish to grasp the complexity of the student's situation in the world through eyes, voice, and bodily attitude that are open, caring, and calm. As the students enter the chaplains' rooms they are exposed to "unusual" or everyday objects, such as small cards with prayers lying on the table, chocolate beans which are on offer, ecological coffee and tea to drink, natural water poured from the tap, small cookies to crunch, plants on the floor, a Jesus-figure wearing boxing gloves on a bookshelf, posters on nature lectures, a chaplain's cyclewear on a chair in the corner, trees, or a dozen tiny birds in a big cage outside the window "participating" in the conversations. The senses are activated by all of the materials—a wealth of human/nature hybrids creates the surroundings for the pastoral care talks/conversations.

With reference to the repertoire of psychology, the first step of the therapeutic process seeks to offer a coherent, closely reasoned, and continuous framework that enables the student to explore their issues in a safe and relatively low-arousal context. That is, a communication is taking place which is personally suited enough to make the student able to feel recognized. The contact provided by the chaplain to the student is to be experienced as personally relevant (Fonagy et al. 2017; Bateman and Fonagy 2019).

The basic contact provided by the professional has, in classic psychoanalytic literature, been compared to a "good enough mother"'s ability to provide "a holding environment" (Winnicott 1965). In McFague's model of the first person in the Trinity, God resembles a mother, not only because she gives birth to the whole universe but also because she is not distant from creation. On the contrary, she is coming near the world, as incarnate God is in the flesh (McFague 1987, p. 110). God as Mother refers to a parent's love—deep and unprejudiced, caring for life in all its manifestations and on all levels, saying: "It is good, that you exist" (ibid., p. 120). It is wishing growth and fulfilment for all, caring for the weak and vulnerable, as well as the strong and beautiful. In her action, Mother God is the life-giver, she is creative power. The metaphor of God as Mother does not build on stereotypes of maternal tenderness, softness, pity, and sentimentality but on women's experience of pregnancy, birth, and breastfeeding (ibid., p. 113). God as Mother is imaging a presence of God signifying a force of action.

Relating this to pastoral care, the above quote reflects Student Chaplain Z's use of maternal mirroring. If the student looks worried, the chaplain feeds back to the student that they are admittedly in a context that is different to what they are used to. Z mirrors the student's bodily reaction with bodily action, meeting the student's expressed feelings of powerlessness with an understanding, maternal voice. The chaplain sends "ostensive cues" to the student, including eye contact, exaggerated facial expressions, use of voice tone, and turn-taking—in a "playing" manner, as Winnicott would have put it (Bateman and Fonagy 2019, p. 16; Winnicott 1971). These cues show that what the caregiver is trying to convey is significant and should be remembered (Bateman and Fonagy 2019, p. 16).

If the student is to get the sense of being understood, the mirroring is to match the student's own experiences of her or his own mental states: the mirroring should be "marked" (Fonagy et al. 2002). There is to be a difference between that which is mirrored and the mirroring itself. At the same time, the mirroring is to be recognized by the student. The chaplain mimes the student's affects. Simultaneously, the chaplain mimes affects that the student does not have. As the chaplain undertakes marked mirroring, the student is capable of relating as a mental actor to the chaplain's mental states and thereby is able to relate to her/his own mental states. The quote indicates how Student Chaplain Z mirrors the student's sobbing by simultaneously reflecting the student's worry and maternally holding her, using calm breathing, and mothering words. Herein, the student gets the feeling that the chaplain really begins to sense how it is to be the student. In short, the chaplain is to recognize the feeling that the student experiences and expresses and mirror it as marked. In this way, the chaplain can appropriately regulate, that is, scale up and down, the feelings expressed by the student and by the chaplain herself. In other words, if students are stressed then this stress needs to be regulated.

In McFague's model of Mother-God as life-giver, that which is most ordinary and close is taken as central. Coincident with the creative force, God as Mother holds justice. As a force involved in the world, she establishes justice and liberates creatures from oppressive structures (McFague 1987, pp. 117–18). This was imaged by Student Chaplain Z too, who was aware of the pressures exerted by escalating climate change insofar as they may be linked to the student's feeling of powerlessness. In this way, the image of Mother-God expands love's different shapes and their meaning—internally, but also beyond our closest family, society—connecting nature and Earth (ibid., pp. 120–21).

It is the contact with the student that always comes first, and it needs to be worked on a lot. If the chaplain gets too occupied with what the problem is or what is to be talked about before establishing personal contact, learning cannot take place. The student who learns is the one whom the chaplain really sees and shows genuine interest in. The chaplain is seeking to form a connection and holds the connections by basic bodily and emotional expression and with the world as the body of God.

6.2. Loving Engagement

"I experience how students stress out about climate change—about eating vegan, food production, recycling—the social control that goes on. It lies implicitly as something stressful, but is expressed directly by saying: 'I am not good enough—because I am not good enough!' It is very difficult for them to be in here. I tell them 'down to Earth'. We wonder if it is okay to put our feet on the ground and live this life. Climate changes are not stopped by not seeing and not living. Creating a peaceful space in the pastoral care room, I attempt to let the student's inner voices be heard so that we can talk with their inner voices, wonder about what the voices are saying. Let voices that control, what they can't stand about themselves, come out. There are voices they are scared of. We try to find out if some of the voices also contain some good. On the positive, the voices are concerned with the climate, but they may have prevailed in the student's mind, shouting too much. Together we wonder about how the inner voices tell us to sustain life—socially and earthly—but wonder if, maybe, the voices need to be calmed down. We say to the shouting voice: 'You are good enough, but now you must lie down a bit'. We treat stress and anxiety a little like a guard dog that needs to be calmed. The voice is to be heard, but needs to be let off a bit sometimes. By doing this we express our trust in it, that there is also something that holds us in the middle of our stress. To have trust in life. To get from control and mistrust—daring to take a few steps and see if it holds. Have faith that life holds us. 'And if it doesn't?', some students ask. There are no guarantees. But the alternative is a life with hands clenched and mistrust. To have faith that something holds me up, that is deeply Christian. We cannot take responsibility for it all. I say sometimes (with a caring smile): 'You don't have that much power'. Otherwise, we must think that we ourselves are God. As chaplain it is about stopping 'private metaphysics'."

Student Chaplain L

The chaplains' interview narratives witness practices which insist on experiencing "present moments" in life (Stern 2004)—both inside and outside the pastoral care room. Drawing from the interviews, the occupation with the presence here and now in the pastoral care work and in relation to the world outside the pastoral care room seems crucial.

The second step in a psychological repertoire is that the chaplain provides the impression that he or she genuinely seeks to understand the student's perspective—this helps enable the student to listen and hear for themselves (Fonagy et al. 2017; Bateman and Fonagy 2019). Actually, the chaplain models this for the student; she demonstrates it by engaging in mentalizing. The pastoral caregiver seeks to make sense of the way the student behaves—and of the way the pastoral caregiver is behaving too. The chaplain looks at the student and looks at herself, asking: "I wonder what the student is doing?", "I wonder what I am doing myself?", "I wonder why you said and did that?", and "I wonder why I said and did that?". The chaplain explores the intentions of what is being said. The chaplain is curious about what she does not know. Then the chaplain and student begin to wonder together why they did as they did—preferably involving some use of delicate humor.

In McFague's model of the Second Person in the Trinity, God as Lover, she points to the act of salvation. This represents a certain approach to the loved one, assuming that the loved one is not bad but that they only love improperly—by loving the self instead of God in the body of the world (McFague 1987, p. 144). This action assumes that the work towards healing the body is the revelation that we are loved deeply and passionately by the force whose love pulses through the universe. This may be a revelation which we are not able to imagine on our own. This knowledge performs what a lover's declaration of love to the loved one can do: to stir up an answer of the same kind. The loved one feels valuable and wishes to repay the love, which is to be closely connected with the other. Interpreted as an image, the Lover, in a climate context, is the world in its many material and non-material forms and shapes, rather than one specific individual (cf. ibid., p. 145).

When we mentalize, we attempt to feel clearly (Allen and Fonagy 2006). Our emotions are then better able to attune us to our surroundings. They enable us to quickly see things precisely as they are so as to be able to react appropriately; our emotions make it possible for us to "get it right" (ibid.). When the chaplain sees a facial expression, the chaplain may create stories about why such a feeling arises (rather than just jumping to a conclusion about the feeling involved). Thus, the chaplain makes use of wondering and imagination without jumping to immediate answers. With this sort of "playing", we can enter into—ideally, at least—an intersubjective community and see ourselves, others, and the world in more nuanced ways.

Connecting mentalizing to the model of God as Lover, salvation is here to be connected with a sense of what is valuable in life and, by extension, with a longing after all kinds of life and creation. Healing, viewed as a way to perceive salvation, emphasizes our opposition to the suffering and destruction of all of creation. This is done by identifying with it (McFague 1987, p. 153). God as Lover says: "You are exceedingly valuable" (ibid., p. 128). Incorporating pastoral care practice into McFague's model, the act of mentalizing can be understood as enabling a feeling of community which connects all life on a deep level. This is by virtue of the powers of imagination that make it possible for us to empathize with all creation despite our differences (ibid., p. 153).

These mentalizing movements create an open and trusting social situation, which can nourish a better understanding of and connection to one's own actions and others. This has the potential to open the student's sense of being related to in a sensitive way by the pastoral caregiver through interpersonal communication. Herein, the student's own ability to mentalize re-emerges. It is a (re-)ignition of the student's wishes to learn about the world.

6.3. Befriending the Environment

"The students are certainly very aware of climate change—at the same time, these are very abstract, because we don't really experience them in Denmark. I mention this, when we are out on our arranged moss and mushroom excursions. We attempt to make the students engage in nature. What you have knowledge about, you care more about. What you care about, you are interested to know more about. You may be able to teach the students to care for biodiversity by teaching them that there exists more than one bird, but many species, by learning their different names, learning that you can find them in our [local] nature and be absorbed in them—or in plants and flowers—and that the life that goes on is of interest. Learning that the way moss grows and reproduces and lives is extremely interesting, although alien to us. To arouse their curiosity in nature by naming all things. To raise questions. To philosophize about them while we walk: does it actually bring a greater understanding of nature and make our relation to nature different, when we are able to say: 'Hey! That was a cormorant', instead of 'I think there was a bird' What it means, when it is named. I think it plays a rather big role. The crisis of biodiversity ... my excitement for such action is related to the Christian idea that it is your duty to save the world. When you get so preoccupied with a bird, well, then love is obliged. When you love something, you cannot help but do acts of good."

Student Chaplain P

Student Chaplain P's interview reflects in different ways a social-minded position to the surroundings and the environment, which they talk with the students about. When trust is present, it creates possibilities for taking in something new, for taking one's understanding further. As one chaplain stated: "there is resurrection in pastoral care conversation"—new beginnings. The new can start in that which is quite basic and ordinary. It can also start in embodiment: holding hands, crying, eating, laughing, maybe praying together.

This is part of the stress relief of a caring community. The third step in a psychological repertoire relates to being able to learn from those who have a precise and personal understanding of you as a person (Fonagy et al. 2017; Bateman and Fonagy 2019). If I feel understood by you, I will open myself up to you, so that I will be able to learn from you about things. This helps change fixed and persisting convictions. The reopening of the potential for understanding by feeling sensitively reacted to may set off more trustful and new relations outside the pastoral care room. This may thereby open the student to new understandings of various social situations when these appear outside the pastoral care room.

When the student relaxes, the ability for trust increases and the student may discover new ways to learn about others and new settings. Such positive social experiences now have the potential to have a positive impact. In other words, the student may begin to experience social interactions in a more benign manner and see their social situation more precisely. The change that happens between the pastoral care sessions is a consequence of changed attitudes towards learning brought about by the pastoral care. In this sense, the changes owed themselves to the transformation of the ways in which the student uses their social environments rather than by things happening in the pastoral care. In the case of Student Chaplain H, this means that the transformations begin in the pastoral care practices and that the students bring them further by expanding their awareness of their entanglements in belonging to the world outside the pastoral care context too—becoming "friends" with birds, moss, and flowers, and learning a praxis of handling plastic, foods, clothes, woods, and so on.

According to McFague, friendship is the most elementary form of bond, a relation created by one's own choice. The image of the third person of the Trinity, "God as Friend", represents a God who sustains, whose immanent presence is the faithful companion, who operates with us in reciprocity in generating healing in all parts of the world's body (McFague 1987, p. 167). We are God's auxiliary force in that mutual project that embraces the whole creation. The basis for friendship is freedom; when friendship is chosen, one of the strongest bonds is created: the bond of trust (ibid., p. 162). Friends are absorbed in a shared interest in the world. However, friends in shared, collaborative projects do represent another aspect of friendly interactions. Collaboration on large projects means that many friends are needed with many different abilities. Of course, one can be friends with anybody across gender, race, class, nationality, age, conviction, and religion (adding species). To be like-minded—across forms of life (and ontological distinctions) is the primary thing. In that sense, one can indeed be friends with God, especially as part of a large-scale collaborative project, such as caring for the Earth really is. In that sense, friendship is the most all-embracing form of love. It means a willingness to take responsibility for the world. Thus, God as Friend can be taken as a model of hope, defying despair (ibid., p. 169).

Enhanced epistemic trust and dismantling of the student's rigidity, by which social experiences are interpreted and reacted to, opens the way for the student to change their views in a safe and secure way; it releases the opening of an "epistemic superhighway" (Fonagy and Allison 2014). All in all, this may serve to nurture a growing resilience in life, whereby the student is able to find new ways of moving forwards through their various difficulties and distress. In short, the experience of feeling understood in pastoral care makes the student feel safe enough to think about themselves in relation to the world. It enables them to learn something new about the world and how to operate in it in a positively responsible manner.

The chaplains' interviews are filled with narratives about students who seek roads to walk by. Student Chaplain C expresses this need for the caregiver to act as a wise person, to give advice on life's conditions, to understand how life is for the young student, and how to take life's problems one piece at a time:

> "I talk with the students about living in the moment and being present instead living only in the future 'Also try to live now and grasp the day instead of just putting all your strength and courage and hope and faith and joy out in the future. You don't know if you are going to be here tonight or tomorrow, and neither do I'. Try to get them to relate to their life. If they constantly try to calculate it in advance, say: 'Are you to figure it out beforehand?' I turn to action: 'Just do it!' 'The plastic wrap is to be saved now!'."

Finally, the core of McFague's model of God as Friend is the joy of being together. An image of eschatological completion is Lord's Supper: sharing a meal. Strangers are welcome. The guest's requirements are what is needed in all human life: food, shelter, clothes, and company. *Koinonia* applies to every life: openness towards what is different, unexpected, and alien (McFague 1987, p. 174). This represents a community of all creation united in the source of life—enacting together just that: food, shelter, cloth, company, birds, moss, and plastic wrap, too.

7. Conclusions

In the present era, the world is undergoing fundamental changes. Thus, our usual understandings of the relationship between humans and our surroundings are changing, too. Based on Danish student chaplains' narratives, this article has attempted to extrapolate a model of "Down-to-Earth Pastoral Care", seeking to build up trust in the process of pastoral care. This is in order to support students suffering from stress by bringing the new climate regime to the foreground.

This practical-theoretical conception for pastoral care conversations has put forward a suggestion regarding how developments within climate anthropology, mentalization-based psychotherapy, and feminist climate/eco-theology may be profitably interwoven. Thereby, through a triune of organizing themes that arose in the course of my chaplain interviews, namely: "Mothering the Content", "Loving Vital Force", and "Befriending the Environment", I have shown how pastoral care conversations transcend differences between everyday language and Christian theological language. They unfold together as a network of deeply interconnected entanglements. This, furthermore, transcends the understanding of each individual theme taken in itself—thus resonating with the image of the Christian Trinitarian God.

The result is a kind of plastic model that seeks to break away from rigidity and monodox thinking within the self, in regard to the world around us, and in relation to God. Ideally, this will give impetus to two movements. Firstly, through its psychological and theological repertoire, the model points towards community, generating resilience against isolation. Secondly, the model puts forward an image of God that, through its feminist framework, insists on an *imago dei* for all—regardless of gender, ethnicity, sexuality, social status, and religion.

Informed by the student chaplains' narratives, this framework model for pastoral care may indicate a practice, actions of taking care, which may contribute to supportive ways of being able to endure the stress of the reality of climate change. This would work by encouraging thinking about belonging to the world and realizing that the world is not just something "out there". In this sense, pastoral care promises a space for students to realize that our planet is full of "agents"—things—which have the power to act according to their own intention, will, force, desire, need, or function—as humans and things are inextricably connected in the body of God.

Funding: This research was funded by Centre for Pastoral Education and Research, Church of Denmark. From 1 October 2019, to 30 September 2023.

Informed Consent Statement: Written informed consent was obtained from all subjects involved in the study.

Data Availability Statement: Not applicable.

Conflicts of Interest: The author declares no conflict of interest.

References

ALLEA. 2017. The European Code of Conduct for Research Integrity. Available online: https://www.allea.org/wp-content/uploads/2017/05/ALLEA-European-Code-of-Conduct-for-Research-Integrity-2017.pdf (accessed on 5 June 2022).

Allen, Jon G. 2013. *Restoring Mentalizing in Attachment Relationships: Treating Trauma with Plain Old Therapy*. Washington, DC: American Psychiatric Association.

Allen, Jon G., and Peter Fonagy, eds. 2006. *Handbook of Mentalization-Based Treatment*. Chichester: John Wiley & Sons.

Allen, Jon G., Peter Fonagy, and Anthony Bateman. 2008. *Mentalizing in Clinical Practice*. Washington, DC and London: American Psychiatric Publishing, Inc.

Appiah-Brempong, Emmanuel, Paul Okyere, Ebenezer Owusu-Addo, and Ruth Cross. 2014. Motivational Interviewing Interventions and Alcohol Abuse Among College Students: A Systematic Review. *American Journal of Health Promotion* 29: e32–e42. [CrossRef] [PubMed]

Bateman, Anthony, and Peter Fonagy. 2019. *Handbook of Mentalizing in Mental Health Practice*. Washington, DC: American Psychiatric Association Publishing.

Budziszewska, Magdalena, and Sofia Elisabet Jonsson. 2021. From Climate Anxiety to Climate Action: An Existential Perspective on Climate Change Concerns Within Psychotherapy. *Journal of Humanistic Psychology* 002216782199324. [CrossRef]

Burke, Susie E. L., Ann V. Sanson, and Judith Van Hoorn. 2018. The psychological effects of climate change on children. *Current Psychiatry Reports* 20: 35. [CrossRef] [PubMed]

Calder, Andy S., and Jan E. Morgan. 2016. 'Out of the Whirlwind': Clinical Pastoral Education and Climate Change. *Journal of Pastoral Care and Counseling* 70: 16–25. [CrossRef] [PubMed]

Campbell, Chloe, Michal Tanzer, Rob Saunders, Thomas Booker, Elizabeth Allison, Elizabeth Li, Claire O'Dowda, Patrick Luyten, and Peter Fonagy. 2021. Development and validation of a self-report measure of epistemic trust. *PLoS ONE* 16: e0250264. [CrossRef]

Campbell-Reed, Eileen R., and Emmanuel Y. Lartey. 2015. Pastoral Theology in the Midst of the Crises of Climate Change, Mass Incarceration and Neo-Liberal Economics. *Journal of Pastoral Theology* 25: 69–70. [CrossRef]

Comtesse, Hannah, Verena Ertl, Sophie M. C. Hengst, Rita Rosner, and Geert E. Smid. 2021. Ecological Grief as a Response to Environmental Change: A Mental Health Risk or Functional Response? *International Journal of Environmental Research and Public Health* 18: 734. [CrossRef]

Cooper-White, Pamela. 2007. *Many Voices. Pastoral Psychotherapy in Relational and Theological Perspective*. Minneapolis: Fortress Press.

Cardoso, Patricia, Laura Thomas, Robyn Johnston, and Donna Cross. 2012. Encouraging Student Access to and Use of Pastoral Care Services in Schools. *Australian Journal of Guidance and Counselling* 22: 227–48. [CrossRef]

Dykstra, Robert C. 1997. *Counseling Troubled Youth*. Louisville and Kentucky: Westminster John Knox Press.

Fabbris, Jéssika Leão, Ana Cláudia Mesquita, Sílvia Caldeira, Ana Maria Pimenta Carvalho, and Emilia Campos de Carvalho. 2016. Anxiety and Spiritual Well-Being in Nursing Students: A Cross-Sectional Study. *Journal of Holistic Nursing* 35: 261–70. [CrossRef]

Field, Tiffany, Miguel Diego, Martha Pelaez, Osvelia Deeds, and Jeannette Delgado. 2011. Breakup distress in university students: A review. *College Student Journal* 45: 461–80.

Fonagy, Peter. 1991. Thinking about Thinking: Some Clinical and Theoretical Considerations in the Treatment of a Borderline Patient. *International Journal of Psycho-Analysis* 72: 639–56.

Fonagy, Peter, and Chloe Campbell. 2015. Bad Blood Revisited: Attachment and Psychoanalysis, 2015. *British Journal of Psychotherapy* 31: 229–50. [CrossRef]

Fonagy, Peter, and Elizabeth Allison. 2014. The role of mentalizing and epistemic trust in the therapeutic relationship. *Psychotherapy* 51: 372–80. [CrossRef] [PubMed]

Fonagy, Peter, Chloe Campbell, and Anthony Bateman. 2017. Mentalizing, Attachment, and Epistemic Trust in Group Therapy. *International Journal of Group Psychotherapy* 67: 176–201. [CrossRef]

Fonagy, Peter, György Gergeley, Elliot L. Jurist, and Mary Target. 2002. *Affect Regulation, Mentalization, and the Development of the Self*. London and New York: Routledge.

Datatilsynet.dk. n.d. The Danish Data Protection Agency. Available online: https://www.datatilsynet.dk/english (accessed on 5 June 2022).

Hai, Audrey Hang, Jennifer Currin-McCulloch, Cynthia Franklin, and Allan Hugh Cole Jr. 2018. Spirituality/religiosity's influence on college students' adjustment to bereavement: A systematic review. *Death Studies* 42: 513–20. [CrossRef] [PubMed]

Haldorsen, Hilde, Nanna Hasle Bak, Agnete Dissing, and Birgit Peterson. 2014. Stress and symptoms of depression among medical students at the University of Copenhagen. *Scandinavian Journal of Public Health* 42: 89–95. [CrossRef]

Hunter, Rodney J., and Nancy Jean Ramsay. 2005. *Dictionary of Pastoral Care and Counseling*. Nashville: Abingdon Press.

January, James, Munyaradzi Madhombiro, Shalote Chipamaunga, Sunanda Ray, Alfred Chingono, and Melanie Abas. 2018. Prevalence of depression and anxiety among undergraduate university students in low- and middle-income countries: A systematic review protocol. *Systematic Reviews* 7: 57. [CrossRef]

Johannessen-Henry, Christine Tind. 2012. Polydox Eschatology: Relating Systematic and Everyday Theology in a Cancer Context. *Studia Theologica. Nordic Journal of Theology* 66: 107–29. [CrossRef]

Johannessen-Henry, Christine Tind. 2013. The Polydoxy of Everyday Christianity. An Empirical-Theological Study of Faith in the Context of Cancer [Danish Publ.: Hverdagskristendommens polydoksi. En empirisk-teologisk undersøgelse af tro i cancerrejsens kontekst]. Ph.D. dissertation, Publikationer fra Det Teologiske Fakultet, Grafisk, University of Copenhagen, Copenhagen, Denmark; 337p.

Johannessen-Henry, Christine Tind. 2017. Listening for Safe Places: Networks of *Playing and Chalcedon* in Disaster Pastoral Care. *Dialogue: A Journal of Theology* 56: 337–51. [CrossRef]

Keech, Jacob J., Martin S. Hagger, Frances V. O'Callaghan, and Kyra Hamilton. 2018. The Influence of University Students' Stress Mindsets on Health and Performance Outcomes. *Annual Behavioral Medicine* 52: 1046–59. [CrossRef]

Keller, Catherine. 2008. *On the Mystery. Discerning Divinity in Process*. Minneapolis: Fortress Press.

Kirkegaard, Tanja, and Svend Brinkmann. 2015. Rewriting stress: Toward a cultural psychology of collective stress at work. *Culture and Psychology* 21: 81–94. [CrossRef]

Klein, L. B., and Sandra L. Martin. 2021. Sexual Harassment of College and University Students: A Systematic Review. *Trauma, Violence and Abuse* 22: 777–92.

Krägeloh, Christian U., Marcus A. Henning, Rex Billington, and Susan J. Hawken. 2015. The Relationship between Quality of Life and Spirituality, Religiousness, and Personal Beliefs of Medical Students. *Academic Psychiatry* 39: 85–89. [CrossRef] [PubMed]

LaMothe, Ryan. 2016. This Changes Everything: The Sixth Extinction and Its Implications for Pastoral Theology. *Journal of Pastoral Theology* 26: 178–94. [CrossRef]
LaMothe, Ryan. 2021. A Radical Pastoral Theology for the Anthropocene Era: Thinking and Being Otherwise. *Journal of Pastoral Theology* 31: 54–74. [CrossRef]
Lancet. 2021. A climate of anxiety. *Lancet Child and Adolescent Health* 5: 91. [CrossRef]
Latour, Bruno. 1993. *We Have Never Been Modern*. Cambridge: Harvard University Press.
Latour, Bruno. 2017. *Facing Gaia. Eight Lectures on the New Climatic Regime*. Cambridge and Medford: Polity Press.
Law, John. 2009. Actor Network Theory and Material Semiotics. In *The New Blackwell Companion to Social Theory*. Edited by Brian S. Turner. Oxford: Blackwell Publishing Ltd., pp. 141–58.
Lazarus, Richard S., and Susan Folkman. 1984. *Stress, Appraisal, and Coping*. New York: Springer Publishing Company, Inc.
Leung, Chi Hung, and Hok Ko Pong. 2021. Cross-sectional study of the relationship between the spiritual wellbeing and psychological health among university Students. *PLoS ONE* 16: e0249702. [CrossRef] [PubMed]
Maymon, Rebecca, and Nathan C. Hall. 2021. A Review of First-Year Student Stress and Social Support. *Social Sciences* 10: 472. [CrossRef]
McBride, Sarah E., Matthew D. Hammond, Chris G. Sibley, and Taciano L. Milfont. 2021. Longitudinal relations between climate change concern and psychological wellbeing. *Journal of Environmental Psychology* 78: 101713. [CrossRef]
McFague, Sallie. 1987. *Models of God. Theology for an Ecological, Nuclear Age*. London: Fortress Press.
McFague, Sallie. 2008. *A New Climate for Theology. God, The World, and Global Warming*. Minneapolis: Fortress Press.
Miller-McLemore, Bonnie J. 1996. The Living Human Web: Pastoral theology at the Turn of the Century. In: Jeanne Steverson-Moessner (red.). In *Through the Eyes of Women: Insights for Pastoral Care*. Minneapolis: Fortress Press, pp. 9–26.
Miller-McLemore, Bonnie J. 2020. Trees and the "Unthought Known": The Wisdom of the Nonhuman (or Do Humans 'Have Shit for Brains"?). *Pastoral Psychology* 69: 423–43. [CrossRef]
Mol, Annemarie. 2002. *The Body Multiple: Ontology in Medical Practice*. Durham: Duke University Press.
Moltmann, Jürgen, and Elisabeth Moltmann-Wendel. 2003. *Passion for God*. London: Westminster John Knox Press.
Moltmann-Wendel, Elisabeth. 1995. *I Am My Body*. New York: Continuum.
Moschella, Mary Clark. 2008. *Ethnography as a Pastoral Practice. An Introduction*. Cleveland: The Pilgrim Press.
Murphy, Joseph, and Linda Holste. 2016. Explaining the effects of communities of pastoral care for students. *The Journal of Educational Research* 109: 531–40. [CrossRef]
Pihkala, Panu. 2016. The Pastoral Challenge of the Environmental Crisis: Environmental Anxiety and Lutheran "Eco-Reformation". *Dialog: A Journal of Theology* 55: 131–40. [CrossRef]
Pihkala, Panu. 2020. Anxiety and the Ecological Crisis: An Analysis of Eco-Anxiety and Climate Anxiety. *Sustainability* 12: 7836. [CrossRef]
Primavesi, Anne. 2009. *Gaia and Climate Change. A Theology of Gift Events*. New York: Routledge.
Regehr, Cheryl, Dylan Glancy, and Annabel Pitts. 2013. Interventions to reduce stress in university students: A review and meta-analysis. *Journal of Affective Disorders* 148: 1–11. [CrossRef] [PubMed]
Ribeiro, Ícaro J. S., Rafael Pereira, Ivna V. Freire, Bruno G. de Oliveira, Cezar A. Casotti, and Eduardo N. Boery. 2018. Stress and Quality of Life Among University Students: A Systematic Literature Review. *Health Professions Education* 4: 70–77. [CrossRef]
Rith-Najarian, Leslie R., Maya M. Boustani, and Bruce F. Chorpita. 2019. A systematic review of prevention programs targeting depression, anxiety, and stress in university students. *Journal of Affective Disorders* 257: 568–84. [CrossRef]
Ruether, Rosemary Radford. 1992. *Gaia and God. An Ecofeminist Theology of Earth Healing*. New York: HarberCollins Publishers.
Russell, Kirsten, Stephanie Allan, Louise Beattie, Jason Bohan, Kenneth MacMahon, and Susan Rasmussen. 2019. Sleep problem, suicide and self-harm in university students: A systematic review. *Sleep Medicine Reviews* 44: 58–69. [CrossRef] [PubMed]
Senbel, Maged, Victor Douglas Ngo, and Erik Blair. 2014. Social mobilization of climate change: University students conserving energy through multiple pathways for peer engagement. *Journal of Environmental Psychology* 38: 84–93. [CrossRef]
Sharp, Jessica, and Stephen Theiler. 2018. A Review of Psychological Distress Among University Students: Pervasiveness, Implications and Potential Points of Intervention. *International Journal of Advanced Counselling* 40: 193–212. [CrossRef]
Smith, Rachel A., and Nigar G. Khawaja. 2011. A review of the acculturation experiences of international students. *International Journal of Intercultural Relations* 35: 699–713. [CrossRef]
Spradley, James P. 1979. *The Ethnographic Interview*. Orlando: Holt, Rinehart and Winston.
Stern, Daniel N. 2004. *The Present Moment in Psychotherapy and Everyday Life*. New York and London: W.W. Norton & Company.
Thai, Chan L., and Julia F. Moore. 2018. Grief and Bereavement in Young Adult College Students: A Review of the Literature and Implications for Practice and Research. *Communication Research Trends* 37: 4–29.
van Nieuwenhuizen, Adrienne, Kelsey Hudson, Xiaoxuan Chen, and Alison R. Hwong. 2021. The Effects of Climate Change on Child and Adolescent Mental Health: Clinical Considerations. *Current Psychiatry Reports* 23: 88. [CrossRef]
Wachholz, Sandra, Nancy Artz, and Douglas Chene. 2014. Warming to the Idea: University Students' Knowledge and Attitudes About Climate Change. *International Journal of Sustainability in Higher Education* 15: 128–41. [CrossRef]
Winnicott, Donald W. 1965. *The Maturational Processes and the Facilitating Environment*. London: Hogarth.
Winnicott, Donald W. 1971. *Playing and Reality*. London: Routledge.

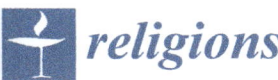

Article

The Body of God, Sexually Violated: A Trauma-Informed Reading of the Climate Crisis

Danielle Elizabeth Tumminio Hansen

Candler School of Theology, Emory University, 201 Dowman Drive, Atlanta, GA 30322, USA; detummi@emory.edu

Abstract: This article employs the body of God metaphor, developed by Sallie McFague, in order to propose that the environmental crisis can be understood as a crisis in which the earth is being subjected to repeated sexual violations. The first section develops what is at stake, theologically, for the climate crisis when utilizing this metaphor. The next considers how applying this metaphor shifts the story of Christianity in ways that illuminate historic hierarchies of creation, as well as shift the way we frame the ecological crisis to one in which sexual harm has occurred. The third section uses trauma theory to understand the earth's response to the climate crisis and proposes a trauma-informed ethic for a revised practice.

Keywords: Sallie McFague; ecotheology; sexual violations; rape; environment

Citation: Tumminio Hansen, Danielle Elizabeth. 2022. The Body of God, Sexually Violated: A Trauma-Informed Reading of the Climate Crisis. *Religions* 13: 249. https://doi.org/10.3390/rel13030249

Academic Editors: Pamela R. McCarroll and HyeRan Kim-Cragg

Received: 6 September 2021
Accepted: 10 March 2022
Published: 15 March 2022

Publisher's Note: MDPI stays neutral with regard to jurisdictional claims in published maps and institutional affiliations.

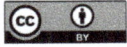

Copyright: © 2022 by the author. Licensee MDPI, Basel, Switzerland. This article is an open access article distributed under the terms and conditions of the Creative Commons Attribution (CC BY) license (https://creativecommons.org/licenses/by/4.0/).

1. Introduction

In August of 2020, the Trump administration authorized oil drilling in the Arctic National Wildlife Refuge, allowing approximately 1.6 million acres, in the coastal plain region of the refuge, to be made available to companies who could extract natural resources from it. While the governor of Alaska hailed the move as an opportunity to create jobs, environmentalists and indigenous activists railed against the decision, arguing that it would devastate a delicate ecosystem and do irreversible damage to a number of species that call the region home.

This is but one anecdote of many in which governments and industries have assumed they have a right to control the earth's body; to understand the earth not as a living, breathing subject, but as an object designed primarily for human use and consumption. Christianity at large has been complicit in the anthropocentrism that permits the objectification and ecological destruction of the earth, thereby also becoming complicit in a seemingly endless climate crisis.[1] As Catherine Keller writes, "One upon a time we had . . . time . . . And now we seem to have lost it" (Keller 2018, p. 1).

Eco-feminists have recognized parallels between the subjugation experienced by the earth and the subjugation experienced by women in ways that mutually enable the perpetuation of patriarchal authority (Warren 2000; Dunayer 1995). These scholars observe that the feminized language used to describe the earth (i.e., Mother Earth/Mother Nature) and the pejorative terms that liken women to animals mutually support epistemic frameworks, as well as practices that allow for the control and manipulation of each (Adams 1990).[2] Both possess, in other words, identities constructed by patriarchal epistemologies that enable their violation. Meanwhile, feminist theologians have been attentive to a number of systemic forms of harm, including traumatic sexual violations inflicted upon human bodies, and while theologians at large are increasingly recognizing the need for theological analysis of the ecological crisis,[3] more work needs to be done, especially by theologians like feminists who are attentive to matters of power. As Rosemary Radford Ruether recognizes, there are "interconnections between the domination of women and the domination of nature" (Ruether 2012), and an awareness of these interconnections not only changes how we think about these relationships but how we inhabit them (Ruether 2012).

This article, therefore, builds upon these interconnections by providing a theological analysis of the climate crisis that emerges when using Sallie McFague's metaphor of the world as the body of God. I propose that this metaphor functions as an important hermeneutic—as well as a deeply challenging one—for theologically framing both the climate crisis, as well as God's identity and relationship to creation. In particular, I elucidate and develop McFague's metaphor to suggest that there are parallels that can be drawn between the sexual violations that the earth experiences and the sexual violations that women's bodies experience. I unpack these challenges and then use this conceptualization as a way to reframe both the dominant denial that characterizes the human response to the climate crisis, and to propose a trauma-informed ethic for moving forward in humans' relationship to creation at large. Such an analysis develops a practical theology of the climate crisis insofar as it both encourages readers to think differently about their relationships to the earth, and to live out that relationship in a way that transforms the earth from object to subject.

Before proceeding further, however, a note of limitation: It is worth naming, at the outset, that women's bodies are not the only human bodies that are subjected to sexual violations. I will be limiting my analysis to women's bodies for the purposes of this article, in part because they constitute the majority of cases of sexual violations, and also because one of the goals of the article is to draw parallels between gender-based sexual violations and the violations inflicted by humans upon the earth.[4] In addition, the role that the systemic oppression of women's bodies plays in the normalization of sexual violations can be paralleled with the systemic oppression the planet faces, resulting in the vulnerability of each to continued harm. Indeed, one might argue that a rise in the awareness concerning the vulnerability of both occurred concurrently in the United States, as the height of the #MeToo movement collided with what might be named as a heightened call to climate action, initiated by Greta Thunberg's school strike. Parallels between the constructed vulnerability of women's bodies, the earth, and the trauma caused to each will be elucidated in what follows.

2. The Body of God, Sexually Violated

Sallie McFague is well-known for the development of metaphorical theology, which is a way of doing theology that considers how words and concepts have come to function as linguistic and conceptual idols, rather than metaphors for the Divine. She proposes in *Metaphorical Theology* that masculine language for God has come to function as such an idol, leading many who employ it to conclude God is essentially male, rather than the recognition that masculine terminology is only a partial and metaphorical representation of the "root-metaphor" of Christianity, the metaphor from which all other Christian metaphorical language ought to emerge (McFague 1982, pp. 28, 194).[5] McFague proposes that the God–human relationship, specifically as represented in the vision of the kingdom of God, ought to ground the root-metaphor (Ibid., pp. 26–28).[6] However, McFague also postulates that the root-metaphor is, essentially, beyond language, which cannot in and of itself encapsulate the divine, because the divine is ontologically more expansive than language, and because language is subject to human influence, including the influence of sin, which distorts it. Language can, therefore, partially represent the root-metaphor but it cannot directly or fully encapsulate it.

McFague proposes linguistic multiplicity as a possible antidote to language's limitations and fallibility, which is why multiple metaphors are important to her. If one metaphor cannot fully represent the Divine, then perhaps many, when used together, can more closely do this linguistic work. Thus, rather than discarding the metaphor of God as a father or the biblical texts that support it, McFague asks readers to consider the extent to which the metaphor—and the biblical texts that name it—may be incomplete or not intended for literal interpretation, even as she simultaneously encourages readers to consider other metaphors that could illuminate previously undeveloped aspects of Christianity's root-metaphor, thereby opening the possibility for humans to deepen their knowledge of, and relationship with, the Divine (TeSelle [McFague] 1975, p. 29). McFague, therefore, suggests that the issue with using masculine language to name the divine is not its existence, but its dominance. In other words, the exclusivity of its use reinforces the power of the linguistic idol, and so the solution is to disrupt the power of that idol by creating more linguistic frameworks which, together, might do a more comprehensive job of representing God.

McFague proposes various metaphors in the corpus of her work, including the metaphor of "friend" (McFague 1989, p. 160; McFague 1982, pp. 178–94) but here I would like to focus particularly on the metaphor of the world as God's body, a metaphor she develops at length in *The Body of God*. McFague argues that the metaphor of the world as God's body is an important supplement to the dominant human male metaphor, because it draws upon the inherent embodiment present in the incarnation itself, such that bodies of all sorts—including the earth's body—matter because God chose to incarnate Jesus into a body. As McFague explains,

> "We will suggest that the primary belief of the Christian community, its doctrine of the incarnation (the belief that God is with us here on earth), be radicalized beyond Jesus of Nazareth to include all matter ... As long as we refuse to imagine God as embodied, we imply ... that the body is inferior" (McFague 1993, p. xi).

The incarnation, therefore, justifies the overall theological import of the body, including the embodiment of the earth upon which Jesus lived and through which he procured sustenance, clothing, and shelter. This does not mean that the earth and its contents can be equated with God, but it does mean that we can know God through the world, the locus where God chooses to self-mediate. As McFague writes:

> "The world, creation, is not identified or confused with God. Yet it is the place where God is present to us. Christianity's most distinctive belief is that divine reality is always mediated through the world, a belief traditionally expressed in the Chalcedonian formula that Christ was "fully God, fully man" ... In both instances, the Word is made flesh, God is available to us only through the mediation of embodiment ... Incarnationalism, radicalized, means that we do not, ever, at least in this life, see God face to face, but only through the mediation of the bodies we pay attention to, listen to, and learn to love and care for" (ibid., pp. 135, 134).

As a result of this fundamental tenet, McFague makes the provocative argument that in destroying the earth, we are participating in the destruction of God, because, while "a panentheistic model does not reduce God to the world ... God is in the young woman killed in the accident and in the baby with birth defects as well as in those who suffer the loss or diminishment of their loved ones" (ibid., p. 176). To that end, God participates in our losses, in suffering, in an embodied, intimate way that not only affects us but also affects God. In turn, the embodied world—creation—becomes not only the site of divine–human suffering, but also of redemption, because if God is in creation, then salvation must take place within it (ibid., pp. 179–80).

McFague's metaphor of the world as God's body has significant implications for both constructing the body theologically and relationally (ibid., p. 101). Because God is part of creation, and because God is, in essence, good, so too are bodies good. To that end, privileging the body's goodness becomes a fundamental priority for McFague, for in the metaphor of the world as God's body, each of our bodies—indeed, the bodies of all creation—are part of God. However, this awareness also means that bodies are connected through their relationship to God, who inheres in each one. As she writes, when one accepts as axiomatic the metaphor of the world as God's body, then it becomes evident that,

> The "God-part" will take care of itself if we can love and value the bodies. That is what an incarnational theology assures us: it is right to have a nature spirituality. In fact, we should have one ... All of us, living and nonliving, are one phenomenon, a phenomenon stretching over billions of years and containing untold numbers of strange, diverse, and marvelous forms of matter—including

our own ... [Therefore] I belong not only to my immediate family or country or even my species, but to the earth and all its life-forms. I know this now. The question is, can I, will I, *live* as if I did? Will I accept my proper place in the scheme of things? Will *we*, the human beings of the planet, do so? (ibid., pp. 97, 113, 211).

The theology that McFague proposes, therefore, maps the body of God metaphor for the purpose of developing a distinctly practical theology. The goal is not just to think about our relationship to the earth differently, but to act differently, because our awareness of that relationship causes us to regard the earth as subject instead of object. Hence, the reader observes how McFague's process of transforming the vocabulary that expresses the divine–human relationship has a broadly performative effect, because it calls us both to experience the ontology of the earth differently and, symbiotically, to act differently.

How, then, might this metaphor of the world as God's body cause us to see ourselves and our relationship to the earth differently, in light of the climate crisis?

3. Assessing the Metaphor

The world as God's body metaphor provokes a number of difficult questions about divine power, the relationship between members of the Trinity, and the dynamics of the God–human relationship. For instance, can humans harm God? Is the first person of the Trinity capable of being harmed? Yet, readers must recall the importance of the word "metaphor" here, before they either raise their hands in despair or abandon McFague entirely because her beliefs seem too radical. Recall that McFague holds that language is imperfect and that God is so vast and beyond linguistic comprehension. I agree with that assertion. Therefore, neither McFague nor I intend for any one metaphor to be a comprehensive representation of the divine, but rather a partial and imperfect reflection that, at best, reveals something of true value that might otherwise go unsaid about the divine–human relationship. The particular metaphor of the world as God's body, then, was never intended to replace or supersede all other representations or beliefs about God, but rather it was meant to supplement those representations that align with the root-metaphor with a vision that adds something new and previously unexpressed.

What is gained theologically by such a metaphor? First, the metaphor of the world as God's body allows McFague to argue that bodies of all kinds matter to God and that any act of violence, injustice, or ecological destruction done to the earth is an act against God. McFague's intention here is not only to draw attention to the theological significance of the harm done to the earth's body, but also to draw attention to the harm done to other objectified bodies, including human ones. In other words, McFague recognizes that while "a panentheistic model does not reduce God to the world ... God is in the young woman killed in the accident and in the baby with birth defects as well as in those who suffer the loss or diminishment of their loved ones" (ibid., p. 176).

To that end, in suggesting that the world is God's body, McFague not only argues that bodies matter, but that any act of violence, injustice, or ecological destruction done to the earth becomes an act against God, and that such harms echo others inflicted upon humans beings whose bodies have been constructed as vulnerable in ways that cause them to become disenfranchised and neglected by those with power in society (ibid., pp. 16–22, 165). Ethical and pastoral implications for ecological theology, and the care of bodies, thus evidence themselves through this metaphor (ibid., p. 186). Insofar as one conceives ecological destruction as a form of sexual violation, then, it becomes possible to argue that McFague's metaphor represents the possibility of divine solidarity with human victims of sexual violations, while simultaneously condemning both the enactment of human and ecological sexual harm on the grounds that both violate the creation in which God embeds. It, therefore, gives a theological warrant for both naming and condemning the sexual violation of the earth, as well as the sexual violation of human bodies.

Second, theologians including Cone, Williams, and Moltmann have convincingly argued that there is value in understanding Jesus' life and death as illuminating the presence of divine solidarity with humans. From an intersectional feminist perspective, solidarity is likewise important, because it calls us to acknowledge the subjectivity of another, such that a relationship between parties is possible. Divine–human solidarity matters, therefore, because it helps humans see that they are not alone in their suffering and that their personhood matters to God. What McFague's metaphor of the world as God's body adds is an additional dimension to divine solidarity, such that solidarity is not just shared with humans, but also shared with the earth. While solidarity alone is not a sufficient telos for the theological project of salvation because it is limited in its ability to actively defeat the given sin or evil at hand, it nonetheless responds to the reality that suffering alone renders a victim more vulnerable and isolated than suffering in a community does.

Relatedly, other theologians have done important work in parsing out how it is possible for Jesus to simultaneously be capable of experiencing embodied vulnerability, while not compromising the divine essence.[8] These conceptions allow for the recognition that Jesus' embodied vulnerability has value, while nonetheless asserting that it is possible for Jesus to have suffered and died on the cross without the simultaneous destruction of the divine essence. Perhaps, then, it is possible to make a similar argument for the first person of the Trinity; to assert that it is possible for the Creator to experience suffering in a way that reconceptualizes and heightens the gravity of the earth's suffering, while also not sacrificing a divine essence that remains inviolable.

Finally, expanding on how and where God engages in solidarity with all of creation has important gendered implications for the environmental crisis as a form of sexual harm, when one considers it in conjunction with the common metaphor that English speakers use to speak of the earth in feminine terms, as "Mother Nature" or "Mother Earth". Ecofeminist philosophers, such as Carol Adams, suggest that the likening of the earth to a woman's body becomes a convenient way to essentialize the earth as an entity that needs to be subdued and controlled, just as women's bodies need to be subdued and controlled (Adams 1990). This gendered metaphorical language itself emerges from the assumption that women's bodies create life, just as the earth creates life, but it also relates to the assumptions about the extent to which either is essentially nurturing, life-giving, and, because of each capacity, mysterious at best, and inferior at worst, to the independent rationality associated with the male mind, as constructed by Enlightenment thought. Language, in other words, frames how we understand the world around such, such that to gender the earth in ways that mirror the subjugation common in women's lives enables the continued subjugation of each, while simultaneously perpetuating patriarchal ways of knowing (Saidero 2017; Gudmarsdottir 2010).

Now, while this language embeds flawed assumptions about gender essentialism and pastoral implications for women whose reproductive organs cannot effect the creation of new life, it also allows theologians to frame the climate crisis in terms of gender-based violence and to query whether the crisis is only a violation of the earth or a violation of women's bodies more generally.[9]

Such a conceptualization also allows theologians to differently frame the earth's response to human actions. At the risk of anthropomorphizing, it allows us to see climate change in terms of sexual violations that can be conceptualized through the lens of trauma.[10] This trauma-informed lens can inform how humans not only see the climate crisis, but also how they respond to it.

4. Applying the Metaphor

First, the application of this metaphor encourages us to consider the role that stories play in how we construct our role in climate change. The metaphor of the world as God's body is but one way to image God's relation to humans, and far from the dominant one. But, by applying the metaphor, we become more attuned to how it causes us to read the climate crisis differently from the way that the dominant metaphor does. Returning again to McFague, she writes in *A New Climate for Christology* that there is indeed a dominant story, a dominant narrative or metaphor about Christianity. She refers to this dominant story as a "model" and explains that much of what we consider undebatable Christian theology is, in fact, "the Western story, anchored by a monarchical, all-powerful God" (McFague 2021, p. 2). McFague goes on to suggest that, truthfulness aside, the usefulness of this particular story has worn thin,[11] and, in turn, it suggests that the Western interpretive story of Christianity is an essentially patriarchal story, one that pits male humans against a male God in a sort of cosmic battle rooted in individualism, Enlightenment ways of knowing, and capitalism (ibid., p. 3).

In terms of inter-human relationships, a consequence of this dominant story is that it allows some bodies to be privileged above other bodies. Humans collectively privilege their own bodies over animal bodies and the body of the earth. More specifically, humans also collectively privilege bodies with lighter skin over bodies with darker skin, as well as the bodies of those who identify as men over the bodies of those who identify as women (ibid., p. 6). Those who find themselves beneath the pinnacle of the most privileged body type therefore find themselves inhabiting a place of vulnerability. This vulnerability, moreover, is socially constructed in such a way that it becomes appropriate to exploit it.[12]

At the same time, it is also a story that allows for the earth's violation. The earth, in this story, is not a body at all, but rather an object and, as such, is designed to be subdued and dominated, in the spirit of a literal reading of Genesis 1:28. There is, in other words, a hierarchy in this story in which God is at the top, humans are directly underneath, and the rest of creation exists to be used at the convenience of these humans. We see the application of this story on a daily basis, in such subtle and insidious ways that we barely notice: Humans choose to drive cars that raise the planet's temperature and destroy its ecosystems. They manufacture and dispose of plastic, to the extent that islands of it have coalesced in the Pacific Ocean. They raise, kill, and consume large numbers of animals, most of whom spend their lives in cramped, contained, and unnatural habitats.

This kind of objectification is precisely the kind seen in inter-human sexual violations in which one human being sees another as an object to be used, rather than a subject with agency that deserves respect. In other words, while the physical forms of harm are not the same, the meaning of them and the goals of them are strikingly similar—to subdue, to dominate, to control. Moreover, that both of these forms of harm exist—and exist in a way that is so normalized—is a symbol of how powerful the dominant story of Christianity is. Applying the metaphor of the body of God becomes one way to disrupt the power of that dominant story, because it brings to light assumptions about the story that may have gone unquestioned by too many for too long.

It also provides a new story of the relationships between God, humans, and the earth that can guide our ethics going forward. In this case, the metaphor of the world as God's body makes it unthinkable to harm the earth, because to harm the earth would be to harm the most generative parts of God's self. To do that would be the very definition of sin, and therefore, the application of this metaphor requires that humans find ways to see the earth as a subject and to treat it with the reverence that we give to God.

5. Ecological Sin as Sexual Selfishness

The second consequence of this metaphor's application is that it allows us to strike a parallel between ecological sin and sexual selfishness. Throughout her corpus, Sallie McFague adheres to the belief that solidarity and relationships are grounding principles of the Christian life, such that the violation of relationships become the basis for her understanding of sin. Phrased differently, if the relationship between God and humans, as modeled in the life of Jesus and the New Testament parables that comprise the root-metaphor of Christianity (the fundamental metaphor through which others derive), then acts that betray the principles of that relationship constitute sin, such that sin becomes the act of ranking oneself above or apart from others, thereby eschewing relationships. Sin, therefore, manifests when individuals refuse to acknowledge that they are in a relationship or refuse to value the other with whom they are in relationship, resulting in their objectification. As McFague summarizes, "Our sin is plain old selfishness—wanting to have everything for ourselves ... Sin is limitless greed" (McFague 1993, pp. 114–15).

McFague describes sin in different ways, depending on the metaphor she is working with, though the priority of selfishness remains consistent between each. When working with her metaphor of God as a friend, she explains sin through the language of betrayal—because loyalty to the friend and the free choice to be in such relationships ground friendships, sin becomes the act of turning away from the relational loyalty to which one is committed (McFague 1989, p. 162). In contrast, when dealing with the metaphor of the world as God's body, McFague suggests that sin involves denying relationships not just with humans, but also with the earth. Indeed, a relationship with the earth is a precondition of human survival, because humans cannot live without certain fundamentals that the earth provides, including food from its soil, heat from its wood, and shelter from its stone. Hence, humans sin when they fail to acknowledge that they are in a relationship with other humans and with nature through virtue of their embodiment. This orientation is also known as speciesism.[13] To that end, McFague writes that:

"It is obvious, then, what sin is in this metaphor of the world as God's body: it is refusal to be part of the body, the special part we are as imago dei. In contrast to the king–realm model, where sin is against God, here, it is against the world. To sin is not to refuse loyalty to the Liege Lord but to refuse to take responsibility for nurturing, loving, and befriending the body and all its parts. Sin is the refusal to realize one's radical interdependence with all that lives: it is the desire to set oneself apart from all others as not needing them or being needed by them. Sin is the refusal to be the eyes, the consciousness, of the cosmos ... If Christian discipleship is shaped by solidarity with the needy, including nature as the new poor, then natural evil is not limited to what happens to me and mine, and sin becomes the limitation of one's horizon to the self" (McFague 1993, pp. 77, 174).[14]

McFague, therefore, concludes that humans make idols of their own identities by limiting their horizon of the self, and by privileging their own subjectivity above the subjectivity of other bodies, or, phrased differently, privileging their own power in a way that constructs the vulnerability of other bodies (McFague 2008, p. 15). Sin, thus, manifests because this form of idolatry refuses to acknowledge the reality that one is in a relationship with others who may have different needs, identities, and values from themselves. This can occur both intra- and inter-species. In cases of misogyny, for instance, men become capable of idolizing their own embodied identity and privileging their own subjectivity above the embodied identity of women, thereby allowing themselves to objectify women, construct women as vulnerable, and enact harm upon them. The corollary in the environmental crisis is that humans, at large, function as men do in misogyny—able to privilege their own subjectivity, to construct the earth as vulnerable by rendering it an object that exists for human use, and to exploit its body without a second thought because we believe that the earth's body belongs to us (McFague 1993, p. 115).

I'd like to build on McFague's conception of sin as selfishness to suggest that the dominant discursive beliefs and practices that humans exercise in their relationship with the earth can be categorized as sin, because they allow humans to objectify and desire the earth in a fundamentally selfish way. The Trump administration's authorization of oil drilling in the Arctic National Wildlife Refuge provides just one of many examples that support this assertion. Lawmakers and other powerful figures in governments and businesses make decisions that are driven by the short-term interests of humans, not of the earth. As a result, a decision like the one to drill in the Arctic is justified by the need for oil to fuel energy-inefficient vehicles that transport humans, as well as arguing that humans need their jobs in the oil and auto industries. Such an argument is, therefore, selfish insofar as it is driven entirely by the needs of human beings—as well as a failure of imagination—without regard for the earth and the damage done to it.

Relatedly, the ecological crisis can be understood not only as a sin but also as an act of sexual violation, because this objectifying orientation allows humans to presume that it is appropriate to penetrate generative parts of the earth's body without the earth's consent.[15] We frack the earth's crust, seizing gas from its innermost parts. We rip trees from soil intended to generate life. We litter the atmosphere with carbon dioxide and methane emissions that pollutes the very air needed for the creation and continuation of life. Humans do this without asking the earth, assuming that it is our right to use the earth's body, including its generative and reproductive capacities, as we please. Indeed, one may go so far as to say that humans have been raping the earth's body.

Now, I recognize that this assertion is, prima facie, problematic in its own right because of the way it anthropomorphizes the earth, constructing it in terms of a subset of human bodies. However, what might be beneficial about attempting, however clumsily, to identify the way in which both women's and the earth's bodies frequently experience a form of sexual violation is that it recognizes that the bodies of each have been constructed as vulnerable in such a way that that the vulnerability can be exploited in ways that become normalized, instead of being identified and responded to as real forms of wrongdoing. Put differently, I am following in McFague's footsteps by proposing a linguistic metaphor that hopefully will not function as an idol, but rather as an important addition that allows us to give speech to forms of harm in new ways. In turn, it also allows us to think about and speak about the relationship between women's bodies and the body of the earth in a new way.

Framing these human acts as rape or as a sexual violation has provocative implications for McFague's metaphor: If we are raping the earth, then are we raping God? What would be at stake were God—and not just the earth—vulnerable to this kind of trauma? This framework challenges us to think afresh about what role vulnerability plays in God's identity, and it also challenges us to consider the possibility that we have become perpetrators who take advantage of that vulnerability.

6. The Dialectic of Trauma and a Proposed Ethic

Sexual violations are, more often than not, traumatic for those humans who experience them. We know this from the numerous studies done on inter-human sexual violations—when one person sexually violates another, it often results in trauma, where the victimized party experiences symptoms of posttraumatic stress, including flashbacks and emotional numbing. These alternating symptoms of hyper-awareness and numbing are known as the dialectic of trauma, meaning symptoms that appear to be antithetical to each other but are, in fact, intimately linked. In the case of trauma, the dialectic symbolizes the desire to both remember the trauma, so it doesn't happen again (as exhibited by symptoms, such as flashbacks and hypervigilance) while also desiring to forget it because of how terrible it was (as symbolized by symptoms, such as numbing or forgetting aspects of the event).

If we apply the metaphor of the world as God's body to the climate crisis and understand the harm we are doing to the earth is a sexual one, in which the agency and generative parts of the earth are being violated by humans, then perhaps there is a traumatic dimension to the earth's violation. Indeed, framing the ecological crisis in terms of a series of sexual traumas undertaken by humans on the earth's body changes how we understand the earth's response, because it causes us to consider the ways in which the earth is a subject and, as a subject, is exerting agency in response to the horror humans are inflicting upon it.

It also calls us to recognize the ways in which trauma—which we often assume is only a human phenomenon—is actually a response that humans share with other parts of creation. Scientists are discovering that animals of all sorts experience traumas in ways that alter brain chemistry and induce posttraumatic stress symptoms, symptoms that include, what trauma theorist Judith Herman calls, a "dialectic" of intrusive and avoidance symptoms (Herman 1997, pp. 47–51). In the Canadian Yukon, for example, the snowshoe hare population rises and falls based not just on how many predators successfully kill the hares, but also based upon the trauma of living among the predators. Ecologists studying the phenomenon have found that snowshoe hare mothers experience such profound stress from living amongst the predators that it causes changes in the brain, including a rise in cortisol levels, that resembles those found present in the brains of humans with PTSD (Sheriff et al. 2010). Interestingly, the researchers also found a generational component to the trauma, as the changes in the brains of the snowshoe hares passed from mother to daughter; both populations produce fewer young as a result of the changes in brain chemistry.[16]

Researchers have hypothesized that trauma works in the wild across species ranging from elephants, to rats, in ways that reminisce the human posttraumatic stress reaction (Zanette and Clinchy 2020). In other words, it appears to be the case that the animal world at large may experience intrusion symptoms—which include recurring memories and dreams about the trauma, flashbacks, emotional distress or flooding when one is reminded of the trauma, and flashbacks—as well as avoidance symptoms, such as attempts avoid locations or people associated with the trauma, as well as dissociation, emotional numbness, attempts to avoid thinking of the trauma, and difficulty remembering the trauma. In addition to those symptoms that are emblematic of the dialectic, posttraumatic stress is also marked by symptoms including guilt, shame, difficulty sleeping, difficulty concentrating, outbursts of anger, and a heightened startle response.

Perhaps most valuably, using a trauma-informed lens to understand climate change as a form of trauma inflicted upon the earth's body allows humans to reframe the events we are seeing in terms of concrete harm: The overall warming of the globe that appears in tandem with periods of striking cold can be understood as a dialectic, an earthquake as an earthly startle response, a hurricane as an outburst of anger. The earth is speaking in its own language, a language of wind, heat, water, and magma. Insofar as we see the world as God's body, this response can also be understood as God speaking through the earth's suffering in order to signal that the violation that humans inflict on the earth breaches the root-metaphor of Christianity and needs to change.

Recognizing earth's speech is essential to responding to the climate crisis for the same reason that it is essential to respond to the speech of other members of creation who experience forms of trauma. It affords them a form of epistemic credibility. By way of an example, research on human traumas shows that affording epistemic credibility to victims is both paramount for their healing and is also countercultural.[17] When victims tell others about traumatic events in their lives, it is not uncommon for witnesses to respond with denial because, as trauma theorists like Judith Herman postulate, it is easier to live in a world where one assumes the victim is lying than to accept the pervasiveness of violence and the reality that we may be complicit in it to some degree (Herman 1997, pp. 7–33). This denial is not helpful to either victims or witnesses. Victims are unable to recover without the ability to speak, to craft a narrative, and to integrate trauma into the reality of their lives. They need witnesses who will listen and respond to isolation with community, to harm with safety (ibid., pp. 155–213). Meanwhile, witnesses who adopt a stance of denial are avoiding both painful truths and the opportunity to serve as supporters and advocates.

If we think about the climate crisis as a form of trauma inflicted upon God's body, then human propensity to deny earth's speech makes more sense. Human denial of the earth's trauma mirrors their denial of the trauma inflicted upon human bodies; in both cases, it remains more convenient to blame the victim than to acknowledge the reality that one lives in a world in which such horrors can occur.[18] Yet, the earth persists in her efforts to be heard, just as human survivors of traumas refuse to be silenced. Melting glaciers, hurricanes, fires, and earthquakes can be read as acts of divine speech that perhaps mirror the words of Jesus on the cross, "Eli, Eli, lama sabacthani?" or "My God, my God, why have you forsaken me?" (Matt. 27:36; Psalm 22:1, NRSV). Ethically, then, we must listen to the testimony of trauma and consider what needs to be done to make things right, because to continue to ignore what is being said is to continue being complicit in the trauma itself.

Lastly, the earth's traumatized speech can be read as an act of resistance undertaken by the earth to draw our attention to the reality of its traumatization, calling humans out of denial to be witnesses. Humans are uniquely responsible for the climate crisis, or, put differently, they are uniquely the perpetrators of the earth's trauma. It is, therefore, imperative that humans find ways to move from a stance of denial to undertake the work of active witnessing and active solidarity. Only by actively witnessing, recognizing, and naming the harm being done can we grow in awareness of it, and awareness is the first step to change, because it allows us to recognize our individual complicity as well as a systemic need for accountability.[19] In other words, if McFague is right in that sin is a form of selfishness, then one way to counteract its power is through a radical practice of empathy that extends beyond our own species and to creation at large, even including the God who made it. Only through that empathy can we begin to comprehend the enormity of the wrong we have done, as well as starting to take concrete steps to listen to what the earth is demanding needs to be done in order to make things right. Such steps would return agency to the earth, and while experiencing the return of agency is a necessary step in healing for any trauma survivor, it takes on a new dimension when we consider its meaning in light of the guiding metaphor of this paper. If, indeed, the world is God's body, then returning agency to the earth is an active step that humans would take to not only make things right for the earth, but also to make things right between themselves and God. It comes as an act of recompense, a form of confession, and a way of atoning for sin.

7. Conclusions

Catherine Keller writes that the earth is "not yielding submissively to the religio-politico-economic schematisms of what we may call anthropic exceptionalism. Earth names do not matter beneath us, not space lying static beneath time, but the teeming sphere of our collectivity" (Keller 2018, p. 6). Humans are, as Keller acknowledges, profoundly dependent on, and connected to, the life of the earth. That recognition of our interdependence is perhaps what led McFague to develop the metaphor of the world as the body of God, a metaphor that supplements the dominant masculine metaphor of the Christian tradition, while raising both relevant and provocative questions about God's identity within the ecological crisis and within the sexual crises facing human bodies. This article sought to parse out some of what might be theologically at stake in this metaphor, suggesting that it has the potential to add theological value and ethical relevance to the current ecological and human crises of our day. The metaphor also parsed out a trauma-informed response that might emerge from reframing the climate crisis as a series of traumatic sexual violations.

McFague, as stated earlier, never intended any of the metaphors she developed to be comprehensive. In this way, she adopted a hermeneutic of humility in her work. This hermeneutic helps readers understand both the significance of her theological contributions, while also orienting them towards a way of living in relation to God that is, in and of itself, humble at its roots. That humility may serve us well as we seek to understand the nature of God and our relationship to the Divine. It may also orient us as we step out of our denial and begin to address the trauma we have inflicted upon the earth.

Funding: This research received no external funding.

Conflicts of Interest: The author declares no conflict of interest.

Notes

[1] Pamela McCarroll writes that theology has been complicit in an anthropocentric focus in its work. Indeed, one could argue that this form of anthropocentrism elevates the status of women's bodies and other minoritized human bodies by denigrating the earth's body, which raises intriguing questions about extending the notion of intersectionality to include systems of power that involve players beyond the human species (McCarroll 2020).

[2] For a helpful primer on the philosophical intersections of feminism and environmental studies, see Warren (2015).

[3] For a particularly comprehensive overview, see the *Routledge Handbook of Religion and Ecology* (Jenkins et al. 2016).

[4] For an extended discussion of how the limits of language enable false or limited assumptions about sexual violations, see Tumminio Hansen (2020); for more on the term "sexual violations" as a preferable alternative to more commonly used terms, including "rape" or "sexual assault" or "gender-based violence", see Alcoff (2018, pp. 12–14).

5   McFague inherits the term "root-metaphor" from Stephen Pepper, who opposes logical positivism, arguing that all data is necessarily subject to interpretation by the interpreter, thereby pressing against the assumption that objectivity exists. In turn, he coins the term "root-metaphor" to mean the guiding principle or the grounding for any interpretation (Pepper 1972).

6   McFague, here, harkens to Earl MacCormac, who defines a root-metaphor as, "the most basic assumption about the nature of the world or experience that we can make when we try to give a description of it" (MacCormac 1976, p. 93).

7   For more of a contrast between McFague's model of a friend and her model of a lover, see McFague (1989, p. 168): "To be friends with God is the most astounding possible, for whereas a mother desires your existence and a lover finds you valuable, a friend likes you". For more on the model of God as a friend, specifically in relation to climate change, see McFague (2021, pp. 69–89).

8   For a book-length consideration of this topic, see Adams (2006).

9   Candida Moss and Joel Baden raise an important biblical challenge to the assumption that women's bodies are essentially reproductive bodies and that their identities ought to be essentially rooted in their reproductive capacities. Relatedly, Danielle Tumminio Hansen develops a practical theology of how the dominant discourse of the biological family functions as something like an idol in the reproductive culture of the United States, to the detriment of those who cannot reproduce via heterosexual intercourse, including those who suffer from infertility or reproductive loss, who are single, or who are in same-sex or transgender relationships. See Moss and Baden (2015) and Tumminio Hansen (2019).

10 I do not mean here to assume that all sexual violations are traumatizing, but rather to say that sexual violations have the potential to be. Indeed, Nicola Gavey has made important contributions from a psychological perspective about how trauma theory has come to be a dominant discourse in evaluating the authenticity of sexual violations, even though it is possible to experience a sexual violation without being traumatized in the aftermath (Gavey 2018, pp. 159–81).

11 As McFague explains, one of the issues with the current interpretation of the Christian story by those in power is that the story does not allow for constructive action in the secular world. As she writes, "A story is most effective when it aligns the religious dimension with the secular: when they are mutually reciprocal and supportive. When the distance between the two interpretations becomes too great, the link between them breaks, and people are left adhering to just one or to none at all. The latter stance is scarcely credible, and folks will fight to hold on to their story, even an "incredible" or mediocre one, rather than be bereft of any story" (McFague 2021, p. 2).

12 McFague writes of vulnerability differently in *A New Climate for Theology*, where she proposes that humans must internalize their own vulnerability to climate change in order to recognize their role in it, their interlocking relationship to the earth, and their responsibility to respond to the harm being done (McFague 2008, pp. 15–20).

13 The term "speciesism" means the privileging of the human species over other forms of creation. The term was popularized by philosopher Peter Singer in the 1970's.

14 The limitation of one's horizon is, likewise, central to McFague's definition of natural evil. Distinguishing between natural evil and sin, McFague explains how they overlap insofar as each roots itself in a kind of selfishness, as defined by being unable to see beyond one's personal horizon. She writes that, "Natural evil and sin join at this one point for both are concerned with a limited horizon, the inability to identify with others outside of the self, the refusal to acknowledge that one is not the center of things. Natural evil is narrowly interpreted as bad things happening to me and sin is the desire to have everything for oneself" (McFague 1993, p. 175).

15 Feminist philosophers and psychologists have raised important questions about the validity of consent as a criterion for evaluating whether a sexual violation has occurred. However, it may still be fair to say that while these scholars express concerns about how it is possible to coerce consent, such that consent can be given when desire is not truly present, they express fewer concerns about instances where consent is explicitly withheld. For a selection of readings that discusses the problems with consent, see Alcoff (2018), Gavey (2018) and Cahill (2014).

16 The authors of the study suggest that there is an adaptive use to the steps taken by the snowshoe hares during this period, as the stress required to survive necessitates that they hide more and eat less in order to survive. Though this causes a reduction in births—as well as in the size of young—it also ensures that the population will continue in the long-term, because the snowshoe hares are taking measures to avoid predators in the short-term (Sheriff et al. 2010).

17 Susan Brison writes at length about how misogyny, a denial of trauma, and our propensity to side with perpetrators affect the epistemic credibility of sexual trauma survivors (Brison 2003).

18 McCarroll suggests that ecoanxiety underlies human denial about the climate crisis, and that this anxiety is grounded emotions like guilt and shame, as well as a sense of psychological paralysis. As she writes, "Perhaps we are so overwhelmed by the enormity of the challenge before us—both as a field rethinking its foundational priorities and as a species in the face of extreme environmental changes—that we would rather close our eyes, close our ears, and carry on as we always have, something like Nietzsche's "last men" seeking to be distracted by trivialities" (McCarroll 2020, p. 44).

19 It is worth naming here that not all humans are equally complicit in the climate crisis and that some have been concrete victims of it. Humans who occupy places of power (as well as the institutions they support) bear a disproportionate amount of responsibility, while the most vulnerable (who are often minoritized bodies) have suffered the greatest impact. As McCarroll summarizes, "While creation is groaning, burdened under the consuming habits of the richest among us, the poorest of the world suffer the

extremes of the environmental crisis" (McCarroll 2020, pp. 30–31). For a book-length exploration of this topic from a womanist perspective, see Baker-Fletcher (1998).

References

Adams, Carol. 1990. *The Sexual Politics of Meat: A Feminist-Vegetarian Critical Theory*. New York: Continuum.
Adams, Marilyn McCord. 2006. *Christ and Horrors: The Coherence of Christology*. Cambridge and New York: Cambridge University Press.
Alcoff, Linda Martín. 2018. *Rape and Resistance*. Cambridge: Polity.
Baker-Fletcher, Karen. 1998. *Sisters of Dust, Sisters of Spirit: Womanist Wordings on God and Creation*. Minneapolis: Augsburg Fortress Publishers.
Brison, Susan J. 2003. *Aftermath*. Princeton: Princeton University Press.
Cahill, Ann J. 2014. Recognition, Desire, and Unjust Sex. *Hypatia* 29: 303–19. [CrossRef]
Dunayer, Joan. 1995. Sexist Words, Speciesist Roots. In *Animals and Women: Feminist Theoretical Explorations*. Edited by Carol J. Adams and Josephine Donovan. Durham: Duke University Press, pp. 11–31.
Gavey, Nicola. 2018. *Just Sex?* 2nd ed. Abingdon and New York: Routledge.
Gudmarsdottir, Sigridur. 2010. Rapes of Earth and Grapes of Wrath: Steinbeck, Ecofeminism and the Metaphor of Rape. *Feminist Theology* 18: 206–22. [CrossRef]
Herman, Judith. 1997. *Trauma and Recovery: The Aftermath of Violence—From Domestic Abuse to Political Terror*. New York: Basic Books.
Jenkins, Willis, Mary Evelyn Tucker, and John Grim. 2016. *Routledge Handbook of Religion and Ecology*. New York: Routledge.
Keller, Catherine. 2018. *Political Theology of the Earth: Our Planetary Emergency and the Struggle for a New Public*. New York: Columbia University Press.
MacCormac, Earl. 1976. *Metaphor and Myth in Science and Religion*. Durham: Duke University Press.
McCarroll, Pamela. 2020. Listening for the Cries of the Earth: Practical Theology in the Anthropocene. *International Journal of Practical Theology* 24: 29–46. [CrossRef]
McFague, Sallie. 1982. *Metaphorical Theology: Models of God in Religious Language*. Philadelphia: Fortress Press.
McFague, Sallie. 1989. *Models of God*. Minneapolis: Augsburg Fortress Press.
McFague, Sallie. 1993. *The Body of God: An Ecological Theology*. Minneapolis: Augsburg Fortress Press.
McFague, Sallie. 2008. *A New Climate for Theology: God, the World, and Global Warming*. Minneapolis: Fortress Press.
McFague, Sallie. 2021. *A New Climate for Christology: Kenosis Climate Change and Befriending Nature*. Minneapolis: Fortress Press.
Moss, Candida R., and Joel S. Baden. 2015. *Reconceiving Infertility: Biblical Perspectives on Procreation and Childlessness*. Princeton: Princeton University Press.
Pepper, Stephen C. 1972. *World Hypotheses: A Study in Evidence*. Oakland: University of California Press.
Ruether, Rosemary Radford. 2012. Ecofeminism—The Challenge to Theology. *Deportate, Esuli, Profughe (DEP)* 20: 12.
Saidero, Deborah. 2017. 'Violence against the Earth Is Violence against Women': The Rape Theme in Women's Eco-Narratives. *Le Simplegadi* 15: 263–73. [CrossRef]
Sheriff, Michael J., Charles J. Krebs, and Rudy Boonstra. 2010. The Ghosts of Predators Past: Population Cycles and the Role of Maternal Programming under Fluctuating Predation Risk. *Ecology* 91: 2983–94. [CrossRef] [PubMed]
TeSelle [McFague], Sallie. 1975. *Speaking in Parables: A Study in Metaphor and Theology*. Philadelphia: Fortress Press.
Tumminio Hansen, Danielle. 2019. *Conceiving Family: A Practical Theology of Surrogacy and Self*. Waco: Baylor University Press.
Tumminio Hansen, Danielle. 2020. Absent a Word: How the Language of Sexual Trauma Keeps Survivors Silent. *Journal of Pastoral Theology* 30: 136–49. [CrossRef]
Warren, Karen J. 2015. Feminist Environmental Philosophy. In *The Stanford Encyclopedia of Philosophy*. Edited by Edward N. Zalta. Palo Alto: Metaphysics Research Lab, Stanford University. Available online: https://plato.stanford.edu/archives/sum2015/entries/feminism-environmental/ (accessed on 1 February 2022).
Warren, Karen J. 2000. *Ecofeminist Philosophy: A Western Perspective on what it is and Why It Matters*. New York: Rowman and Littlefield.
Zanette, Liana Y., and Michael Clinchy. 2020. Ecology and Neurobiology of Fear in Free-Living Wildlife. *Annual Review of Ecology, Evolution, and Systematics* 51: 297–318. [CrossRef]

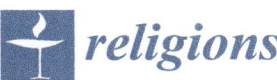

Article

Climate Emergency as Revelation: The Tragedy and Illusion of Sovereignty in Christian Political Theologies

Ryan Williams LaMothe

Pastoral Care and Counseling, Saint Meinrad Seminary and School of Theology, St. Meinrad, IN 47577, USA; rlamothe@saintmeinrad.edu

Abstract: In this article, the realities of the climate emergency reveal that human beings, especially those of us in the grips of capitalism, imperialism, and nationalism, have little control over nature and we are inextricably a part of nature. This revelation further exposes the tragedy and illusions of sovereignty, which is produced and maintained, in part, by Judeo-Christian scriptures and political theologies. While this revelatory event is disruptive, it also invites us to reimagine political theologies without the belief that sovereignty is existentially or ontologically necessary for political belonging. This includes embracing the revelation of the infinite, non-privileging care of a non-sovereign God for all creation.

Keywords: climate emergency; belonging; political theology; revelation; sovereignty

Citation: LaMothe, Ryan Williams. 2022. Climate Emergency as Revelation: The Tragedy and Illusion of Sovereignty in Christian Political Theologies. *Religions* 13: 524. https://doi.org/10.3390/rel13060524

Academic Editors: Pamela R. McCarroll and HyeRan Kim-Cragg

Received: 25 February 2022
Accepted: 1 June 2022
Published: 7 June 2022

Publisher's Note: MDPI stays neutral with regard to jurisdictional claims in published maps and institutional affiliations.

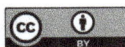

Copyright: © 2022 by the author. Licensee MDPI, Basel, Switzerland. This article is an open access article distributed under the terms and conditions of the Creative Commons Attribution (CC BY) license (https:// creativecommons.org/licenses/by/ 4.0/).

1. Introduction

In the last several years, the discourse around climate change has shifted to climate emergency. There is growing realization of an existential threat regarding the long- and short-term impacts of climate change. At an international conference on climate change, a reporter cornered two scientists, wanting to know their thoughts about the causes of climate change and the possibility of effective responses by nations to slow or stop the destructive trajectory of climate change. The scientists looked at each other. One of the scientists turned back to the reporter and succinctly said, "We're fucked" (Dufresne 2019, p. 93). I imagine that the "we" the scientist referred to is human beings. However, "we" are not alone. As Elizabeth Kolbert (2014) and Naomi Klein (2014) note, the earth is in the midst of a sixth extinction event,[1] which they and others call the Anthropocene Era[2]—an era of mass extinctions caused by human beings. Famed Harvard biologist E. O. Wilson (2005) predicts that by the end of this century, over half of all known species will be extinct, leaving a less biodiverse earth and the very real possibility of the eventual extinction of human beings.[3]

In this article, I consider the climate emergency as a revelatory event that exposes the tragedy and illusion of sovereignty, which is produced and maintained, in part, by Judeo-Christian[4] scriptures and political theologies (and philosophies[5]). This revelatory event, while painfully disruptive, invites us to reimagine political theologies without the belief that sovereignty is existentially or ontologically necessary for political belonging. To make my case I first identify and discuss the meaning and attributes of sovereignty, as well as the negative impacts on subordinated and subjugated human beings and more-than-human beings. This sets the stage to argue that sovereignty is a central belief in Judeo-Christian scriptures and Western political theologies (and philosophies), shaping political subjectivities and relations. Put differently, I contend that scripture and political theologies operate as apparatuses[6] that secure the belief in sovereignty vis-à-vis human dwelling as existentially and ontologically necessary. I then move to depict how our climate emergency reveals the tragedy and illusion of our belief in human and divine sovereignty. The last section depicts how this revelation, when acknowledged and embraced, renders human and divine sovereignty inoperative, which invites forms of political belonging that affirm (1) the infinite, indiscriminate, non-privileging care of a non-sovereign God for all creation and, correspondingly, (2) the categorical political demand to care for all human beings, other-than-human species, and the earth.

Before beginning, it is necessary to offer five clarifications. First, theological renderings of the notion of "revelation" reveal varied characteristics of God with regard to creation and, in particular, human beings. While biblical revelations can be experienced as affirming and pleasantly appealing (e.g., God's love for creation), they can also be understood as psychosocially disruptive and painful. A revelatory event is disruptive in that it can unsettle our unquestioned and unquestionable "normative" ways of being in the world, rendering inoperative[7], in this case, human apparatuses of political belonging that depend on beliefs in human and divine sovereignty. In this article, it is the latter that is my focus. A second point concerns the traditional relation between revelation and sin. In one sense, the harm to human beings, more-than-human beings, and the earth by human participation in the construction of ecologically destructive systemic apparatuses such as capitalism, imperialism, and nationalism—which intersect with and depend on the idea of sovereignty—can fall under the heading of social sin, with some human beings bearing more accountability than others. However, my focus is not moralization but instead on depicting the tragic nature of the human theological and philosophical beliefs associated with human and divine sovereignty. Third, the general claims made regarding scripture and Western political theologies regarding the issue of sovereignty are intended to be heuristic rather than definitive or reductive about scripture or political theologies. A fourth and related clarification concerns the heuristic use of scripture to reimagine the revelation of a non-sovereign God. As Roland Boer (2009) notes, Ernst Bloch (and others; Benjamin, Adorno, Althusser, and Žižek) was "enthusiastic about the revolutionary possibilities of certain types of biblical myth" (p. 27). Thus, in critiquing and rendering inoperative scripture and political theologies vis-à-vis sovereignty, an emancipatory space is created wherein we reimagine human belonging in the Anthropocene Age. Finally, focusing on sovereignty is not meant to suggest that this is the only artifice that has moved us into the Anthropocene Age. Clearly, there are other social imaginaries (e.g., capitalism, imperialism) that have contributed to climate change and serve as obstacles to climate action.

2. Sovereignty: Meaning and Attributes

Jean Bodin (1530–1596), a French jurist and political philosopher, was interested in explicating the nature of sovereignty, perhaps because of the political instability resulting from the Protestant Reformation. Of course, sovereignty and its varied forms had been discussed and argued since Plato and Aristotle (Grayling 2019, pp. 35–39), if not before. However, Bodin (2009) sought to identify its fundamental attributes. There are, for Bodin, four essential features of sovereignty, namely, supreme power (no superior), absolute, indivisible and perpetual. One can easily imagine these traits fitting best in relation to God, but, for Bodin, they are features of human sovereignty. The king has no superior (except God); is absolute in his rule; his power and rule cannot be divided; and his rule is perpetual, handed down to his sons (in rare cases, daughters). In the 20th century, German jurist Carl Schmitt (2005) picked up on Bodin's work, pointing out that it is widely referenced in previous political philosophical works on sovereignty. Schmitt writes:

Bodin asked if the commitments of the prince to the states or people dissolve his sovereignty. He answered by referring to the case in which it becomes necessary to violate such commitments. To change laws or to suspend them entirely according to the requirements of a situation, a time, and a people. If in such cases the prince had to consult a senate or the people before he could act, he would have to be prepared to let his subjects dispense with him. Bodin considered this an absurdity because, according to him, the estates were not masters over the laws . . . Sovereignty would thus become a play between two parties. (pp. 9–10)

What Schmitt is pointing to is the idea of "the state of exception" as a central feature of sovereignty. "The sovereign", he writes, "is he who decides on the state of exception" (p. 5). He adds, "What characterizes an exception is principally unlimited authority, which means the suspension of the entire existing [juridical] order. In such a situation it is clear that the state remains, whereas the law recedes" (p. 12). The law and the state, in other words, are subordinate to the absolute authority of the sovereign.

Philosopher Giorgio Agamben (2005) further clarifies the state of exception. "The state of exception", he writes, "is not a dictatorship (whether constitutional or unconstitutional, commissarial or sovereign) but a space devoid of law, a zone of anomie in which all legal determinations—and above all the very distinction between public and private—are deactivated" (p. 50). One immediately can see the paradox here. For Agamben (1998), the "paradox of sovereignty consists in the fact that the sovereign is, at the same time, outside and inside the juridical order. The sovereign, having the legal power to suspend the validity of the law, legally places himself outside the law" (p. 15). "The sovereign", Sergei Prozorov (2014) remarks, "remains a borderline or threshold figure at the limit of order" (p. 99). As a threshold figure, the sovereign "is both the sign of the rule and the jurisdiction of law, and supervenes the law" (Brown 2001, p. 59). What is interesting and important here is that the sovereign possesses the supreme (legal) authority to set aside laws because they are given the legal power to determine the exception. Add to this the idea that the state of exception is at play in the very creation of the law itself. Put another way, the establishment of the law already reveals the state of exception. I stress here that the state of exception does not make the law invalid, but rather that in the exception, the law is simply not applicable. The law remains in effect, but is set aside.

Naturally, the sovereign need not act on the state of exception. It can simply be potential, which is nevertheless powerful. Prozorov (2014) writes, "even when exceptional or emergency measures are not actualized in policies, they remain potentialities of state action and may indeed be more effective as potentialities, capable of regulating conduct by sheer threat of their actualization" (p. 101). This is analogous to the U.S. Internal Revenue Service (IRS) having the power to audit someone but choosing not to exercise it. The threat of being audited motivates many people to make sure they pay their taxes.

Wendy Brown (2010), surveying classical theorists of modern sovereignty such as Thomas Hobbes, Jean Bodin, and Carl Schmitt, summarizes the core attributes of sovereignty: "supremacy (no higher power), perpetuity (no term limits), decisionism (no boundedness by or submission to law), absolutism and completeness (sovereign cannot be probable or partial), nontransferability (sovereignty cannot be conferred without cancelling itself), and specialized jurisdiction (territoriality)" (p. 22). Given this, I want to elaborate further on other attending features of sovereignty.

First of all, there is no such thing as a sole sovereign. Sovereignty exists because of the construction of social and political apparatuses that produce and maintain the idea of sovereignty and the belief in its necessity for political belonging and stability. Thomas Hobbes' leviathan is, perhaps, the most obvious depiction of the absolute belief in the necessity of sovereignty—lest we sink into social chaos and brutality. The social contract citizens make with the all-powerful leviathan provides society with peace and stability so that citizens can, within limits, pursue their individual desires. The apparatuses that produce the belief in the necessity of a sovereign also reveal the presence of sovereign classes. A sovereign or leviathan, then, cannot exist without sovereign classes that support and advance supremacy, the state of exception, perpetuity, etc.

Another key feature of sovereignty's state of exception is its dependence on force/violence or the threat of violence. Agamben (2005) addresses both law-making and law-preserving violence, and he asserts that what the "law can never tolerate . . . is the existence [of violence] outside the law" (p. 53). Violence outside the law "neither makes nor preserves law, but deposes it." As I understand this, sovereignty accompanies and depends on legitimate violence exercised by the apparatuses that produce and maintain the sovereign. Sovereign violence is never outside the law, even though the law is set aside. Violence outside the law is a threat to the sovereign because the sovereign and sovereign classes possess the sole legitimacy with regard to the exercise of political violence. To return to Hobbes' leviathan, the leviathan—a construction of human beings—retains the only capacity for legitimate violence.

Of course, history is replete with stories of violence perpetrated by those who question, reject, or rebel against the sovereign. Even those in sovereign classes can join in the violence to overthrow the sovereign. Yet, as Saul Newman (2019) notes, "[R]evolutions and counterrevolutions often share the same structure—both gravitate around sovereignty and both affirm its place of transcendence and authority. While counterrevolution safeguards the constitutional state order by suspending it in the state of exception—thus creating, artificially, a situation that resembles a revolution—a revolution destroys an existing constitutional state order only to erect a new one in its place. The core of sovereignty is retained in both" (p. 106). The violent overthrow of the sovereign simply shifts the legitimacy of violence to the revolutionary group. Sovereignty and political violence remain unquestioned and unquestionable.

A related feature of sovereignty and violence is that it is founded on relations of subordination and, more often than not, subjugation. All residents are subordinate to the sovereign, including those of the sovereign classes. Residents who disobey or reject the sovereign are subject to the sovereign's disciplinary apparatuses. For Hobbes, citizens willingly accept subordinate status for the sake of the political security and stability that are needed for the freedom to pursue their individual desires. Indeed, most people internalize the beliefs that subordination to the sovereign is natural or existentially necessary. There are also numerous examples in history of sovereigns and their sovereign classes subjugating people (e.g., enslaving people, jailing dissidents, terrorizing persons, colonization).

Relations of subordination also point to the hierarchical nature of sovereignty, which is accompanied by beliefs in exceptionalism and beliefs in superiority and inferiority. To exercise the state of exception necessarily accompanies the belief that sovereigns (and sovereign classes) are exceptional (in their beingness). The apparatuses that produce and maintain sovereignty also carry this belief in exceptionalism, which is buttressed by the social, economic, and political privileges that accrue to the sovereign and elite sovereign classes. This exceptionalism is joined to the beliefs in the superiority of the sovereign and sovereign classes and the inferiority of non-sovereign classes.

One might question this by suggesting that democracy as the rule of the people is egalitarian, thus eschewing relations of subordination and beliefs in exceptionalism, superiority, and inferiority. First, the notion of democracy retains the belief in sovereignty as necessary for ordering political belonging. In a "democracy" the "people" have supreme power, exercise the state of exception, legitimate the use of political violence, and the indivisibility of the people's rule. If everyone is sovereign, then no one is subordinate, exceptional, and superior. Of course, reality reveals something different. In one of the earliest democracies—Athens—it is clear that adult male citizens were the sovereign class, while non-citizens (barbarians) and women were constructed as subordinate and inferior classes. This group of men exercised the state of exception and political violence by sentencing Socrates to death for corrupting the youth. Leaping to the 21st century and the putative U.S. democracy, sovereign elites (political and economic classes) believe and act out their exceptionalism and beliefs in their superiority. People of color, poor persons, incarcerated persons, and immigrant persons without documents are examples of those deemed to be inferior, especially in relation to white citizens (see Desmond 2016; Wilkerson 2020).[8]

Implicit in the attributes of relational subordination/subjugation, violence, and beliefs in exceptionalism, superiority, and inferiority are two other features of sovereignty, namely, instrumental knowing and relating. The obvious and egregious illustration of instrumental knowing and relating is found in the term "bare life", which, for Agamben, refers to persons "caught up in the sovereign ban . . . stripped of all protections and abandoned to the force of law" (Prozorov 2014, p. 102). Stated more starkly, "The sovereign sphere is the sphere in which it is permitted to kill without committing homicide" (Agamben 1998, p. 83). That is, "it is the sovereign who, insofar as he decides on the state of exception, has the power to decide which life may be killed without the commission of homicide" (p. 142). All of this comes across as pretty drastic and dramatic, perhaps referring to a tiny segment of the population that have committed crimes, but this is not the case. Bare life can be seen in instrumentalizing African Americans (Alexander 2010; Anderson 2016), and is produced by apparatuses that deny or disrupt the distribution of the resources needed to live well (Fraser and Honneth 2003). An example of this is the rise of the "Black Lives Matter" movement, which rose in response to the killing of African Americans by police (an apparatus of sovereign's violence)—killings that are not considered to be homicides. Instrumental knowing and relation are also evident in innumerable examples of how, in a market society, those who are employed are constructed in terms of the demands of the capitalistic system (global sovereign) and those who are poor (Marx's reserve army of labor) are disparaged and denied resources, which undermines their well-being (Lukács 1968). An additional example of the instrumental knowing and relating vis-à-vis sovereignty is the categorization and objectification of so-called illegal immigrants who are residents of the society without rights of citizenship.

The final attribute of sovereignty, which is tacitly evident in the discussion above, is its inherent exclusivity. This exclusivity can be seen within the borders of a nation. The sovereign and the sovereign classes exclude or restrict non-sovereign classes from participating in public spaces of speaking and acting together. Ancient Athens excluded women and resident "barbarians" from engaging in political spaces of speaking and acting together. Today, voter suppression laws, laws regarding those who have committed felonies, and immigration laws exclude millions of persons from political spaces. Sovereignty is also exclusionary when it comes to those who reside outside the boundaries/borders, which are constructed by the sovereign and the sovereign classes. Wendy Brown (2010), for instance, notes the proliferation of nation-states that are building walls to ensure the exclusion of those deemed to be threats (e.g., U.S. southern border wall, Israel's wall separating themselves from Palestinians).

Thus far I have focused primarily on sovereignty and its relation to human beings and their political belonging. I want to extend these attributes of sovereignty to our relations to more-than-human species and the earth. Colby Dickinson (2015), referring to the work of Giorgi Agamben, contends that in Western political philosophies (and their affirmations of sovereignty), there is a "deep ontological rift ... between animal and human" (p. 173). Agamben (2004) writes:

> It is as if determining the border between human and animal were not just one question among many discussed by philosophers and theologians, scientists and politicians, but rather a fundamental metaphysico-political operation in which alone something like 'man' can be decided upon and produced. If animal life and human life could be superimposed perfectly, then neither man nor animal—and, perhaps, not even the divine—would any longer be thinkable. (p. 92)

The ongoing drive in the West to differentiate between human beings and animals, which is a project of philosophy, theology, and some of the sciences, leads to "a radical and total discontinuity between human and nonhuman" (Kompridis 2020, p. 252) and, consequently, privileging human beings over all other species—anthropocentrism. In short, these political theologies and philosophies produce the belief in the sovereignty of human beings over other-than-human beings and the earth. Human beings have supreme power. We believe we are superior and exceptional (anthropocentrism). Our power vis-à-vis other species and the earth is absolute. We exercise "legitimate" violence toward other species who are deemed subordinate and can be legitimately subjugated for human benefit, which accompanies a disavowal of the singularities and needs of other species and the earth. If other species and the earth are considered in terms of the political, it is almost always instrumentally for the sake of human political belonging, which also means that the needs of other species are considered to the degree that they benefit human beings.

Evidence for this abounds: factory farming, the use of other-than-human beings in scientific experiments, the removal of, if not extinction of species for the sake of human land use, mining operations such as mountain top removal, which also undermines the well-being of local human beings.[9]

In summary, sovereignty comprises a number of interrelated features. Jean Bodin identified four features, namely, supreme power (no superior), absolute, indivisible, and perpetual. An aspect of supreme power is the sovereign's state of exception, which entails the capacity to decide to set aside laws. Sovereignty and the state of exception are founded on political violence or the threat of political violence, which is part of possessing supreme power. I also noted that a sovereign exists by virtue of sovereign classes and the attending apparatuses that produce and maintain a belief that sovereignty is existentially necessary for political belonging. Included in this are the beliefs in superiority and exceptionalism of the sovereign and sovereign classes, as well as the inferiority of subordinate and subjugated others (which includes other species). Three other attending features I identified were exclusivity, objectification or instrumentalization, and the disavowal of the needs and singularities of othered human beings and other species and the earth.

3. Sovereignty, Scripture, and Political Theologies

Carl Schmitt believed that "all significant concepts of the modern theory of the state are secularized theological concepts" (Brown 2010, p. 59). Similarly, Wendy Brown (2010) notes that "sovereignty, secularized for political purposes, does not lose its religious structure or bearing, even as it ceases to have the direct authority of God at its heart" (p. 70). In the West, this religious structure is rooted in Judeo-Christian scriptures, which are foundational for the construction of political theologies. The stories in scripture consistently and unquestioningly affirm the ontological sovereignty of God. The attributes of sovereignty are clearly present in the belief that God is sovereign over all creation. God is superior, all creation is subordinate. God's power is absolute, indivisible, and eternal, which is evident in the creation stories, as well as miracle stories. That is, as part of God's absolute power, God can exercise the state of exception, setting aside natural and divine laws. Having heard the laments of the Israelites in Egypt, for example, God performed a series of violent miracles, killing untold numbers of Egyptians and devastating the land. More miracles took place during the Israelites sojourn in the desert, and when it came to entering the promised land, God, the ultimate sovereign, commanded the Israelites, in what today we would call ethnic cleansing, to remove the inhabitants—apparently setting aside previous commandments regarding killing, coveting, and stealing. God's exercise of the state of exception also means that God's political violence, whether performed through miracles or commanded, is legitimate. We read, "Shall not the Judge of all the earth do right?" (Gen 18:25). This means that God's commands are unfailingly just and those who obey the divine sovereign do right, which accompanies absolute disavowal of the suffering inflicted on subordinate and subjugated othered human beings, other species, and the land. The sovereign and those who obey the sovereign's order to kill are without remorse. It is also important to note that the stories in Genesis and Exodus are devoid of the voices of those who were subjugated. Harm inflicted on othered human beings, othered animals, and the earth goes unremarked. The silence reveals the din of the sovereign's commands and a disavowal of the singularities, needs, and sufferings of subjugated others.

The attributes of divine sovereignty are also evident in God's relation to the Israelites as the chosen people. By virtue of God choosing the Israelites, they retain the belief in their exceptional status, which is reflected in their God-given "right" to inhabit the promised land. Of course, this exceptional status comes with the demand to obey the covenant and God uses political violence or the threat of physical violence to punish those who resist. Consider that the Israelites (read men), who were subordinate to God, were repeatedly called a stiff-necked people, usually by God (Ex. 32:9, 33:3, 5; 34:9; Deut. 9:6, 13; 10:16). Synonyms of stiff-necked are obstinate, headstrong, strong-willed, obdurate, and bull-headed. This suggests that not everyone was happy to submit to divine or a human appointed sovereign. The response to obdurate Israelites entailed varied forms of punishment (or threat of punishment) by God—political violence. Of course, the ultimate exercise of political exclusionary violence toward members of the community was death or bare life. God, for instance, commanded Moses to kill those Israelites who had rebelled by fashioning a golden calf (Ex. 32:25–29). Absent in the narrative is Moses' hesitation or remorse, which again points to the state of exception, righteous violence, and bare life (killings were not considered sacrifices or homicides).

While God's sovereignty is unquestioned and unquestionable, things become more complicated when it comes to human beings and the Israelites in particular. First, it is important to mention that in Genesis (1:26, 28) God gives human beings dominion over nature. Indeed, God as sovereign has created animals and plants for use by human beings. Of course, one may interpret dominion to mean that God commands human beings to care (stewardship) for nature and for other animals. Even if this is correct, a belief in human sovereignty over nature is retained and has been a pervasive feature of Western political philosophies and theologies, leading to the ontological rift mentioned above.[10] It is more complicated when we turn to sovereignty among the Israelites. Initially, the Israelites viewed God as their sovereign, which meant that any leader (e.g., Moses) appointed by God was subordinate to the sovereign, though not sovereign himself (see Walzer 2012, p. 53). As noted above, in terms of the state of exception, this meant that the Israelites could exercise political violence at God's command. This arrangement, though, proved to be unsatisfactory for these "stiff-necked people." After defeating the Midianites, the elders asked Gideon to be their ruler. Gideon responded, "I will not rule over you, and my son will not rule over you; the Lord will rule over you" (Judges 8:23). Gideon was adhering to the traditional story that God is the only sovereign. Later we learn that the desire to be ruled over by a king continued. The elders of Israel asked Samuel to "appoint for us a king to govern us like other nations" (1Sam. 8:5). God commanded Samuel to go to the people and warn them of the consequences of having a human as their sovereign. Samuel told them that:

> These will be the ways of the king who will reign over you: he will take your sons and appoint them to his chariots and be his horsemen, and to run before his chariots; and he will appoint for himself commanders of thousands and commanders of fifties, and some to plow his ground and to reap his harvest, and to make his implements of war and equipment of his chariots. He will take your daughters to be perfumers and cooks and bakers. He will take the best of your fields and vineyards and olive orchards and give them to his courtiers. He will take one-tenth of your grain and of your vineyards and give it to his officers and his courtiers. He will take your male and female slaves, and the best of your cattle and donkeys and put them to his work. He will take one-tenth of your flocks, and you shall be his slaves. (v.11–17)

As Samuel predicted, a human leviathan possesses the state of exception, establishes relations of subordination and subjugation, and rules through actual or threatened political violence. The elders remained adamant, perhaps because having a king would result in the elders' elevation to the sovereign class. God, we read, accepted and fulfilled their request, though God remained sovereign.

Christian scriptures also repeatedly affirm the sovereignty of God, though I will qualify this below. Jesus, as the son of God, tells Pilate that his kingdom is not of this world (John 18:36). The kingdom of God is referenced throughout the Gospels, which only reinforces the idea of God's sovereignty. Perhaps, though, the revelation of the incarnation is a different kind of sovereign God than that of Jewish scriptures, namely, the sovereignty of God's love for all of humanity. Yet, if we turn to the last canonical text, we see an orgy of political violence in heaven and on earth. There is no spoiler alert here since it is fairly obvious how this story of political violence will end. God, the absolute sovereign, prevails by way of violence, leading to a new heaven and a new earth.

The sovereignty of God is lauded in Christian rituals, in the hymns people sing, in sermons, etc. Roman Catholics, along with other denominations, celebrate Christ the King Sunday. Even the monarchical structure of the Roman Catholic polity parallels and looks to the sovereignty of God for its legitimacy. Add to this the innumerable theological texts over the centuries that overtly proclaim God's sovereignty. My point here is threefold. First, scripture, Christian rituals, theologies, and, often, Judeo-Christian polities unquestioningly proclaim the sovereignty of God/Jesus Christ. Second, all of these serve as apparatuses to produce and maintain the idea of and belief in God's sovereignty, as well as the sovereignty of human beings over more-than-human species and the earth. Put another way, these apparatuses produce a belief, often unstated, that sovereignty is necessary for maintaining the polis/ekklesia. Without a leviathan, whether that is God or God's representative on earth, life would be nasty, brutish, and short. Third, scriptural stories of sovereignty, whether human or divine, possess the attributes identified above.

4. Climate Emergency and Revelation of Non-Sovereign Humanity and a Non-Sovereign God

At the beginning of this article, I mentioned Naomi Klein's (2014) and Elizabeth Kolbert's (2014) survey of the data about climate change, as well as E. O. Wilson's (2005) prediction that at least half of all known species will be extinct by the end of this century. When considering the present and future realities of the climate emergency, it is, in my view, an obfuscation to simply say that climate change is caused by human beings, as if all human beings share equal responsibility. It is instead more important to identify particular systems and apparatuses constructed by human beings that lend themselves to harming other human beings, other species, and the earth, and to consider how these apparatuses deflect accountability for the consequent harm. Jason Moore, for instance, coined the term "capitalocene age" to highlight the role of capitalism in climate change. Capitalism, however, is not simply an economic system. It is inextricably tied to political systems, which created (Woods 2017) and maintain it (Brown 2015). Western imperial nation-states, also, were and are largely responsible for globalizing capitalism (Klein 2007). The apparatuses of capitalism, imperialism, and nationalism are intertwined. One thing that binds them together is the notion of sovereignty and its attending attributes. For instance, capital is sovereign in that it rules over workers and nature, though regulations and protections mitigate some of capitalism's excesses. In addition, capitalism as sovereign is produced and maintained by sovereign political classes (Piketty 2014, 2020; Reich 2007; Woods 2017), who make laws that legitimate the dominion of capitalists. Moreover, the sovereign political classes of imperial nation-states are sovereign over subordinate and subjugated countries. The intersection and interplay of these apparatuses produce and maintain the belief in individual sovereignty over "nature", as well as the belief that the sovereignty of these apparatuses is necessary for human life and political belonging. This belief in the necessity of sovereignty is noted in Frederick Jamison's (2016) remark that "it is easier . . . to imagine the end of the world than to imagine the end of capitalism" (p. 3 or nationalism).

The realities of climate change reveal that human beings, especially those of us in the grips of capitalism, imperialism, and nationalism, have little control over nature and we are inextricably a part of nature. Yes, we obviously do have some control, and many of us have used this control to exploit other-than-human beings and the earth for our short-term benefits; yet, we are not sovereign over the earth. Climate devastation, in other words, demonstrates that the earth is not subordinate to human beings and we cannot subjugate the earth without undermining human and other-than-human existence. We are limited in knowledge and in our ability to manage the earth and the climate. Of course, some scientists and engineers are seeking to develop macro geoengineering solutions to mitigate the destructive aspects of climate change. Meanwhile, human sovereignty with regard to capitalism, nationalism, and imperialism remains unquestioned and unchanged by billions of people. The claim here is that although we can continue to try to control, subjugate, and subordinate other species and the earth, climate change reveals the tragic and illusory nature of this belief and the actions that stem from it. In short, human sovereignty and its attributes are illusory precisely because the likely possibility of human extinction demonstrates an end to human political power, whether it is understood as necessary for human belonging or in relation to other species and the earth. Extinction, in other words, negates any relation of subordination and subjugation, as well as any belief in human superiority and other-species inferiority.[11] Jonathan Schell (2020) summarizes this well, remarking, "If we conquer nature, we will find ourselves among the defeated" (p. 19; see also Wallace-Wells 2020).[12] Moreover, we will have defeated ourselves by refusing to let go of our belief in sovereignty—both human and divine.

Perhaps a religious reader will concede that human beings are not sovereign over nature and that the belief in human sovereignty over nature has led to ecological disasters, yet continue to affirm God's sovereignty. The climate emergency as a revelatory event may show human hubris, ignorance, and greed, but it does not, in and of itself, negate God's sovereignty. My response to this is to first note how persistent the belief in the idea and necessity of a sovereign God is. Maybe we feel a need to believe that, despite the mess many of us have created and despite the possibility of human extinction, God is and will be in control, enacting miracles when needed. This said, the climate emergency as a revelatory event cannot definitively reveal the non-sovereignty of God, but it can invite us to imagine a non-sovereign God, and, for Christians, a non-sovereign Christ (Caputo 2006). Put another way, the climate emergency can move us to realize that the idea of sovereignty and the belief that it is necessary for human dwelling are strictly speaking human constructions, which ultimately say nothing about God or Being. Second, if one can argue that political belonging does not depend, necessarily, on human or divine sovereignty, then would we really need to believe in the sovereignty of God? Or, relatedly, does our "belonging" to God and belonging to each other (polis) require belief in God's sovereignty? More specifically, can we turn to scripture for help in considering a non-sovereign humanity and a non-sovereign God? Moreover, what would human dwelling or belonging mean without a sovereign or sovereign classes—divine or human? Will all of this result in changing how we relate to each other, to other species, and the earth?

As to the question about scripture and sovereignty, Jacob Taubes (2004) provides an interesting and important interpretation of Paul's epistle to the Romans (see also Crossan 1995, 2007; Horsley 2003, 2011). Commenting on Taubes' work, Hartwich et al. (2004) write that the Epistle to the Romans was "directed against Rome and relativizes Rome's world imperialism ... and directed against Jerusalem in that it relativizes the limits of Israel's self-definition, which are founded on *nomos* and *ethnos*" (p. 117). Stated differently, Jesus "frees himself from the determination of *ethnic* ties and the Roman idea of empire" (p. 119; emphasis mine) as a condition of belonging vis-à-vis the *ecclesia* or *polis*. Hartwich et al. explain further that Paul, from Taubes' perspective, "doesn't oppose a political theology of the Torah to the Roman nomos of the earth in order to establish a new national form of rule. He fundamentally negated the law as a force of political order. With this, *legitimacy is denied to all sovereigns of this world, be they imperatorial or theocratic*" (p. 121). The Epistle, then, "undermines the function of the law as ordering power, be it in the context of political order, church order, or a natural order" (p. 122). The messiah does not and cannot represent or legitimate institutions of earthly sovereignty nor political violence used to establish belonging. Instead, the messiah "can only make them irrelevant and ultimately replace them" (p. 142). I add here that this new political order of love of neighbor and enemy is further understood as based on the revelation of Jesus as the incarnation of the infinite, indeterminate care of a non-sovereign God (Caputo 2006). Put another way, political dwelling vis-à-vis the *ecclesia* is not dependent on relations of subordination/subjugation or beliefs in superiority and inferiority, which are inherent in any iteration of sovereignty. Likewise, the *ecclesia* does not rely on the threat or use of political violence to order belonging and cooperation. That said, Hartwich et al. (2004) point out that the "position of Paul doesn't imply any positive political form" (p. 121), though, the principles of dwelling are identified, namely, care, mercy, compassion, and forgiveness.[13] They continue by arguing that the "ecclesia understands itself, not as an autarchic polis that separates itself militantly from other communities, but as a new universal world order" (p. 130). "The new political order", they continue, "is constituted by love in its two forms: love of neighbor (inward love) and love of enemy (outward love)" (p. 130).

Giorgio Agamben (2013), who is familiar with Taubes' work, provides a philosophical view of this form of political belonging without sovereignty. In the coming community, he argues, human beings can "co-belong without any representable condition of belonging", "without affirming identity" (p. 5). According to Agamben, "What the State (or sovereign) cannot tolerate in any way is that the singularities form a community without affirming an identity, that human beings co-belong without any representable condition of belonging" (p. 5). Using Agamben's notion of inoperativity, identity that is rooted in and dependent on sovereign apparatuses (Jewish or Roman in the case of Paul), is deactivated with regard to who belongs and who merits care. It is possible to hear echoes of Agamben's coming community in Galatians (3:28 NRSV): "There is no longer Jew or Greek, there is no longer slave or free, there is no longer male and female; for all of you are one in Christ."

Taubes and Agamben envision political belonging that does not depend on the belief in the necessity of human or divine sovereignty. As a result of shedding this belief, interhuman relations are altered, as well as the possibility for more just and caring relations between human beings, other species, and the earth. First, let me return to Agamben and sovereignty. Above I noted Agamben's contention that Western political theologies and philosophies produce and maintain an ontological rift—"a radical and total discontinuity between human and nonhuman" (Kompridis 2020, p. 252). This ontological rift privileges human beings over all other species.[14] Agamben (2004) asserts further that when we render these apparatuses of sovereignty inoperative, it will "show the central emptiness" of the proposition that human beings are superior and privileged beings (p. 92). Rendering these apparatuses inoperative creates space for relating to other species and earth in ways that respect the singularities of other species and the earth.

The coming community, then, establishes belonging that does not depend on a sovereign state constructing and legitimizing particular identities vis-à-vis belonging. Those human and other-than-human species that are present belong and, therefore, are due care—a categorical demand to care for all who belong. At the same time, the deactivating apparatuses that produce a belief in human sovereignty over other species, makes possible the realization that other-than-human species are necessary for human belonging—the very existence of a polis depends on a biodiverse earth. Lest one believe that this is an unattainable utopian idea, we need only turn to the Norwegian town of Longyearbyen[15] that requires no visa to belong and is not "ruled" by an individual or a group.[16] It is a town without visas and there are over 50 nationalities represented. It is an inclusive community that seeks to care for and respect its residents—human and other-than-human (and the earth). I add that in the last 30 years, there has been a growing trend toward creating eco-villages throughout the world (U.S., Chile, Canada, Japan, etc.),[17] where people live in cooperation with nature. These eco-villages are diverse, but they are not organized by apparatuses of capitalism and nationalism or the attending illusions of human dominion, exceptionalism, superiority, and entitlement. There are also efforts by some Christian communities to find ways for more sustainable living. "Eco-Church" was started by the Diocese of London in 2016 and now has over 1500 member churches. In the U.S., Robert Shore-Goss (2016) has been the senior pastor of MCC United Church of Christ in California since 2004. During his pastoral leadership, he and other pastoral leaders have listened to congregants and facilitated the congregation's discernment about climate change and how to respond (see also, Antal 2018; Spencer and White 2007). This said, it is not entirely clear that these Christian communities, while ecologically minded, have shed beliefs that are embedded in scripture and theologies regarding human and divine sovereignty. Nevertheless, they are pursuing forms of political dwelling that take into account the needs of other human beings, other species, and the earth.

If climate change is a revelatory event that invites human beings to render inoperative the apparatuses that produce and maintain beliefs in human sovereignty, then this event may similarly disclose the revelation of a non-sovereign God's indeterminate, and infinite care of all creation—not simply privileging human beings. Given this, we may turn to scripture and the revelation of Jesus Christ, not as a confirmation of divine or human sovereignty, but rather as the possibility of belonging based on non-sovereign care for all those who reside, which today includes the recognition of other-than-human species and the earth as the material foundation of human belonging and flourishing.

5. Conclusions

Albert Camus ([1947] 2002) remarked that "[W]hen an abstraction starts to kill you, you have to get to work on it" (p. 69). In this article I have claimed that climate change reveals that sovereignty is the abstraction that is killing us and millions of other species. To "work" on this abstraction includes first acknowledging it. Only then can we begin to envision how we might live and relate to each other and other species without this abstraction. As Clayton Crockett (2012) suggests, "We need to experiment radically with new ways of thinking and living, because the current paradigm is in a state of exhaustion, depletion, and death" (p. 165). I also argued that the revelation of climate emergency invites us to reimagine the Christian revelation as one that invites believing and living together without the apparatuses of human and divine sovereignty. It is altogether another question whether this will be enough.

Funding: This research received no external funding.

Data Availability Statement: Not applicable.

Conflicts of Interest: The author declares no conflict of interest.

Notes

1. There is considerable debate about the idea of a sixth extinction event and, if so, what date is to be used to mark the beginning of this event. See Northcott (2017) and Nichols and Gogineni (2020).
2. Scientists Crutzen and Stoermer (2000) coined the term "Anthropocene Age" to indicate that we are now out of the Holocene Age.
3. The scientific data regarding global warming is mountainous and easily attainable, which is why I have decided not to take it up here. I am presuming that readers are already acquainted with some of the research since it is part of the news nearly every day. However, for those who may be interested in some of the recent research, I suggest the following websites: Sixth Assessment Report (ipcc.ch) accessed 8 February 2022; NASA: Climate Change and Global Warming accessed 8 February 2022.
4. The use of this appellation is simply to identify the scriptural sources used for some of the beliefs associated with the notion of sovereignty that emerge from Western Christian political theologies and philosophies. To use an alternative term, such as Abrahamic scriptures, would incorrectly imply my familiarity with Islamic scriptures and political theologies.
5. The idea of sovereignty is not simply a concern of political theologians. Secular political philosophers have, since the Enlightenment, argued about various iterations of sovereignty being necessary for political dwelling. While this paper concerns political theologies that promulgate notions of human and divine sovereignty, I contend that the climate emergency reveals the illusions and tragedy of sovereignty promulgated by Western political philosophies.
6. For Giorgi Agamben (2009) the term "apparatus" refers to "a set of practices, bodies of knowledge, measures and institutions that aim to manage, govern, control, and orient—in a way that purports to be useful—the behaviors, gestures, and thoughts of human beings" (p. 13). Referencing Foucault, Agamben writes that "in a disciplinary society, apparatuses aim to create—through a series of practices, discourses, and bodies of knowledge—docile, yet free, bodies that assume their identity and their 'freedom' as subjects" (p. 19).
7. For Agamben "inoperativity" means to deactivate the functioning of apparatuses, which does not mean that these apparatuses do not continue to operate or do not continue to have effects (Prozorov 2014, pp. 31–34).
8. Let me complicate this a bit further. Western nations affirm democracy, yet, in reality, democracy is mostly a mirage—a seemingly unattainable ideal. Wendy Brown (2015), in a nod to Agamben, notes that "capital takes shape as an emerging global sovereign. Capital alone appears perpetual and absolute, increasingly unaccountable and primordial, the source of all commands, yet beyond the reach of *nomos*. Capital produces life absent provisions of protection and ties of membership, turning population around the world into *homo sacer* (bare life)" (p. 64). More particularly, "states are subordinated to the market, govern for the market, gain and lose legitimacy according to the market's vicissitudes" (p. 108). Taking this further, Sheldon Wolin (2008)

argues that the dominance of neoliberal capitalism has resulted in an inverted totalitarian system in which the state is used to legitimate and extend the power of the market (the new sovereign with political and economic elite sovereign classes), through legal privatization of previously public institutions, deregulation, austerity measures, and the expansion of money's influence in the political process. Moreover, non-state institutions such as corporations, think tanks, lobbying groups, etc., (sovereign classes) work closely with the state to deregulate and privatize the common. Inverted totalitarian systems, Wolin argues, project power inward by "combining with other forms of power, such as evangelical religion, and most notably encouraging a symbiotic relationship between traditional government and the system of 'private' governance represented by the modern corporation" (p. xvi). The accumulation of the various forms of power means there is no clear leader or sovereign of the system, as there would be in a totalitarian system (p. 44). In totalitarian states, there is a dictator who is sovereign, while in inverted totalitarian societies there are many leaders from different parts of society (e.g., political, economic, religious—sovereign classes) who support and shape the totalitarian system. Because there is no clear, single institution or person involved in using the state, it becomes impossible to locate the leaders who are responsible, heightening a sense of helplessness and futility among many citizens. I would add that while the center of power is difficult to locate, citizens may continue to believe in democracy and believe that the power resides in traditional government institutions and in the democratic citizenry when, in fact, it is diffused over a wide area and subservient to the needs of the market god (Cox 2016).

9 Of course, one can cite numerous examples of human beings caring for other species and the earth, but the long history of human sovereignty over "nature" and systemic disavowal of the singularities and needs of other species are evident in the destructive realities of climate change.

10 It is not simply theology and philosophy that affirm human sovereignty over nature. Devout Anglican, philosopher, and scientist Francis Bacon (1561–1626), for example, claimed that "the practical aim of improving humanity's lot [depended on] the increased understanding and *control* of nature" (in Grayling 2019, p. 197). There are numerous instances of scientists tacitly claiming sovereignty over other animals and the earth (e.g., experimenting on other animals, developing technologies for fracking, mountain top removal mining, etc.).

11 The possible extinction of human beings does not mean "nature" is sovereign. Applying the notion of sovereignty to nature is a category mistake. Sovereignty is a human concern and pertains only to human beings.

12 Alan Watts (1957) also points out Western preoccupations with conquering nature, as if nature is an object to serve the needs of humanity or that "nature" can actually be conquered (pp. 174–75).

13 Arendt (2005) argues that, because of human limitations and failings, forgiveness is necessary for a viable polis.

14 Philosophers Deleuze and Guattari (2003) agree with Agamben's claim, arguing that "We make no distinction between man and nature . . . man and nature are not like two opposite terms confronting each other . . . rather they are one and the same essential reality" (pp. 4–5). These philosophers argue that the ontological rift is a human construction and one that is, in the end, deadly for human beings and other species. Interestingly, earlier echoes of this are evident in Ralph Waldo Emerson's (1849) writings about nature.

15 https://en.visitsvalbard.com/visitor-information/destinations/longyearbyen (accessed on 28 July 2021).

16 Another illustration is noted by Bryant Rousseau (2016), who points out that New Zealand has two representatives in Parliament whose duty is to represent the lands and rivers of particular areas of the country. Granted, New Zealand is a democracy, which still retains the notion of sovereignty. Yet, there is a realization that nature and other species are integral to the political well-being of the people and therefore need to be represented.

17 Ecovillages: definition, examples and characteristics—Iberdrola accessed 11 February 2022.

References

Agamben, Gilles Deleuze Felix Guattari. 1998. *Homo Sacer: Sovereign Power and Bare Life*. Translated by D. Heller-Roazen. Stanford: Stanford University Press.
Agamben, Gilles Deleuze Felix Guattari. 2004. *The Open: Man and Animal*. Translated by K. Attell. Stanford: Stanford University Press.
Agamben, Gilles Deleuze Felix Guattari. 2005. *State of Exception*. Stanford: Stanford University Press.
Agamben, Gilles Deleuze Felix Guattari. 2009. *What Is an Apparatus? And Other Essays*. Stanford: Stanford University Press.
Agamben, Gilles Deleuze Felix Guattari. 2013. *The Coming Community*. Translated by M. Hardt. Minneapolis: University of Minnesota Press.
Alexander, Michelle. 2010. *The New Jim Crow*. New York: The New Press.
Anderson, Carol. 2016. *White Rage*. London: Bloomsbury.
Antal, Jim. 2018. *Climate Church, Climate World: How People of Faith Must Work for Change*. New York: Rowman & Littlefield.
Arendt, Hannah. 2005. *The Promise of Politics*. New York: Schocken Books.
Bodin, Jean. 2009. *On Sovereignty: Six Books on the Commonwealth*. Seven Treasures Publishing.
Boer, Roland. 2009. *Criticism of Heaven*. London: Haymarket.
Brown, Wendy. 2001. *Politics out of History*. Princeton: Princeton University Press.
Brown, Wendy. 2010. *Walled States, Waning Sovereignty*. New York: Zone Books.
Brown, Wendy. 2015. *Undoing the Demos*. New York: Zone Books.

Camus, Albert. 2002. *The Plague*. London: Penguin. First published in 1947.
Caputo, John. 2006. *The Weakness of God: A Theology of the Event*. Bloomington: Indiana University Press.
Cox, Harvey. 2016. *The Market as God*. Cambridge: Harvard University Press.
Crockett, Clayton. 2012. *Radical Political Theology*. New York: Columbia University Press.
Crossan, John. 1995. *Jesus: A Revolutionary Biography*. New York: HarperOne.
Crossan, John. 2007. *God and Empire*. San Francisco: HarperSanFrancisco.
Crutzen, Paul, and Eugene Stoermer. 2000. The "Anthropocene". *IGB Global Change Newsletter* 41: 17–18.
Deleuze, Gilles, and Felix Guattari. 2003. *Anti-Oedipus: Capitalism and Schizophrenia*. Minneapolis: University of Minnesota Press.
Desmond, Matthew. 2016. *Evicted: Poverty and Profit in the American City*. New York: Crown Publishers.
Dickinson, Colby. 2015. The absence of gender. In *Agamben's Coming Philosophy: Finding a New Use for Theology*. Edited by Colby Dickinson and Adam Kotsko. Lanham: Rowman & Littlefield, pp. 167–82.
Dufresne, Todd. 2019. *The Democracy of Suffering: Life on the Edge of Catastrophe, Philosophy in the Anthropocene*. Montreal: McGill-Queen's University Press.
Emerson, Ralph. 1849. *Nature*. E-Book. Minneapolis: James Monroe and Company.
Fraser, Nancy, and Axel Honneth. 2003. *Redistribution or Recognition?* London: Verso Books.
Grayling, Anthony. 2019. *The History of Philosophy*. New York: Penguin Press.
Hartwich, Wolf-Daniel, Aleida Assmann, and Jan Assmann. 2004. Afterword. In *The Political Theology of Paul*. Edited by Jacob Taubes. Stanford: Stanford University Press, pp. 115–42.
Horsley, Richard. 2003. *Jesus and Empire*. Minneapolis: Fortress Press.
Horsley, Richard. 2011. *Jesus and the Power: Conflict, Covenant, and the Hope of the Poor*. Minneapolis: Fortress Press.
Jamison, Fredric. 2016. *An American Utopia: Dual Power and the Universal Army*. Edited by Slavoj Žižek. London: Verso.
Klein, Naomi. 2007. *Shock Doctrine: The Rise of Disaster Capitalism*. New York: Henry Holt and Company.
Klein, Naomi. 2014. *This Changes Everything: Capitalism vs. the Climate*. New York: Simon and Schuster.
Kolbert, Elizabeth. 2014. *The Sixth Extinction: An Unnatural History*. New York: Henry Holt.
Kompridis, Nikolas. 2020. Nonhuman agency and human normativity. In *Nature and Value*. Edited by A. Bilgrami. New York: Columbia University Press, pp. 240–60.
Lukács, Georg. 1968. *History and Class Consciousness*. Cambridge: MIT Press.
Newman, Saul. 2019. *Political Theology: A Critical Introduction*. Cambridge: Polity Press.
Nichols, Kyle, and Bina Gogineni. 2020. The Anthropocene dating problem. In *Nature and Value*. Edited by Akeel Bilgrami. New York: Columbia University Press, pp. 46–62.
Northcott, Michael. 2017. On going gently into the Anthropocene. In *Religion in the Anthropocene*. Edited by C. Deane-Drummond, S. Bergmann and M. Vogt. Eugene City: Cascade Books, pp. 19–34.
Piketty, Thomas. 2014. *Capital in the 21st Century*. Cambridge: Belknap Press.
Piketty, Thomas. 2020. *Capital and Ideology*. Cambridge: Harvard University Press.
Prozorov, Sergei. 2014. *Agamben and Politics*. Edinburgh: Edinburgh University Press.
Reich, Robert. 2007. *Supercapitalism: The Transformation of Business, Democracy, and Everyday Life*. New York: Vintage Books.
Rousseau, Bryant. 2016. In New Zealand lands and rivers can be people too (legally speaking). *The New York Times*, July 13. Available online: https://www.nytimes.com/2016/07/14/world/what-in-the-world/in-new-zealand-lands-and-rivers-can-be-people-legally-speaking.html (accessed on 4 February 2022).
Schell, Jonathan. 2020. The human shadow. In *Nature and Value*. Edited by A. Bilgrami. New York: New Columbia University Press, pp. 13–24.
Schmitt, Carl. 2005. *Political Theology: Four Chapters on the Concept of Sovereignty*. Translated by G. Schwab. Chicago: University of Chicago Press.
Shore-Goss, Robert. 2016. *God Is Green: An Eco-Spirituality of Incarnate Compassion*. Eugene City: Cascade Books.
Spencer, Nick, and Robert White. 2007. *Christianity, Climate Change, and Sustainable Living*. London: SPCK.
Taubes, Jacob. 2004. *The Political Theology of Paul*. Translated by Dana Hollander. Stanford: Stanford University Press.
Wallace-Wells, David. 2020. *The Uninhabitable Earth*. New York: Dugan Books.
Walzer, Michael. 2012. *In God's Shadow: Politics and the Hebrew Bible*. London: Yale University Press.
Watts, Allan. 1957. *The Way of Zen*. New York: Vintage Books.
Wilkerson, Isabel. 2020. *Caste: The Origins of Our Discontents*. New York: Random House.
Wilson, Edward. O. 2005. *The Future of Life*. London: Abacus.
Wolin, Sheldon. 2008. *Democracy Incorporated*. Princeton: Princeton University Press.
Woods, Ellen. 2017. *The origins of Capitalism*. London: Verso.

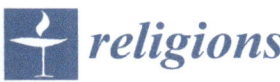

Article

Unshakeable Hope: Pandemic Disruption, Climate Disruption, and the Ultimate Test of Theologies of Abundance

Tallessyn Zawn Grenfell-Lee

Climate Resilience Leadership, LLC, Marlborough, MA 01752, USA; tallessyn@climategrace.com

Abstract: Leaders on the forefront of the rapidly escalating climate crisis continually seek effective strategies to help communities stay engaged without burning out or spiraling into despair. This paper examines the concept of adaptive change for its potential to reframe disruption and intentionally harness its potential for building resilience in both practical and psychological ways. In particular, social science suggests that secure communal bonds lay the foundation for the adaptive ability to build resilience through and from disruption. Swiss history offers an intriguing example of this phenomenon: held up as a model for its social, political, and ecological resilience, Swiss democracy evolved as part of the restructuring of society after a series of disruptive historical pandemics. This paper uses the Swiss example and the current COVID-19 (Coronavirus Disease) pandemic in order to explore the potential of transcendent and adaptive sociological and theological frameworks for the development of robust concepts of resilience in the face of climate destabilization. It further argues that a wide theological interpretation of Eucharistic abundance offers a lens through which to claim the liberative resurrection of disruptions, even, or perhaps especially, in the extreme case of human or planetary annihilation.

Keywords: climate change; adaptive change; climate resilience; climate theology; climate ethics; ecojustice; political theology; liberation theology; pandemic resilience; empathy; hope

Citation: Grenfell-Lee, Tallessyn Zawn. 2022. Unshakeable Hope: Pandemic Disruption, Climate Disruption, and the Ultimate Test of Theologies of Abundance. *Religions* 13: 404. https://doi.org/10.3390/rel13050404

Academic Editors: Pamela R. McCarroll and HyeRan Kim-Cragg

Received: 23 March 2022
Accepted: 26 April 2022
Published: 28 April 2022

Publisher's Note: MDPI stays neutral with regard to jurisdictional claims in published maps and institutional affiliations.

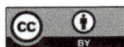

Copyright: © 2022 by the author. Licensee MDPI, Basel, Switzerland. This article is an open access article distributed under the terms and conditions of the Creative Commons Attribution (CC BY) license (https://creativecommons.org/licenses/by/4.0/).

1. Introduction

In the midst of the already highly disruptive and destructive era of climate change, the global COVID-19 pandemic has added an additional, smaller scale but more distinctly defined disruption. In cases of sufficient stability and support, societies can take advantage of these disruptions: with new awareness around social inequity, many communities have responded with new creative solutions to address gaps in access to societal security and safety nets. This particular pandemic effect channels sudden, disruption-driven changes in awareness into high impact momentum for the common good (Stiglitz 2020; Liu et al. 2020).

How can societies better understand, prepare for, and utilize disruption more intentionally, in order not only to reduce and prevent suffering but also to create a more resilient future? Social scientists note that cycles of adaptive change, in societies, smaller human organizations, and in ecosystems, require certain levels of connective stability in order for a disruption to yield an overall increase in function, for the good of the overall system (Holling 2001). Stable human communal connections provide the foundation for the mindfulness, empathy, and altruism required to transcend, alleviate, and prevent future suffering.[1] Such a transformation occurred in Switzerland in the late 19th Century, where growing networks of social solidarity took advantage of a series of epidemics to spur the development of what is now considered the most robust form of democracy in the world (O'Sullivan 2020).

This paper begins with a general overview of socioecological cycles of adaptive change, specifically the need for connectional foundations that allow disruptive change to bring about greater resilience. It then uses the historical example of Swiss democracy to examine the ways such communal connections provided the theological and socioecological foundations necessary for resilient adaptation in response to various disruptions. It further explores the ways theological ethics intentionally draws upon both connection and disruption as a way to formulate strategic approaches to the unprecedented disruption of the climate crisis. It argues that non-attached approaches to survival, such as from wilderness skills practitioners, provide an important piece of the connectional foundation needed to formulate climate change frameworks of adaptive change that offer resilient kinds of hope in the face of possible human extinction. In particular, it explores the ways in which the climate crisis presents a kind of acid test of the application of disruption-based theological frameworks of hope: for example, the viability of the transcendent promise of resurrection in the face of human annihilation. It argues that close examination of biblical narratives and theologies of disruption and hope reveals their appropriateness and utility for contemporary applications to today's greatest disruptive challenges.

2. The Ambivalence of Disruption: Destruction as an Essential Part of the Creative Cycle

The word 'disrupt' includes the idea of 'rupture,' to break apart. Though we instinctively shy away from disruption due to its inherently destructive nature, we also recognize the necessity for disruption, or change, in order to achieve growth. The amniotic sac literally ruptures to allow a woman to birth a child. Disruption—rupture—must continually occur, in some form, for life to exist; in other words, the moment we let go of disruption is the moment we die.

Social scientists note this dual, cyclic nature of social and ecological disruption and change in the development of models of adaptation and resilience.[2] These models recognize the destabilizing nature of disruption as an essential precursor for the possibility of rapid social and ecological—and thus, interconnected socioecological—restructuring that integrates needed forms of resilience. C. S. Holling measures socioecological sustainability based on the resilience of what he calls a 'panarchy': the interconnected cycles of disruption and reorganization within larger ecosystems and in societies, "interlinked in never-ending adaptive cycles of growth, accumulation, restructuring, and renewal" (Holling 2001, p. 392). In a panarchy, periods of stability actually lay the groundwork for future disruptive phases, which in turn lead to highly resilient periods of reorganization, tolerant of novel arrangements and the possibility of failure (see Figure 1). Holling further argues that this model reconciles nature's dual conservative and creative functions into a comprehensible system; periods of restructuring—such as following a wildfire—provide the most resilient moments:

> [A] fertile environment for experiments, for the appearance and initial establishment of entities that would otherwise be outcompeted . . . many will fail, but in the process, the survivors will accumulate the fruits of change. It is a time of both crisis and opportunity.
> (Holling 2001, p. 395)

Holling notes various ecological, economic, and political examples of this phenomenon; for example, habitat disruption, such as the wildfire mentioned above, suddenly releases the "resources accumulated and sequestered in vegetation and soil", such that "the tight organization is lost". Social systems, such as large corporations, can over-accumulate stability; in such cases, their overly rigid structures require disruption in order to spur reorganization and therefore build new resilience, a process economists call "creative destruction".[3] Importantly, systems cannot always recover in this model; panarchic adaptation relies on a critical mass of the previously laid foundations of stability in order for a system to withstand severe disruption well enough to reorganize and function, rather than collapse (Holling 2001, pp. 394–96, 399–400).

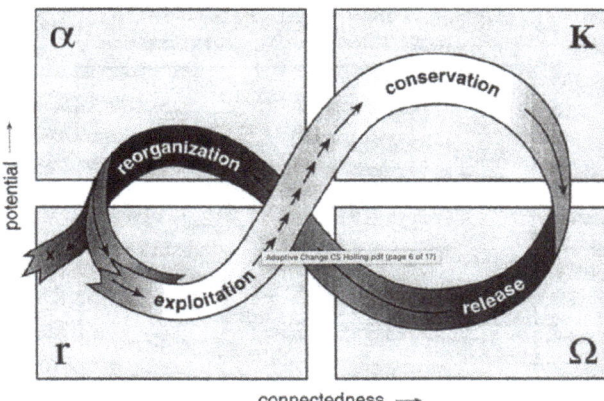

Figure 1. Stylized representation of Holling's Adaptive Cycle for ecological, economic, social, and cultural change. Four distinct sectors (α, r, K, and Ω) represent phases of greater and lesser stability and disruption, with corresponding variations in connectedness and potential: the more connectedness a system builds during periods of heightened implementation (r) and codification of efficient functionality (K), the greater the potential for disruptions, or crises (Ω), to build new forms and levels of resilience during periods of reorganization (α).[4]

To apply this model to human communities, the stable connectivity Holling mentions could correspond to the secure attachment required for proper development of empathy and the ability to transcend and withstand disruption and crisis. The "empathy–altruism" hypothesis describes the ways that securely attached relationships in early childhood lay the foundation for the later ability to turn toward suffering with a sense of kinship and an understanding of the wider context in which crises occur (Davies and Frawley-O'Dea 1994, p. 65). In other words, a foundation of secure emotional connection allows people to view crises from a more mindful perspective.

This application of the empathy–altruism framework draws upon the three "stances of the self" described by psychologist David Wallin: people respond to difficulties with either an embedded, reflective, or mindful approach. Children who have experienced abuse and neglect often exhibit the rigid, chaotic 'embedded' stance, which conflates reality with the crisis: the self remains trapped in and controlled by the crisis, unable to escape its influence or envision alternative meaning constructs (Schore 2001, p. 237). The 'reflective' stance is able to see the wider context in which difficulties unfold and reflect on possible interpretations and contributions to the crisis or challenge, from an often defensive but more stable mental state. Lastly, the 'mindfulness' stance integrates full awareness of the challenges of the present moment with a neutral curiosity toward whatever unfolds; without any external change, mindfulness carries a sense of both connection and even contentment (Wallin 2007, pp. 137–39).

These contributions from social psychology show how Holling's model of adaptive change can work in individuals and societies: communities that include sufficiently stable and healthy relational bonds build the psychological foundations through which to transcend suffering and embrace a vision of meaning and purpose beyond specific moments of disruption. With sufficiently connected foundations, the greatest disruptions actually have the potential to allow forces to emerge that transcend the greatest forms of human suffering and create space for evolved organizational forms. Biehl and Locke describe this sociological approach in ethnographic studies with poor urban communities in Brazil and Bosnia-Herzegovina: notably, this empowering lens respects the agency and potential in these communities for the process of 'becoming':

individual and collective struggles [can] come to terms with events and intolerable conditions and [can] shake loose, to whatever degree possible, from determinants and definitions ... [I]n contexts of clinical and political-economic crisis ... the unexpected happens every day, and new causalities come into play [for] human efforts to exceed and escape forms of knowledge and power and to express desires that might be world altering. (Biehl and Lock 2010, p. 317)

These cycles of disruption and adaptive change offer a useful lens through which to examine crises and resilience; but how helpful are they in the face of the unprecedented disruptions of today? The combination of the COVID-19 pandemic and escalating climate change have left the entire world reeling. To explore the potential for this approach to deal with current crises, this paper will first more thoroughly analyze a specific successful example: how the country of Switzerland used pandemics of the past to forge a notably resilient, stable, and functional democracy.

3. A Contextual Example: How Switzerland Used Historic Pandemics to Build Socioecological Resilience

In discussions of modern democracies, Switzerland always emerges as a shining example. Nestled at the crossroads of Germanic, Latin, and Slavic cultures, this tiny country somehow manages to perform astonishingly well on index after index: among the very highest for political rights, civil liberties, freedom of the press, wealth per capita, economic competitiveness, human development, quality of life, ecological sustainability, and political transparency (and, therefore, lowest for political corruption).[5] Switzerland's unique system uses a political economy that combines direct democracy, multi-party collaborative political coalitions, and an approach to capitalism that prioritizes access, transparency, and the middle class (Lucchi 2017). As a result, Switzerland represents the kind of adaptive panarchy described above: it has experienced relatively less COVID-19 disruption and a comparatively fast economic recovery (SWI 2021). How did Switzerland develop such a robust, resilient society?

Although a combination of factors contributed to modern day Swiss democracy, a large part of the credit apparently goes to past pandemics. In 1867, a cholera epidemic spread rapidly in Zurich, particularly in the poorest areas. The new public health authorities tried to contain the spread and unite the community, but wealthier residents fled to the countryside, and nearly 500 people died. Zurich citizens had prided themselves on their just and equitable society; many were truly shocked at the actual disparity in health and economic vulnerability that cholera had uncovered. The resulting demonstrations led to a power shift away from wealthy families and toward more democratic rule.[6] Zurich implemented a new local constitution that allowed for direct democracy through referendum; soon other cantons followed suit, ending with a new federal constitution in 1874 that lasted until 1999 (O'Sullivan 2020).

Not far away, in Basel, cholera and then typhus had recently claimed the lives of thousands. Similar to Zurich, reform included a collaboration between former conservative elites and the new, more liberal centers of gravity; in efforts to promote both health and equity, medieval city walls came down, open gardens sprung up, and primary schools eliminated tuition and added large windows for plenty of fresh air and sunlight. By the late 19th Century, organized labor had helped end child labor and established workers' rights and other socialist reforms, which spread across the whole country (Habicht 2008, pp. 129–37).

Importantly, both of these cities embraced the interplay among various centers of power—merchant guilds, wealthy dynastic families, workers unions, and Protestant and Catholic religious bodies.[7] Within the context of a strong sense of connectedness for the wider community, the evolution of Swiss democracy included a push and pull in which governance regularly shifted from election to election. Key leaders gracefully—albeit reluctantly—relinquished their power and respected this ebb and flow as part of a larger picture of change over time. In Zurich, Alfred Escher had established some of the most important institutions for modern day Swiss technology and economics before he was forced to give way to new liberal leaders (FDFA 2020). On the other side of the political spectrum in Basel, Wilhelm Klein's far-sighted vision for social equity simply overwhelmed conservative concerns, such that he lost his position to more conservative and religious leaders (Habicht 2008, p. 135). In 1918, the Swiss intentionally implemented proportional representation rather than majority voting, thus solidifying their system of compromise and collaboration among many political parties (Nappey 2010, pp. 68, 78).

The traditionalism of Swiss culture must remain front and center in this picture. As another example of connectional stability, Swiss culture rejects progress for its own sake. Women did not achieve suffrage, for example, until 1971, with the most conservative areas holding out until forced to concede in 1990 (Nappey 2010, p. 78). Even today, Swiss people prioritize traditional, closely knit family culture as a primary source of social support (SWI 2017). Their skepticism is understandable: in a carefully engineered society that ticks along like a well-made watch, why fix something that is not demonstrably broken? Somehow, the Swiss embody the panarchy—integrating both protest and conservatism, innovation and slow deliberation—with an eye toward overall socioecological resilience.

Interestingly—and not accidentally—these historical pandemics also unfolded in a theological context of comparative tolerance and notable humanism, a sense of connection with all humanity. Various influential thinkers from Erasmus to Calvin found both physical and intellectual refuge in cities like Basel, Zurich, and Geneva, partly through open-minded universities and an enthusiasm for the access offered by the printing press. A true cultural crossroads, Basel in particular tended toward tolerance over bloodshed (Habicht 2008, p. 64–84). Prior to the brutal Thirty Years' War, the loosely connected cantons of Switzerland had already gone through their own, comparatively mild upheaval and hammered out a way for each canton to choose its Protestant or Catholic identity (Nappey 2010, pp. 30–37). The evolution of its contextual theology clearly played a significant role in Switzerland's ability to withstand, manage, and benefit from disruption.

4. Connectional Theological Ethics That Transcend Disruption

As a foundational part of the human experience, disruption naturally plays a central role in theological meaning constructs for human societies. Prophets of the Hebrew Bible recognize disruption in the cosmos, in communities, and in the form of intentional sign act protests, as both indictment of current injustice and the inbreaking promise of future justpeace.[8] Frequently using birth symbols, these prophets, along with psalmists and other biblical writers, holistically capture the inequitable and devastating impacts of crises, while they simultaneously situate disruption within a larger theological and metaphysical frame in which the Sacred Cosmos unfolds through a power greater than any individual moment of suffering, liberation, or healing. This section explores the ways disruption theologies have offered meaning constructs that transcend the destructiveness of disruption and how to apply this approach more broadly to climate disruption.

4.1. Disruption Theologies of Healing and Abundance

The cosmic frame mentioned above, within which earthly disruptions occur, offers a meaning construct that includes human suffering and yet transcends it. Ancient and modern theologians continually explore the various dimensions of the inherent challenge of human and earthly suffering, tackling its thorny complexities head on: Can suffering ever be considered inherently good? If healing follows pain, does that end 'justify the means,' making the pain ethically 'good'?[9] What ethics apply when one person's struggle represents another's healing liberation? How do ancient and modern martyrs achieve such deep inner peace that they joyfully embrace what normally looks like traumatic tragedy? Are experiences of suffering and transcendence therefore mutually exclusive, or a matter of interpretation, spiritual maturity, or even choice?[10] How do these interpretations of human suffering—and healing—integrate with and/or apply to the rest of Creation?[11] Lastly, how can we apply the theological ethics of disruption to the wider issue of climate disruption and its role in human meaning?[12]

As these important questions show, theology must offer frameworks that incorporate both the destructive and creative aspects of disruption in order to offer ultimate meaning and hope in the face of humanity's great challenges. The following two examples show how models of adaptive change can apply in the exploration of some of these theological questions.

Calling today's landscape of intersectional oppression and socioecological destruction "radical evil", Christine M. Smith draws upon themes from liberation theology to argue for the potential of preaching to create connective space that allows for deep transformation. She contends that a combination of homiletical weeping, confession, and resistance builds a communal foundation strong enough to carry both the fullness of suffering and the possibility of hope. Faithful weeping, like biblical lament, offers an expression of radical faith, a proclamation of "life in the midst of death ... hope in the midst of despair". Likewise, confession that embraces the full truth of our diverse, complex, challenging reality leads to resilient forms of hope that "resist the seductions of segmenting life, reducing life's complexities to false simplicity, or collapsing life's paradoxes to immobilizing moralisms". Lastly, faithful resistance intentionally turns toward the most difficult challenges of our time; the transcendent frame in this example relies on openness to the movement of the Spirit through all persons and creatures. Beyond "truthful speech", homiletical resistance confronts radical evil with integrity by inspiring acts of courageous discipleship that transcend the fear that disruption can bring based on a sense of trust in a larger historical and pneumatological paradigm (Smith 1992, pp. 4–5).

Like Smith, Traci C. West also explores the ethics of resistance in the face of massive forces of societal oppression. For West, suffering caused by intentional disruption counterbalances existing, oppression-based suffering; therefore, a larger vision of ultimate justice both motivates and transcends individual moments of suffering. West urges an intentionally disruptive social ethic, "to find a way to force a rupture between prevailing cultural arrangements of power that reproduce oppressive conditions, like poverty, and communal tolerance for permanently maintaining such conditions" (West 2006, p. xviii). She suggests the intentional use of diverse resources to forge stronger communal connections that reveal and reshape unexamined theological assumptions:

> Multicultural theoretical approaches can assist Christians in making liturgical choices that enhance their recognition of human diversity as good, as well as their intolerance for unjust social relationships among diverse human communities. Multicultural understandings can offer guidance in creating worship rituals where Christians are more likely to be offered the chance to participate in disrupting a commitment to white dominance than encouraged in going along with it and similar repressive social practices. (West 2006, p. 134)

Both Smith and West intentionally utilize strategic disruption as a way to address other forms of oppression-based disruption. This approach harnesses the adaptive potential of connectional bonds by introducing targeted disruption into the overall communal system, as a way to spur reorganization for the goal of new levels of socioecological justpeace. They employ theologies that include and transcend disruption, such as the integration of lament as an expression of radical faith, and the call to turn toward suffering with a moral courage that arises from a wider vision more powerful than human fears.

In terms of climate disruption, people understandably often assume the goal for adaptive change to include humanity's survival; yet scientific and ethical honesty compels us to consider the possibility of human annihilation and to examine whether these adaptive models and related theological meaning constructs still hold. To explore this challenge, we turn next to concepts that arise from a community that regularly and intentionally faces the question of survival: those who practice and teach survival skills.

4.2. The Contributions of Survival Non-Attachment to a Climate Resilience Mindset

Wilderness and disaster survival practitioners offer a useful approach through which to consider human and planetary survival because they have long studied the factors that make the difference between life and death in extreme situations. In addition to obvious preparatory and response skills, they work to build a foundational source of survival resilience: the 'Survival Mindset.' Without this mindset, people cannot effectively utilize the practices and resources available to them in survival situations. In short, the mindset itself often plays the biggest role in whether or not someone survives, and a key part of this mindset includes letting go of the fear of death. To put it another way, true survivalists practice non-attachment about survival itself as a way to survive (McMahon 2010; Pollard 2012).

Survival 'non-attachment' can feel counterintuitive or confusing unless carefully distinguished from either 'detachment' or 'attachment.' In 'detachment,' people respond to frustration or suffering by complete withdrawal from the pursuit of temporal goals, effectively 'giving up.' Unlike the secure attachment bonds described above, survival 'attachment' involves the fixation on temporal goals in the hopes that their achievement will bring fulfillment. In contrast to both alternatives, 'non-attachment' involves "a transcendent evenness of mind which enables one to participate in the temporal process without attachment". In other words, release of attachments to specific goals, through the focus on a larger frame that transcends those smaller goals, paradoxically enables a fuller engagement in their pursuit, and therefore, a higher chance of actually achieving the goals (Nagley 1954, p. 307). The concept of 'transcendence,' both as used here and in this overall discussion, does not have to include specific theological commitments, but simply a wider understanding or framework that allows individual events to continue to 'make sense' and even contribute toward a broader purpose or meaning construct.

Despite the widespread popularity of both the concept and practice of non-attachment, it seems to hit a wall when confronted with its ultimate test. Applying it to the largest climate issues generates an explosion of resistance. Is it possible to expand survivalist approaches to non-attachment to include climate devastation, our children's future, and the survival of all humankind? Ironically, the great difficulty in letting go of these attachments indicates the even greater importance for developing the Climate Resilience Mindset through non-attachment to these exact ideas and outcomes. Moreover, non-attachment addresses the demands of compassion: it effectively both embodies and reinforces our commitment to the places of deepest suffering.

Frances Moore Lappé describes this counterintuitive effect in *Eco-Mind: Changing the Way We Think, to Create the World We Want* (Lappé 2011). Lappé argues that certain modes of thought around climate change—what she calls "Thought Traps"—appear helpful and logical on the surface, but they actually reinforce a sense of isolation and scarcity that freezes us in overwhelming despair:

> It's too late! Human beings have so far overshot what nature can handle that we're beyond the point of no return. Democracy has failed—it's taking way too long to face the crisis. And because big corporations hold so much power, real democracy, answering to us and able to take decisive action, is a pipe dream. (Lappé 2011, p. 145)

While she acknowledges the stark reality of climate disruption, Lappé uses the present reality of suffering to challenge the utility of narratives of scarcity:

> Half the world is getting by right now on a daily sum equal to the price of a single American latté—or less. About 1 billion of us lack the food and water we need. In the Global North, millions are struggling and stressed as well. Even before the Great Recession, it was estimated that almost 60 percent of Americans will live in poverty for at least a year during their adult lives. In short, catastrophe is already the daily experience of huge numbers.
>
> So here's my question: Too late for what? (Lappé 2011, p. 146)

In contrast, she advocates an intentional shift to narratives that face our current reality with a focus on connection, which generates resolve, joy, gratitude, and abundance:

> I agree ... it is too late to prevent massive change in the climate we humans have taken for granted for thousands of years. Erratic, extreme, and destructive weather is already with us. It is too late to prevent suffering. Terrible suffering is already with us.
>
> But it is not too late for life. Life loves life ... That's just what we do. In other words, the very essence of life, including the version we call human, isn't changed by climate chaos. It is not too late to be ourselves. In fact, for our species, with its passion for shared action toward common ends, maybe now is the time to be alive.
>
> When facing staggering setbacks ... most human beings don't end up ruing life. What makes us miserable isn't a big challenge. It's feeling futile, alone, confused, discounted—in a word, powerless. By contrast, those confronting daunting obstacles, but joined with others in common purpose, have to me often seemed to be the most alive. (Lappé 2011, p. 146)

Importantly, Lappé demonstrates not only acceptance of the realities of the climate crisis but also a practical approach that does not rely on limited definitions of success. Through these thought traps and their alternatives, Lappé points to the possibility of a wider, more resilient vision: the possibility of unshakeable hope as part of a transcendent socioecological framework large enough to include even worst-case climate futures.

4.3. Non-Attached, Unshakeable Hope as an Adaptive Framework for Climate Theology

Discussions of the climate crisis inevitably include the question of hope. Common interpretations of hope hinge on the 'success' of certain tangible goals—hope *for* specific outcomes; yet as noted above, determination of adaptive 'success' depends on the definition of success. In the survivalist mindset, ultimate 'success' does not necessarily require survival itself but rather the ability to maintain intentional, mindful, grounded internal focus, regardless of the external outcome. The ability to be mindful in survival situations arises from an unshakeable connection to concepts of success that transcend survival for both self and other. These understandings of success reflect the 'most alive' feeling Lappé notes, which come from the conviction that there are things worth doing, regardless of the outcome. In the doing itself, with the sense of shared purpose toward a noble cause, a seemingly doomed event transforms into a 'finest hour.'[13]

This discussion highlights the need to reclaim wider conceptions of hope itself. The word 'hope' has always included multiple meanings. The most common usage, attached to specific outcomes, helps clarify goals, inspires a sense of excitement, and focuses efforts, yet it also carries a downside. When a situation does not work out the way people hope it will, they can feel destabilized, like the sense of a rug being pulled out from underneath. This externally-dependent, fragile kind of hope can plummet quickly into a sense of failure, depression, and despair.

An older definition of hope conveys a 'hopefulness,' or 'trust,' not necessarily associated with any particular outcome.[14] This non-attached hope arises out of a deeper sense of meaning and purpose: the determination to remain faithful to shared principles and a wider vision, no matter what happens.[15] It embodies the sense of the greater worth of a life well-lived, regardless of what happens. This kind of hope transcends attachment to specific outcomes; therefore, in theory, it persists regardless of survival, even the survival of all humankind.[16] It inspires the ability to 'go for broke': as Lappé describes above, the sense that these intense moments can enable us to reach deep inside ourselves and find the hopeful place that nothing can touch—even death.[17] This kind of hope is truly unshakeable.

Ethically speaking, the concept of unshakeable climate hope arises through deontological faithfulness, 'doing what is right,' rather than as the result of teleological survival. Theologically, it suggests the necessity of letting go of the attachment to survival in order to find true liberation, or salvation. Many biblical stories reflect this call for faithfulness, such as to a larger vision and covenant for justpeace, over attachment to survival; these stories used community narratives to invite readers to find that kind of unshakeable vision and hope in their own times of disruption and despair.[18] In the face of climate despair, these narratives can be applied interpretively today in similar ways: for example, Moses faithfully led the people to the Promised Land, knowing he would not enter it; in today's terms, can the reader, too, work for the healing of Earth, even if humanity as a species will no longer dwell there? As the early church knew, Jesus and Paul each chose to journey to Jerusalem knowing full well the powerful forces that threatened their lives. The authors of the gospels had already experienced the utter devastation of the Jewish War, yet they still held to the transcendent purpose of Jesus and Paul, a vision greater than survival: a healing rebirth, resurrection, or liberation, from brokenness and oppression. Can the reader, too, choose faithfulness and liberation over survival?

These narratives are not outdated, limited examples of smaller crises and disruptions. Rather, they arise out of overwhelming suffering and destruction and unflinchingly face the hardest questions of what it means to be human: when push really, truly comes to shove, where is a larger vision and purpose? How can communities find it, and how can it offer divine salvation? The book of Revelation offers yet another example even in the midst of the most terrifying situation imaginable—where "nations will be in anguish and chaos at the roaring and tossing of the sea ... People will faint from terror, fearful of what is coming on the world, for the powers of the heavens will be shaken"—the author urges the readers to "stand up and lift up your heads. New life, redemption, is drawing near".[19] These passages speak *precisely* to very human attachments, fears, and suffering in the face of planetary annihilation.

These disruption-based narratives present three main ideas to the reader. First, they offer understanding and compassion: they validate the overwhelming fear, suffering, chaos, and destruction of crises. Second, they offer a theological framework, or container, big enough to carry the crisis, no matter how big it is. They repeatedly situate end-of-the-world scenarios into a larger vision of cosmic justpeace, which calls humanity to faithful participation in a hope grounded in something bigger than our own survival.[20] Lastly, they personally invite the reader into the vision.

Eucharist theologies provide a good example of such a broad, invitational vision: the brokenness of crucifixion, symbolized in the broken bread and poured-out cup, offers validation and compassion for the suffering, fear, and sense of chaos experienced within disruptive crises. The larger resurrection vision of cycles of death and rebirth, as part of the liberative salvation process of a Divine Creation, offers the container of meaningful hope that interprets crises as part of cycles of adaptive change that ultimately bring the Cosmos closer to the Divine kin-dom. Finally, Eucharist narratives also invite the reader to participate in this courageous, hopeful vision, embodied in the communal ritual itself. They offer the disrupted, broken bread and poured-out cup to the reader, as if to say, here, amidst brokenness, is a communion, a connection, that yields abundant life: will you receive it?

As with the disruptive theological ethics described earlier, a theology of unshakeable hope does not passively accept suffering, deny it, sanitize it, or condone it. It does not rest upon simple reassurances of a happy afterlife. It does not flow from places of privilege, shielded from the worst effects of disruption. These expressions of transcendent peace and courage arise from the oppressed margins, as from generations of brutally enslaved Africans who insist, 'This little light of mine, I'm gonna let it shine,' and, 'I ain't gonna let nobody turn me 'round.'[21] In popular culture examples, they urge us to *run toward* what is coming, shouting, "Death! Ride, ride to ruin and the world's ending!" (Tolkien 1995, p. 826). They sing, "Let the sky fall; when it crumbles, we will stand tall, face it all together" (Adkins et al. 2012).

These examples show how other generations have also faced the possibility of annihilation and still found sources of unshakeable hope. We must also find a way through this climate crisis that not only acknowledges the real possibility of human annihilation but also uses this possibility as a powerful resource for even greater inspiration, resolve, and courage—as Tinyiko Maluleke says, "to make peace with death, not merely to accept its inevitable approach, but to actually meet death halfway" (Maluleke 2021, p. 338). These narratives invite the following question: can we, like those who came before us, embrace the healing liberation of our planet, work for it with all our strength, even if we as a species will not survive?

5. Conclusions: Are We Able?

In the face of accelerating climate destabilization, efforts to halt and mitigate climate change often try to motivate more engagement through an increasingly determined insistence that if everyone pitches in, we can 'still turn this ship around.' These noble efforts to unite and inspire nonetheless cannot adequately address the mounting concerns of more and more citizens, people who want to do their part but feel increasingly terrified and hopeless.[22]

Socioecological models of adaptive change offer a helpful way forward, providing frameworks for non-attached hope that enable us to transcend the question of our own survival. These adaptive models illustrate how resilience can evolve through cycles of disruption and reorganization. As illustrated by the positive consequences of historic Swiss pandemics, successful adaptive change requires robust connectedness as both the foundation for successful recovery and the source of potential for new concepts and structures of resilience. Thus, in terms of planetary climate disruption, humanity's role contributes just one part of a larger picture of planetary adaptation: rather than fixation on survival, we can mindfully redefine 'success' as the greatest possible human contribution to the overall socioecological connectivity and therefore adaptive resilience of the planetary panarchy. By providing this larger framework, these models offer a non-attached, mindfulness-based process through which to transform burnout, overwhelming feelings, anxiety, and despair into resources for motivation, courage, and resolve.

These sociological frameworks go hand in hand with many theologies of disruption, which also offer unshakeable hope in a vision larger than human survival. As Cornel West says, "These oppressive systems are mighty; but they are never almighty. What breaks the back of fear? Love. And love is the ability to learn how to die" (West 2017). These theologies insist that humanity already bears witness to the labor, travail, and birth pangs of Creation's Promised Land. Whether we survive to participate in it or not may depend on our ability to call forth a sacrifice of praise for something bigger than our own survival, thereby setting us free to work for this greater vision with bottomless wells of courage and hope. This audacious kind of liberation theology invites us not just to face our own annihilation, but to do what seems impossible: to embrace this moment, and sing.

From a foundation of powerful, enduring connections, with one another, their shared vision, and the Creation, our biblical faith ancestors clearly found the courage to do the impossible. They let go of survival for something bigger, an enduring vision of cosmic justpeace. Their stories invite us to ask ourselves the same, age-old question as well, which still 'whispers down eternity': are we able?

Funding: This research received no external funding.

Institutional Review Board Statement: Not applicable.

Informed Consent Statement: Not applicable.

Data Availability Statement: Not applicable.

Conflicts of Interest: The author declares no conflict of interest.

Notes

1 For an overview of the empathy–altruism hypothesis, see (Davies and Frawley-O'Dea 1994, p. 65); for secure attachment and mindfulness, see (Wallin 2007, p. 4).
2 For example, the socioecological theories of Deleuze and Guattari on synergistic, interconnected becoming (esp. Deleuze and Guattari 1987), (see Michon 2021), and the socioecological resilience theories of adaptive change (Holling 2001).
3 Holling quotes Schumpeter here (Holling 2001, p. 395), who actually argued that capitalism would eventually destroy itself through this process; see (Schumpeter 1950, pp. 82–83, 139).
4 From *Panarchy* edited by Lance H. Gunderson and C.S. Holling. Copyright© 2002 Island Press. Reproduced by permission of Island Press, Washington, DC (Gunderson and Holling 2002).
5 For various indexes, see (Schwab and Zahidi 2020, p. 15; TEIU 2020, p. 9; RWB 2021; FH 2020; TI 2021; Mercer 2019; UNDP 2020; Mulhern 2021). Note that like everywhere, Swiss history includes success and failure: for example, the cautionary tale of the effective but highly toxic pesticide DDT, for which a Swiss scientist received the Nobel Prize. Subsequent use in warfare and awareness of its danger to human ecological health helped give the Swiss their understandable ambivalence about scientific and technological 'progress' (Buschle and Hagmann 2015, pp. 103–7).
6 Many authors have noted the opposite scenarios, in which pandemics result in, or are exploited for, further power imbalance and oppressive or exploitative social structures, e.g., (Maluleke 2021, pp. 328–30; Klein 2007, pp. 8–20).
7 Although it is tempting to view Swiss banking as an aberration, its mixed history reflects the same push and pull among the values of neutrality, protection of privacy, conservatism, innovation, equity, and democracy, such that despite valid criticisms, Swiss people do not view their banks and banking history in a simple and negative light; for a good summary, see (Thomasson 2013).
8 For example, see (Alter 2019, e.g., pp. 617–20).
9 As noted, many scholars have offered theological frameworks that harmonize this apparent paradox; see particularly (Sölle 1975, e.g., p. 164) and a more recent comprehensive overview (Merrigan and Glorieux 2012). Others have explored the idea of suffering as much broader than pain and requiring physical, psychological, and spiritual resources; see (Amato and Morge 1990, e.g., p. 15).
10 Biblical writings obviously vary; in addition to ideas of Divinity as 'Love, broadly defined,' other passages depict a Divine Sovereign who intentionally inflicts vengeful suffering on both humans and Creation, and not always for the sake of justice. Understandably, such narratives cause confusion: is not every divine act necessarily 'good'? Some scholars argue that these texts satirically describe a 'Monster God,' as a way to criticize unjust human rulers by disguising them as Yahweh in the narratives. Simple interpretations nonetheless lead to theologies of inherently redemptive suffering, which cause highly problematic religious frameworks. Beyond simple comfort in divine omnipotence, such ideas have been used to justify, perpetuate, and even glorify the unjust suffering of children, women, enslaved peoples, and otherkind. The idea that Jesus *willingly* bore the cross—a symbol of unjust torture and execution—gets twisted around and used to pressure people to feel grateful for trauma. For the Monster God hypothesis, see (Fretheim 1994, pp. 361, 364; Crenshaw 2005, p. 179; Penchansky 1999, pp. 5–17); for a summary of the problematic of redemptive suffering, see (Trible 1984, pp. 2–5; Fitzpatrick et al. 2016).
11 Of course, Leonardo Boff addresses this question exquisitely (Boff 1997, esp. pp. 104–14); for climate change specific discussions, see also (Estok 2019; Wapner 2014; Berzonsky and Moser 2017, e.g., pp. 163–64).
12 Susanne C. Moser discusses this issue in terms of new leadership strategies needed today (Moser 2012).
13 A recent article about pandemic resilience references the film *Apollo 13*, which depicts the incredible series of challenges that were overcome in order to bring the astronauts back to Earth alive. The author suggests that this historic moment offers "a great example of how to rise to a challenge for which there was no playbook or blueprint, with resourcefulness and determination". In particular, he notes the powerful impact of narratives and frameworks: this space mission "could be the worst disaster NASA's ever experienced", vs. "With all due respect, sir: I believe this is going to be our finest hour" (Eriksen 2020). These examples allude to Winston Churchill's speeches during World War II, which relied on wider concepts of success to inspire common purpose toward noble causes, his definition of a 'finest hour' (for a good summary analysis, see HOTN 2000).
14 This somewhat archaic usage can be found in many dictionaries; for example, see (Merriam-Webster 2022). For an overview of different understandings of hope, see (McCarroll 2014, pp. 7–16).
15 Sometimes these two ideas are distinguished by the terminology of 'hopes' (attached to outcomes) vs. 'hope' (larger sense of hopefulness); see (McCarroll 2014, p. 24).
16 Alexander Hampton talks about the need to reconsider the role of humanity in nature in order to implement the highly effective solutions we already have at our disposal; the pandemic and the climate crisis disrupt our assumptions about human agency and authority and offer opportunities to consider more eco-centric perspectives that may have felt unimaginable in the past. See (Hampton 2021, pp. 17–9, 57). In the same volume, Lisa Sideris describes ways to decenter humanity that yield both humility and courage (Sideris 2021, pp. 202–3, 209–10, 214–15).
17 Jürgen Moltmann attributes this kind of eschatological despair to the human tendency to want to be in control, or godlike; this desire stems from the sin of pride and thus results in the sin of despair, in which we no longer engage in what we are called to do

18   and become. To escape this eschatological despair, we give up and try to reconcile ourselves to, or rationalize, the status quo. See (Moltmann 1993, pp. 20–22).

18   For a summary of the role of the reader in biblical narratives, see (Ska 1990, pp. 61–63). For an example of the application of a biblical, cosmic frame in which to situate the current pandemic and other crisis, see (Claassens 2021, esp. pp. 271–75).

19   My interpretive translation of Luke 21: 25–28.

20   See (Vaai 2021, pp. 213–14) for a blended Wesleyan and Samoan example of a cosmic-centered, rather than human-centered, theology of pandemic and climate disruption.

21   Lyrics from African American spirituals; Howard Thurman writes about this present moment-focused eschatological hope, based on knowledge of the sacredness of the inmost self (Thurman 1979, pp. 217–18). For more examples of theologies of hope in the face of death, see (McCarroll 2014, esp. pp. 35–37).

22   The New York Times just published yet another article about the epidemic of climate anxiety (Barry 2022).

References

Adkins, Adele Laurie Blue, Paul Epworth, and J. A. C. Redford. 2012. *Skyfall*. London: Abbey Road Studio, XL Columbia/Melted Stone.

Alter, Robert. 2019. Prophets. In *the Hebrew Bible: A Translation With Commentary*. 3 vols. New York: W. W. Norton & Company, vol. 2.

Amato, Joseph Anthony, and David Monge. 1990. *Victims and Values: A History and a Theory of Suffering, Contributions in Philosophy*. New York: Greenwood Press.

Barry, Ellen. 2022. Climate Change Enters the Therapy Room. *New York Times*. February 6 Health. Available online: https://www.nytimes.com/2022/02/06/health/climate-anxiety-therapy.html?searchResultPosition=1 (accessed on 6 February 2022).

Berzonsky, Carol L., and Susanne C. Moser. 2017. Becoming homo sapiens sapiens: Mapping the psycho-cultural transformation in the anthropocene. *Anthropocene* 20: 15–23. [CrossRef]

Biehl, João, and Peter Lock. 2010. Deleuze and the Anthropology of Becoming. *Current Anthropology* 51: 317–51. [CrossRef]

Boff, Leonardo. 1997. *Cry of the Earth, Cry of the Poor, Ecology and Justice*. Maryknoll: Orbis Books.

Buschle, Matthias, and Daniel Hagmann. 2015. *How Basel Changed the World*, 1st ed. Basel: Christoph Merian Verlag.

Claassens, L. Juliana. 2021. An Infinite Present: Theology as Resistance Amid Pandemics. In *Doing Theology in the New Normal: Global Perspectives*. Edited by Jione Havea. London: SCM Press, pp. 265–78.

Crenshaw, James L. 2005. *Defending God: Biblical Responses to the Problem of Evil*. Oxford and New York: Oxford University Press.

Davies, Jody Messler, and Mary Gail Frawley-O'Dea. 1994. *Treating the Adult Survivor of Childhood Sexual Abuse: A Psychoanalytic Perspective*. New York: Basic Books.

Deleuze, Gilles, and Felix Guattari. 1987. *A Thousand Plateaus: Capitalism and Schizophrenia*. Minneapolis: University of Minnesota Press.

Eriksen, Brion. 2020. I Believe This Will Be Our Finest Hour. A Medium Corporation. Available online: https://medium.com/elexicon/i-believe-this-will-be-our-finest-hour-98649e23dc99 (accessed on 19 February 2022).

Estok, Simon C. 2019. Suffering and climate change narratives. *CLCWeb: Comparative Literature and Culture* 21. Available online: https://docs.lib.purdue.edu/cgi/viewcontent.cgi?article=3259&context=clcweb (accessed on 8 February 2022).

FDFA. 2020. Alfred Escher: A Visionary of Modern Switzerland. Federal Department of Foreign Affairs. Available online: https://www.houseofswitzerland.org/swissstories/history/alfred-escher-visionary-modern-switzerland (accessed on 10 February 2022).

FH. 2020. Freedom in the World 2020: Switzerland. Freedom House. Available online: https://freedomhouse.org/country/switzerland/freedom-world/2020 (accessed on 11 February 2022).

Fitzpatrick, Scott J., Ian H. Kerridge, Christopher F. C. Jordens, Laurie Zoloth, Christopher Tollefsen, Karma Lekshe Tsomo, Michael P. Jensen, Abdulaziz Sachedina, and Deepak Sarma. 2016. Religious Perspectives on Human Suffering: Implications for Medicine and Bioethics. *Journal of Religion and Health* 55: 159–73. [CrossRef] [PubMed]

Fretheim, Terrence E. 1994. Genesis. In *The New Interpreter's Bible: A Commentary in Twelve Volumes*. Nashville: Abingdon Press, Available online: https://www.logos.com/product/8803/new-interpreters-bible-a-commentary-in-twelve-volumes (accessed on 15 December 2021).

Gunderson, Lance H., and C. S. Holling, eds. 2002. *Panarchy*. Washington, DC: Island Press.

Habicht, Peter. 2008. *Basel—A Center at the Fringe: A Concise History*. Basel: Merian, Christoph Verlag.

Hampton, Alexander J. B. 2021. Pandemic, ecology and theology: Perspectives on COVID-19. In *Routledge Focus on Religion*. Abingdon and New York: Routledge.

Holling, C.S. 2001. Understanding the Complexity of Economic, Ecological, and Social Systems. *Ecosystems* 4: 390–405. [CrossRef]

HOTN. 2000. "The Finest Hour Speech", History on the Net. Salem Media. Available online: https://archive.org/details/finesthourwinsto0000gilb/page/566/mode/2up (accessed on 25 February 2022).

Klein, Naomi. 2007. *The Shock Doctrine: The Rise of Disaster Capitalism*. London: Penguin Books.

Lappé, Frances Moore. 2011. *EcoMind: Changing the Way We Think, to Create the World We Want*. New York: Nation Books.

Liu, Amy, Alan Berube, and Joseph Parilla. 2020. *Rebuild Better: A Framework to Support an Equitable Recovery from COVID-19*. Washington, DC: Brookings Institution.

Lucchi, Micol. 2017. This Is How Switzerland's Direct Democracy Works. World Economic Forum. Available online: https://www.weforum.org/agenda/2017/07/switzerland-direct-democracy-explained/ (accessed on 15 December 2021).

Maluleke, Tinyiko. 2021. Beyond the Graveyard and the Prison, a New World is Being Born. In *Doing Theology in the New Normal: Global Perspectives*. Edited by Jione Havea. London: SCM Press, pp. 327–43.

McCarroll, Pamela R. 2014. *The End of Hope—The Beginning: Narratives of Hope in the Face of Death and Trauma*. Minneapolis: Fortress Press.

McMahon, Kathy. 2010. The Survival Mindset. Post Carbon Institute. Available online: https://www.resilience.org/stories/2010--03-15/survival-mindset/ (accessed on 18 February 2022).

Mercer. 2019. Quality of Living City Ranking. Mercer. Available online: https://mobilityexchange.mercer.com/insights/quality-of-living-rankings (accessed on 13 February 2022).

Merriam-Webster. 2022. Hope. Encyclopedia Britannica, Inc. Available online: https://www.merriam-webster.com/dictionary/hope (accessed on 21 February 2022).

Merrigan, Terrence, and Frederik Glorieux. 2012. *"Godhead Here in Hiding": Incarnation and the History of Human Suffering, Bibliotheca Ephemeridum Theologicarum Lovaniensium*. Leuven and Walpole: Peeters.

Michon, Pascal. 2021. Gilles Deleuze & Félix Guattari and the Rhuthmoi of Thought—Part 2. *Rhuthmos*, July 20.

Moltmann, Jürgen. 1993. *Theology of Hope: On the Ground and the Implications of a Christian Eschatology*. Translated by James W. Leitch. Minneapolis: Fortress Press.

Moser, Susanne C. 2012. Getting Real about it: Meeting the Psychological and Social Demands of a World in Distress. In *Environmental Leadership: A Reference Handbook*. Edited by Deborah Rigling Gallagher. Thousand Oaks: SAGE Publications, Inc, pp. 900–8.

Mulhern, Owen. 2021. Switzerland—Ranked 20th in the Global Sustainability Index. Earth.org. Available online: https://earth.org/global_sustain/switzerland-ranked-20th-in-the-global-sustainability-index/ (accessed on 8 February 2022).

Nagley, Winfield E. 1954. Thoreau on Attachment, Detachment, and Non-Attachment. *Philosophy East and West* 3: 307–20. [CrossRef]

Nappey, Grégoire. 2010. *Swiss History in a Nutshell*. Translated by Histoire Suisse. Original edition, Histoire Suisse. Basel: Bergli Books.

O'Sullivan, Domhnall. 2020. How A Zurich Epidemic Helped to Birth Swiss Direct Democracy. Swiss Broadcasting Corporation. Swiss Broadcasting Corporation. Available online: https://www.swissinfo.ch/eng/directdemocracy/viral-history_how-a-zurich-epidemic-helped-to-birth-swiss-direct-democracy/45708992 (accessed on 15 December 2021).

Penchansky, David. 1999. *What Rough Beast?: Images of God in the Hebrew Bible*, 1st ed. Louisville: Westminster John Knox Press.

Pollard, Dave. 2012. Preparing for Collapse: Non-Attachment, NOT Detachment. Dave Pollard. Available online: https://howtosavetheworld.ca/2012/12/20/preparing-for-collapse-non-attachment-not-detachment/ (accessed on 19 February 2022).

RWB. 2021. World Press Freedom Index. Reporters Without Borders. Available online: https://rsf.org/en/ranking (accessed on 12 February 2022).

Schore, Allan N. 2001. The Effects of Early Relational Trauma on Right Brain Development, Affect Regulation, and Infant Mental Health. *Infant Mental Health Journal* 22: 201–69. [CrossRef]

Schumpeter, Joseph A. 1950. *Capitalism, Socialism and Democracy*. New York: Harper & Row.

Schwab, Klaus, and Saadia Zahidi. 2020. *The Global Competitiveness Report: How Countries Are Performing on the Road to Recovery*. Geneva: World Economic Forum.

Sideris, Lisa H. 2021. Listening to the Pandemic: Decentering Humans through Silence and Sound. In *Pandemic, Ecology and Theology: Perspectives on COVID-19*. Edited by Alexander J. B. Hampton. New York: Routledge, pp. 201–19.

Ska, Jean Louis. 1990. *"Our Fathers Have Told Us": Introduction to the Analysis of Hebrew Narratives, Subsidia Biblica*. Roma: Editrice Pontificio Instituto Biblico.

Smith, Christine M. 1992. *Preaching as Weeping, Confession, and Resistance: Radical Responses to Radical Evil*, 1st ed. Louisville: Westminster/John Knox Press.

Sölle, Dorothee. 1975. *Suffering*. Philadelphia: Fortress Press.

Stiglitz, Joseph. 2020. Conquering the Great Divide: The pandemic has laid bare deep divisions, but it's not too late to change course. *Finance and Development*, 17–19. Available online: https://www.imf.org/external/pubs/ft/fandd/2020/09/COVID19-and-global-inequality-joseph-stiglitz.htm (accessed on 8 February 2022).

SWI. 2017. "Swiss Youth Remain Conservative". Swiss Broadcasting Corporation. Available online: https://www.swissinfo.ch/eng/family-values_swiss-youth-remain-conservative-/43629840 (accessed on 8 February 2022).

SWI. 2021. "Swiss Economy Tipped for Stronger Rebound from Pandemic". Swiss Broadcasting Corporation. Available online: https://www.swissinfo.ch/eng/swiss-economy-tipped-for-stronger-rebound-from-pandemic/46706226 (accessed on 11 February 2022).

TEIU. 2020. *Democracy Index 2020: In Sickness and in Health?* London: The Economist Intelligence Unit.

Thomasson, Emma. 2013. Special Report: The Battle for the Swiss Soul. *Reuters*, April 18.

Thurman, Howard. 1979. *With Head and Heart; The Autobiography of Howard Thurman*, 1st ed. New York: Harcourt Brace Jovanovich.

TI. 2021. Corruption Perceptions Index: Switzerland. Transparency International. Available online: https://www.transparency.org/en/cpi/2021/index/che (accessed on 9 February 2022).

Tolkien, John Ronald Reuel. 1995. *The Lord of the Rings*. London: Harper Collins Publishers.

Trible, Phyllis. 1984. *Texts of Terror: Literary-Feminist Readings of Biblical Narratives, Overtures to Biblical Theology*. Philadelphia: Fortress Press.

UNDP. 2020. The Next Frontier: Human Development and the Anthropocene. In *Human Development Report 2020*. New York City: United Nations Development Programme.

Vaai, Upolu Lumā. 2021. Lagimālie: COVID, De-Onefication of Theologies, and Eco-Relational Well-being. In *Doing Theology in the New Normal: Global Perspectives*. Edited by Jione Havea. London: SCM Press, pp. 209–21.

Wallin, David J. 2007. *Attachment in Psychotherapy*. New York: Guilford Press.
Wapner, Paul. 2014. Climate Suffering. *Global Environmental Politics* 14: 1–6. [CrossRef]
West, Traci C. 2006. *Disruptive Christian Ethics: When Racism and Women's Lives Matter*, 1st ed. Louisville: Westminster John Knox Press.
West, Cornel. 2017. *Faith in Action: Poverty and the Racialization of Economy*. Boston: Boston University School of Theology.

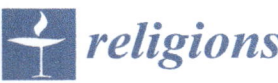

Article

The Environmental Activism of a Filipino Catholic Faith Community: Re-Imagining Ecological Care for the Flourishing of All

Jeane C. Peracullo [1,*] and Rosa Bella M. Quindoza [2]

1. Department of Philosophy, De La Salle University, Manila 2401, Philippines
2. Department of Communication Research, Polytechnic University of the Philippines, Manila 01008, Philippines; rbmquindoza@pup.edu.ph
* Correspondence: jeane.peracullo@dlsu.edu.ph

Abstract: Extensive open-pit mining activities in the Philippines since the 1970s up to the present confront the meaning of the "Church of the Poor", a description that the Catholic Church in the Philippines uses to visualize its prophetic mission. Alongside mining, many more environmentally destructive industries are present in the poorest areas in the country, even though the Philippines is disaster-prone and one of the world's most vulnerable countries to the devastating effects of the climate crisis. The environmental degradation has prompted many Filipino Catholic organizations and communities to act together through various campaigns to address the problem. The article examines a case of a faith-based community that rose to the challenge to address various environmental issues their community has encountered and continues to experience. The community's environmental activism presents a viable model for a re-imagined ecological care towards the "flourishing of all" as a response to Pamela McCarroll's call to action to continue conversations on the many ways practical theology can move beyond anthropocentrism while focusing on social justice.

Keywords: ecological activism; practical theology and environmental crisis; ecological care; action research

Citation: Peracullo, Jeane C., and Rosa Bella M. Quindoza. 2022. The Environmental Activism of a Filipino Catholic Faith Community: Re-Imagining Ecological Care for the Flourishing of All. *Religions* 13: 56. https://doi.org/10.3390/rel13010056

Academic Editors: Pamela R. McCarroll and HyeRan Kim-Cragg

Received: 10 December 2021
Accepted: 4 January 2022
Published: 7 January 2022

Publisher's Note: MDPI stays neutral with regard to jurisdictional claims in published maps and institutional affiliations.

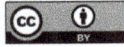

Copyright: © 2022 by the authors. Licensee MDPI, Basel, Switzerland. This article is an open access article distributed under the terms and conditions of the Creative Commons Attribution (CC BY) license (https://creativecommons.org/licenses/by/4.0/).

1. Introduction

Lynn White's article, which came out in 1967, made a controversial claim. According to White, the root cause of the environmental crisis is religion, specifically Christianity, which privileged the human person over animals and other nonhuman beings in the world (White 1967). Towards the end of the article, however, White discloses that the remedy for the crisis is also religious. After that, he cites Buddhism and St. Francis of Assisi as exemplars of a deep understanding of our connection with nature. The Filipino Catholic bishops in 1988 declare that a particular task, the stewardship of creation, was given to humans by God based on their reading of Gen. 1: 27–28. Stewardship points to an ethic of responsible management or stewardship of these natural resources so that the next generations of humans can have continued access to these resources. The stewardship ethic is a response to White's claim that religion could offer remedies against the environmental crisis. It uses the language of conserving resources for future generations—an implicit acknowledgment of its usefulness to human beings. The 1988 pastoral letter refers to this notion of stewardship as an act of Christian duty.

For the Filipino Catholic bishops, stewardship is the approach for viable resource management that aims to restore the beauty of the Philippine natural environment and serve the needs of the future generations of Filipinos. The environmental actions that the Catholic bishops have inspired manifested an anthropocentric dimension of stewardship, even though the environmental issues and concerns were massive, like mining and deforestation. In 1998, they called for the repeal of the Mining Act of 1995.

William Holden (2012) documents the Catholic response to large-scale mining in the Philippines. The global mining industry has taken note of the Church's opposition to mining. According to Holden (2012, p. 852), for the Catholic Church in the Philippines, environmental issues such as mining must not be seen as purely environmental issues, but also as human rights issues because mining not only disrupts the biophysical environment, but degrades natural resources upon which many poor people rely; it further impoverishes them.

In 1991, the Catholic Bishops Conference of the Philippines (henceforth CBCP) convened the 2nd Plenary Council (PCP II). The "Church of the Poor" became the blueprint for the Catholic Church's renewal in the country. The Basic Ecclesial Communities (BECs) or Catholic faith communities in the rural areas of the country were instrumental in translating the ideas of being the "Church of the Poor" into concrete actions (Dagmang 2015). Some BECs widely interpreted one of the visions of the 2nd Plenary Council of the Philippines, "a Church is a community of disciples", as about a spirituality of stewardship (Picardal 2013). This interpretation enabled some BECs to incorporate environmental campaigns into their action platforms. However, it is worth noting that there is no provision in the Acts and Decrees of the PCP II, published in 1992, that specifically mentioned the environmental crisis (Peracullo 2020). The localization of efforts towards addressing environmental issues and concerns is sustainable because local Catholic communities and progressive groups are invested in these issues, specifically mining, deforestation, and increasingly by 2015, climate change. After all, these issues impact their vulnerable communities significantly.

The study participates in the conversation by reflecting on two questions: (1) Can care be re-imagined as a non-anthropocentric response to the environmental crisis? (2) What model for ecological care beyond anthropocentrism arises from the environmental activism of a faith-based community in the Philippines? The study examines Marinduque Council for Environmental Concerns (MaCEC)'s notion of ecological care. Moreover, the study investigates how the organization's concepts or ideas of care go beyond anthropocentrism. Finally, the study proposes a model of ecological care that promotes the flourishing of all in ecological communities. Cultural values such as *pagtutulungan* (service), *pakikiisa* (solidarity), and *pananampalataya* (faith) are features of the model of ecological care beyond anthropocentrism.

1.1. From Stewardship to Ecological Care

Since its publication in 2015, *Laudato Si* (Francis 2015) became a model of doing theology that engages with the scientific community, the faithful, and the nonhuman members of the biotic community. Rolando Tuazon (2018, p. 198) claims that Pope Francis rejects the dominant view about environmental stewardship as dominion. *Laudato Si* provides a new way of regarding nature largely absent in many encyclicals in the past, even though those advocated for sustained economic and political justice towards the poor in society (Eballo 2018). For Wolfgang Sachs (2017, p. 2583), *Laudato Si* pillories excessive anthropocentrism and emphasizes relationships with nature, others, oneself, and God (Sachs 2017, p. 2580). This intertwining relationship calls for an integral ecology (Francis 2015). Integral ecology corrects that binarism or dualism (Canceran 2018, p. 9).

For the CBCP (2019, par. 23), echoing Pope Francis, there is a need for a paradigm shift to reestablish our sacred relationship with nature and not just for a token of environmental protection and stewardship. The Catholic bishops seemed to underscore the language of care from the language of stewardship. Nonetheless, the language of care still evokes anthropocentrism because, as Wickman and Sherman (2020) emphasize, the scope of the Anthropocene is essentially planetary. Whatever it means, it refers to the enormous influence of human beings upon the entire terrestrial system and thus the historical emergence of the *Anthropos* as a geological agent. Anthropocentrism refers to the idea that only human beings possess inherent worth and moral standing. Anthropocentrism's literal or etymological meaning is "human-centered". This concept asserts that the human being—as an individual or species—stands at the center of existence in descriptive and normative modes (Beever 2018, p. 39).

The influence extends to the kinds of response to the environmental degradation that is largely human inflicted. Sally McFague points out: "It is hard to care for the Earth when one has never cared for a piece of it" (McFague 1997, p. 155). In using the analogy of a gardener, McFague points to the gardener who cares as pragmatic, practical, immersed in trying to look for local solutions to make the garden flourish, and in so doing, able to distinguish suitable interventions from bad ones in gardening.

Caring for a garden is a case of making the personal political (McFague 1997). McFague argues that this particular activity of caring can motivate groups of gardeners to lobby for inner-city parks where poor people in urban areas can commune, appreciate, learn to care for the environment; to work for a community where people and nature can co-inhabit; and lastly to advocate for a simpler, limited lifestyle, in which a sense of community, a high literacy rate, the emancipation of women, preventive medicine, and ample green space are considered the good life. She cites examples of such communities, both rich and poor.

The ecological ethic of care suggests relating to nature-appreciation and not domination. For McFague (1997), the former is the crucial point we have missed from Genesis. God appreciates what God created, and as beings made in God's image, our attitude toward nature should also be valued. She also points out that this attitude toward nature is in keeping with the commandment to love God and neighbor. McFague (1997, p. 166) puts it this way:

"God is the ultimate Subject: we love God (or should love) because God is God and deserves our adoration. We love our neighbor (or should) because we see human beings as ends in themselves, as valuable. After all, they are. A human being is good, period. Gen. 1 says that we should extend the way we relate to God and neighbor to nature: nature is good, period."

For Pamela McCarroll, though, McFague's recommendation belongs to the efforts in religious ethics and systematic theology "to replace the image of the human as "master", and maker of history with the image of the human as caretaker, steward, custodian, and fellow creature upon the Earth, created to love, reverence and care for the planet, its animals and processes" (McCarroll 2020, p. 35), and this can be problematic. McCarroll continues that "until the living web of humanity can be conceptualized within the more extensive live web of creation, our research and practice cannot help but serve human-centric ways of being in the world. Ultimately, it re-inscribes and normalizes human-centricity, the fundamental cause of the environmental crisis (McCarroll 2020, p. 36).

1.2. Small Island Communities in the Philippines

The Philippines' archipelagic nature and its location in the most disaster-prone region in the world and the Pacific 'Ring of Fire' make it even more critical for this calamity-prone country, particularly for small island communities. The Philippine Department of the Interior and Local Government (DILG) enumerates the following factors to describe small islands: (1) Physical dimension, e.g., the land area of less than 10,000 sq km; (2) distance from the mainland; (3) geo-physical profile; (4) substrate or origin; (5) population density; (6) resource limitations, usually resulting in food insecurity and chronic poverty; (7) dependence on the mainland; (8) lack of access and links to market institutions and technology; (9) political/social marginalization due to the existing governance structure; (10) lack of alternative sustainable livelihoods to complement farming and fishing; (11) direct exposure to climate-related hazards, especially typhoons and storm surges; (12) lack of risk assessment, early warning, and search and rescue capacity; and (13) isolation, especially when disasters hit (CCS et al. 2011, p. 3).

Thousands of small islands with fragile ecosystems and populated by communities heavily dependent on natural resources are highly exposed to natural and human-induced hazards. As such, these small islands become the most vulnerable to risks because they face multiple threats and the possibility of isolation from the mainland (CCS et al. 2011, pp. 125,

130). Nevertheless, these communities most susceptible to environmental challenges and climate risks also have the most potential to advocate a response concretely and appropriately, and act on these risks and challenges.

1.3. Profile of the Island Province of Marinduque

Marinduque is situated about 170 km south of Metro Manila at the eastern portion of Luzon, Philippines. Tayabas Bay on the north, Mongpong Pass on the northeast, Tayabas Strait on the southeast, and the Sibuyan Sea on the southbound Marinduque bound the province. It comprises the main island and 17 islets and spans 959,000 sq. km. Approximately 83% are hills and mountains, while 17% are coastal, swamps, and marshy areas (UP PLANADES 1999; Province of Marinduque 2011, p. 2).

It has pristine biodiversity and ecosystems of natural forests, agricultural fields, seas, coastlines, thirty-two (32) river basins, and copper, copper concentrate, copper metal, iron, manganese, limestone, gold, and silver. The region is primarily agricultural. The sector provides 48% of employment, while approximately 53% of the total land area is devoted to crop production, mainly coconut and copra (Province of Marinduque 2011, p. 5). Figure 1 presents the location map of the island-province map of Marinduque.

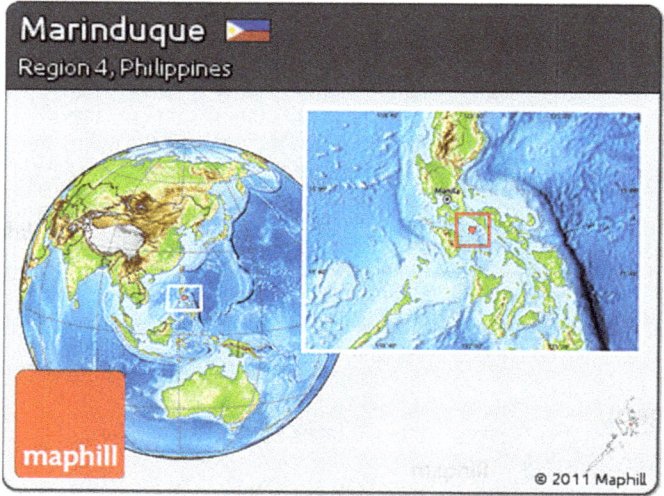

Figure 1. Location map of Marinduque Philippines. Original image from ©Maphill (2011) distributed under license CC BY-ND.

Historical studies on disaster pointed to several environmental, tragic, and climate risks faced by the island province (Magalang 2010; Formilleza 2010). Marinduque's geographical feature makes it an earthquake-prone area. It is home to a dormant volcano, Mt. Malindig, located in the municipality of Buenavista, and is situated along the Boac River Fault line. The island province is considered the 7th landslide-prone province in the country, with the heavy disturbance of its mountains' physical base caused by large-scale mining operations. According to the Department of Environment and Natural Resources Mine and Geosciences Bureau (DENR-MGB), the province has a high risk for landslides during earthquakes and large-scale flooding. Marinduque's location in the country's typhoon belt means that it is either directly hit or affected by an average of twelve typhoons each year which caused devastating damage to properties, infrastructure, agriculture, livelihoods, and living conditions (Province of Marinduque 2011, p. 7; Magalang 2010).

For over 30 years until 1996, the Marinduque Copper Mining (Marcopper) operations served as a source of livelihood for some residents. However, the mine operations have caused innumerable threats, particularly health, environmental problems, and risks. Mining has polluted waterways, killed fish, and flooded agricultural fields. With poverty incidence moved from 12.5% in 2015 to 10% in 2018, almost 24% of its population is still under poverty, even after hosting mining operations for three decades (PSA 2020, p. 45; Salvacion and Magcale-Macandog 2015, p. 28).

A cumulative effect of the mine tailings dumping occurred when the Mogpog and Boac Rivers overflowed the banks during a typhoon in 1993. On 24 March 1996, the pit, which used to hold the wastes of the Marcopper, failed and caused a massive spill of mine tailings into the Boac River and other bodies of waters traversing three towns. The mining spill destroyed a significant water artery in the capital town of Boac that brought about further environmental, health, social, and economic problems. In addition, flooding in the island-province's coastal and flood plain areas aggravates the increasing effects of sea-level rise due to climate change and climate variability.

The flow of mine tailing deposits from impounding pits that collapsed in 1993 and 1996 placed many communities along the riverbanks and low-lying areas vulnerable to flood-related risks. The possible collapse of at least six abandoned and unmaintained mine tailing dams located up in the mountains and above the primary fault line and still contain contaminated liquid and solid materials pose a severe disaster threat even after the close of mining operations in the province (Magalang 2010; Province of Marinduque 2011, p. 10).

Moreover, water quality and hydrology analysis in Boac River indicates that "water conductivity is higher than the acceptable values for a freshwater body and that concentrations of arsenic, lead, mercury, manganese, and copper with the first three as highly toxic are 'above their threshold limits'" (Cruz et al. 2020, p. 152).

One of the many Basic Ecclesial Communities that mainly attend to environmental issues is the Marinduque Council for Environmental Concerns (MaCEC) that Rev. Rafael M. Lim, the first bishop of the Diocese of Boac, established in 1978. The initial advocacies of MaCEC focused on the struggle of the fisherfolks against the surface dumping of mine tailings at Calancan Bay and Boac River by the Marcopper Mining Corporation (Magalang 2010). With support from national organizations such as CBCP's National Secretariat for Social Action (NASSA), Luzon Secretariat for Social Action (LUSSA), and *Lingkod Tao Kalikasan* (Service, People, Nature), the struggle took the form of pressing legal and administrative charges against the mining firm. However, the environmental disaster due to the mine tailings spill in 1996 brought together residents of the province, non-governmental organizations, local Church organizers, and local public officials in a collective and integrated advocacy and action (Quindoza 2015).

2. Methods

The study is essentially participatory action research that uses a qualitative approach and documents review, interviews, and observation as data collection methods. It is limited to the case of the Marinduque Council for Environmental Concerns (MaCEC) involving several faith communities, community chapters, or members. The participants in the interviews were purposively selected using the following criteria: (1) living in the community/province for ten years or more; (2) a member/leader of MaCEC community/chapter; (3) resident of capital town villages with high 'risks' based on Provincial Disaster Risk Reduction and Management (PDRRM) Plan; (4) willingness to participate in the interview; and (5) access to digital/online platform for data gathering activities. While MaCEC has village and town chapters in all six towns of the province, the interviewees selected were limited to village-level formations in the capital town of Boac, as this was the most accessible to the researcher at the time. Documents reviewed included MaCEC plans and reports, press statements, online information, and documentation of events from its official social media, training modules, and relevant local policies and programs.

The study observes ethical considerations of ensuring voluntary participation and withdrawal, informed consent, and the health and safety of the research community. With the observance of government quarantine and mobility restrictions during the field research schedule, the researchers modified the interviews into paper/online interviews with follow-up phone calls arranged based on the availability of the interviewees and contingent on the health situation and connectivity access households/villages. The discussions proceeded with an interview guide that grouped questions into the participants' understanding of how cultural and religious aspects figure into their work as environmental stewards, the cultural and religious elements in the risk and resilience messages, results, and recommendations. In coordination with MaCEC staff, the researchers identified a total of nine (9) informants: four (4) of which are community/chapter leaders, four (4) are community/chapter members, and one (1) is the head of the MaCEC. The researchers then contacted them and sent printed copies of the interview guide. After two weeks, the researchers retrieved the filled-out interview guides. The researchers did some follow-up phone calls during data processing to validate or probe the recorded responses.

The organization permitted the researchers to conduct an online observation of a MaCEC Leaders' Discussion scheduled during their meeting on 7 October 2021. It informed the researchers of the process and content of organizational ecological discussions, planning, and evaluation. The validation session proceeded with emails and scheduled phone calls with MaCEC leaders and staff.

3. Results

The Significance of Cultural and Religious Aspects of Resilience

Resilience, in the context of risk, refers to the "ability of a system, community or society exposed to hazards to resist, absorb, accommodate, adapt to, transform and recover" from the effects of a hazard (UNGA 2017, p. 22). A community's resilience depends on the degree of availability of resources and capacity to organize itself before and during times of need (UNISDR 2009, p. 24; 2017). Participants regarded resilience as *pagbawi* or *pagbangon* (the ability to rise beyond adversity). The participants compared themselves to the "bamboo which bends with the wind but never breaks". The description is apt because the participants believed that they could rise above the adversities they regularly experience and could even face the danger of a looming environmental disaster if the abandoned dams that hold toxic mine tailings would give way.

The participants, living in Marinduque, understood that the precarity of their existence could lead to negative consequences such as "something bad happening", "*panganib* (danger)", which affect people, property, communities, environment, livelihood, and even cause "fear" or "phobia" related to disaster, calamity, and climate emergency. In these instances, most participants turned to family and community support and prayer and devotion, especially among the Roman Catholics, to the *Ina ng Biglang-Awa* (Our Lady of the Prompt Succor), the Patroness of the Diocese of Boac. The prayer and devotion are part of the coping process of some of the participants as they navigate their lives around the risks posed by natural and human-made challenges.

MaCEC members and leaders underscored that the concepts of *pagtutulungan* (service to one another), *pakikiisa* (solidarity), and *pananampalataya* (faith) are significant manifestations of resilience. Participants stated that close family ties, formations, and support in the neighborhood (*kapitbahayan*) and community (*pamayanan*) and faith are vital in addressing, responding to, and coping with risk, disaster, or disaster adversity.

Moreover, the community expanded its Basic Ecclesial Community (BEC) program to address environmental issues and concerns. It conducted the activity, *Bahaginan ng Pamayanang Kristiyano sa Salita ng Diyos* (Sharing of the Word of God among Christian Communities) in villages for their members to become what they call the "basic faith communities of environmental stewards" (BFC-ES). The spiritual-ecological course, *Batayang Pag-aaral Pangspiritwal at Pangekolohiya* (Learning Modules on Spirituality and Ecology), youth environmental camps, youth and adult leaders ecological learning exchange, among others, are some environmental education formats implemented to enhance and sustain ecological awareness and action.

4. Discussion

Vera Files, an independent news organization in the Philippines, featured a story on the continuing ill-effects that the people of Marinduque suffer from as a result of the disastrous spilling of the mine tailings into the Boac River in 1996. Twenty-three years later, the people are still trying to rebuild their lives (Dizon 2019), while the Boac River remains biologically unable to sustain life (DENR 2020). Without adequate support from the local and national governments to rehabilitate the poisoned land and waters, it would be up to the people in Marinduque to find ways to help one another. Against this backdrop, MaCEC drafted its members' mandate to be environmental stewards.

In its 25th year of existence, MaCEC demonstrates how a local, faith-based organization can effectively respond to the risks and challenges of living in a place where natural and human-induced disasters occur. While it started as a social action environmental arm of the local Church, which supported fisherfolks who suffered from surface dumping of mine tailings into their traditional fishing areas, it expanded into a significant partner of local and national organizations that oppose large-scale mining operations in the country. At present, MaCEC provides the bulk of environmental advocacy in the province of Marinduque by its work on climate emergency mitigation and response, disaster management, environmental justice, and care. In the various campaigns, advocacy work, and mobilizations, MaCEC's core environmental advocacy framework flows from three program components: ecological literacy, ecological actions, and ecological ethics. Literacy and steps lead to public awareness and knowledge; literacy and ethics produce socio-environmental values and ethics and actions that result in desired environmental behavior changes in its members. It hopes to do the same in the greater public.

MaCEC operations envisioned a clean, bountiful, and life-giving environment in the Island Province of Marinduque, which will benefit the present and future generations. In fulfilling this vision, it adheres to democratic processes, collective actions, the inspiration of Gospel values, and the Social Doctrine of the Church (MaCEC 2021). The Social Doctrine of the Church includes the CBCP pastoral letters that are typically read on Sunday services for the Catholic community.

MaCEC's initial understanding of environmental stewardship is a blend of the Catholic bishops' view of stewardship as resource management for the future generations of *Marinduquenos* and the members' awareness of the responsibility of rehabilitating the poisoned waters and land of the province and restoring the livelihood of those who were greatly affected by environmental disasters. The first logo of MaCEC in Figure 2 reflects this view of stewardship.

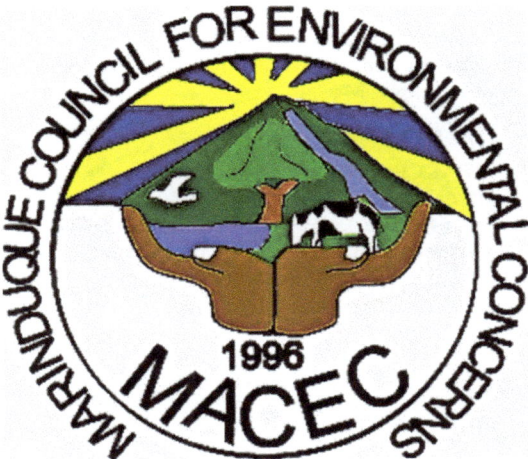

Figure 2. The original logo of MaCEC.

The older logo features an oversized pair of hands that holds the entire province, particularly rivers, trees, mountains, and cows. The natural world is now under the care of humans, the *Marinduquenos*. The disembodied hands accentuate the outsize responsibility of MaCEC to aid, support, and care.

Over time, the notion of stewardship expanded to include environmental justice. According to the 2021 Press Release of the organization, in 2003, Bishop Jose Oliveros of the Diocese of Boac headed the first Diocesan Synod that led to the ratification of decrees that became the pillars for the local Church in Marinduque. Part of the document included *Katarungan* or Justice. MaCEC expanded its mission to have "a firm stance on the explicit objection over any forms of large-scale mining and other similar industries and activities that can cause serious effects on the environment and ecology of the province" (MaCEC 2021).

MaCEC has since launched massive campaigns and advocacies on the environment, climate justice, and disaster risks following the spirit of social justice and guided by the local Catholic Church, specifically, its mission of being the "Church of the Poor". It successfully lobbied at the *Sangguniang Panlalawigan* or the Provincial Assembly to declare a 50-year large-scale mining moratorium in the entire island through legislative enactments by the *Sangguniang Panlalawigan*. It also successfully lobbied to remove the San Antonio Copper Project from the national government's list of priority mining areas (Magalang 2010, p. 73).

MaCEC began as a Basic Ecclesial Community that grew stronger over time. The BEC members had reached a more sophisticated level of conscientization and organizing. They wanted to address more fundamental issues confronting their precarious life like the security of land/housing tenure and disaster risk engaging the community (Holden et al. 2017, p. 41). Over the years, long-time members have begun to deepen their ecological consciousness, as evident in expanding their environmental education courses to include the rights of nature, *Kalayaan ng Kalikasan* (freedom of nature), and, following Pope Francis, care for our common home, Earth.

In the Philippines, Christianity came through colonization. This sobering truth has led to more disquieting reflections in recent years on the many ways religion sustains epistemic violence by those in power. The presence of Christianity in the Philippines is always problematic from a postcolonial perspective. The Philippine Catholic Church has tried to address this problem. Karl Gaspar cited the 2010 Episcopal Commission on Indigenous Peoples' statement that essentially asks for forgiveness from indigenous peoples for the "historical wounds" that were inflicted for the time when "[the Church] entered indigenous communities from a position of power, indifferent to their struggles and pains. We ask forgiveness for moments when we taught Christianity as a religion robed with colonial cultural superiority, instead of sharing it as a religion that calls for a relationship with God and a way of life" (Gaspar 2010). Like the other pastoral letters or messages, the concrete calls to action are localized through the endeavors that directly impact vulnerable communities, such as MaCEC.

4.1. The Three Dimensions of Ecological Care

In 2017, MaCEC updated its logo that captured the essence of the organization. MaCEC patterns the evaluation of the stages of village chapters, from formation to maturity, after the four stages of development of a butterfly, namely: egg, larva, pupa, and adult. The butterfly hovering above the heart-shaped Marinduque is a symbol in the official logo of MaCEC. Figure 3 presents the ecological ethic of care and its three features.

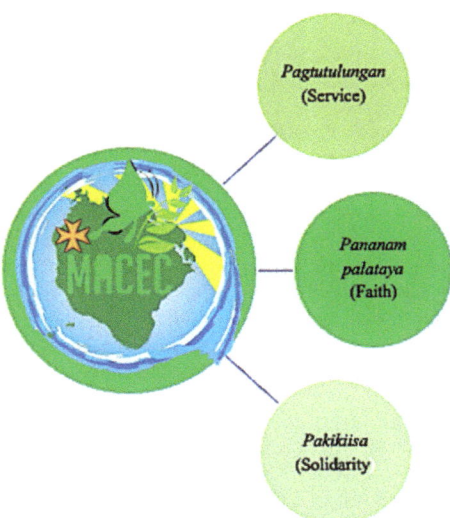

Figure 3. The conceptual framework of ecological care.

The new organization logo adopted in 2017 has some elements: The green heart in the blue circle symbolizes the island province, the home of all those living in its ecological communities. The six rays of the sun represent the six towns where local chapters are located and reflect light and hope to the members and all Marinduque, especially the poor, living in the present and the future. Circling white and blue colors refer to the cleanliness and clarity of its ecological vision and mission for caring and protecting God's creation, based on the principles of social justice. The butterfly resting on a green stem is likened to the clean, healthy, and bountiful ecosystem and life support that reminds the organization of its mandate to care for God's creations and of the challenge to protect, cultivate, and restore the damaged ecosystem to health.

The parallelism between the butterfly and MaCEC cannot be more evident. As the pupa emerges from the cocoon, it faces several challenges that it must overcome to progress into an adult butterfly. The butterfly lives precariously and, like the pupa, must learn to navigate the world it inhabits to be healthy enough to lay eggs. Additionally, the cycle continues.

The use of nature imagery to describe the journey of the village chapters manifests the full ecological consciousness of the members that displaces human superiority and affirms the value of the natural process. Like fireflies, they are reflections of a healthy ecosystem for the members. Robyn Eckersley (1992) puts the basic tenets of ecocentrism based on an ecologically informed philosophy of internal relatedness. All organisms are not simply interrelated with their environment but are also constituted by those environmental interrelationships. Like the butterfly, the life cycle of village chapters undergoes the organic process towards maturity.

While most of the work that MaCEC is doing is gardening, tree-planting, and cultivating land to be a viable source of food for its members and the people of Marinduque in general, MaCEC did not use the image of a gardener or a resource management officer to describe what it does. From an ecocentric perspective, singling out only our unique attributes as a basis of our exclusive moral considerability is simply human chauvinism that conveniently fails to recognize the unique characteristics of other life forms. The use of nature imagery to capture what the organization, at its core, does, is ecocentric.

4.2. To Care Is to Be Human in the Complex Web of Creation

For MaCEC members, the cultural values are *pagtutulungan* (service to one another), *pakikiisa* (solidarity), and *pananampalataya* (faith). Humans undoubtedly do activities above, but they do not necessarily point to human exceptionalism or superiority. The lived experiences of the MaCEC members gave rise to the cultural values that guide their work and reflect their mission.

Pagtutulungan or service to others. Several Filipino scholars point to *pagtutulungan* or service to others as a Filipino value akin to a similar value, *Bayanihan*. For Eade and Su (2018, p. 334), *Bayanihan* is the Filipino principle of mutual effort. *Bayanihan* was a term that originated in farming communities. It worked within the rhythm of harvests and the weather and was based upon common expectations, benefits, and trust (Eade and Su 2018, p. 342). *Bayanihan* is translated to helping each other in a time of crisis (Soriano et al. 2021, p. 91). In the studies cited above, *Bayanihan* reveals uneven power dynamics. The more desperate for help and assistance become dependent on the dole-outs of those who control the goods and services, often local and national leaders, aid and grant agencies, and wealthy individuals in the wake of the devastating damage due to typhoon Haiyan in 2013 (Eade and Su 2018, p. 334). *Bayanihan* is especially important amongst poor communities lacking other forms of capital (Jocson and Ceballo 2020). In the context of digital labor in the platform economy, those who dispense advice become social media influencers who attract desperate subscribers eager to participate in a largely unregulated industry (Soriano et al. 2021).

Pagtutulungan, literally translated to "helping one another", points to a more egalitarian relationship among participants, who are either the donor or recipient and vice versa. *Pagtutulungan* underscores the members' affinity to each other as all of them experienced the ill effects of various environmental disasters in one form or the other. Each of them faces the dangers and risks together. Based on the interviews and documents review, abandoned and unmaintained mine structures, including the open pit and dams of the closed mining site, are a source of disaster risks in the entire province. MaCEC leaders pointed to interconnected environmental and climate change risks for the island province, mainly coastal and riverside communities. While MaCEC members believe that people and communities in the island province can recover, the process takes time. *Pagtutulungan* highlights the eco-anxieties (McCarroll 2020) that environmental activists feel due to the seemingly slow-moving pace of ecological rehabilitation while living under the constant threat of *panganib* or danger. However, helping one another overcome despair is one of the ways that help sustain their energy and commitment.

Pagtutulungan parallels the dynamics in the ecosystems of the planet. Ecologists point to the mutual interdependence at play because the environment is both dynamic and diverse, ecologists recognize that there is no single set of ecological attributes or strategies that make an organism "the best". All living populations and species continuously change in response to pressures from other organisms and variability in Earth's geology and climate. Over time, this dance of evolving interactions has produced a fantastic array of organisms that depend upon and compete across the surface of the planet (Malmstrom 2010, p. 88).

Pakikiisa or solidarity. *Pakikiisa* or solidarity is a common feature in Philippine social movements that address social and political inequalities in society. At the community level, women workers in the informal economy, when organized and galvanized through collective forms of action in peri-urban areas stricken by disasters related to climate change, produce and sustainable ways of surviving and adapting (Ofreneo and Hega 2016, p. 180). There is a strong link between poverty and environmental degradation in the climate crisis, making poor people more vulnerable to climate-change-related disasters (Holden et al. 2017, p. 8). *Pakikiisa* or solidarity occurs when there are shared experiences among the actors, such as the case of women workers above and the members of MaCEC.

Pakikiisa or solidarity highlights relational ethics more than the individualistic ethics that have long governed how we relate to other people. In the ecological sense, solidarity "means a relationship of care and concern for the Other. The Other can be fellow human beings and the natural environment. We should correct the tendency to see humans as ontologically separate and above nature" (Jennings 2015, p. 6). Thompson et. al echo the same sentiment:

"When we come together to study environmental issues and concerns and work together to find viable and sustainable solutions to the problem, we can support one another. What will emerge from the connection and support is an ecological ethic of solidarity, which mirrors the interconnectivity and reciprocal interdependence of beings in the world" (Thompson et al. 2011, p. 144).

The coming together to support each other is evident in MaCEC's core values of environmental advocacy, environmental literacy, and environmental education towards what they termed "ecological care".

Households, particularly in riverside barangays, use bamboo materials for disaster preparedness as a native life raft (*timbulan ng buhay*) like the image above in Figure 4. *Timbulan* or a bamboo raft is a lifesaving device that you hold onto when you are in the middle of the sea, ocean, lake, or river.

Pakikiisa resonates with what Jennings and Gwiazdon call "The Principle of Solidarity Respect and Equity" that should be pursued with a recognition of the limits of everyone's ability to determine the conditions of their own lives and our mutual interdependency and reliance on outside support, care, and assistance. The notion of solidarity and interdependence applies in a social context among individuals and groups. Still, it applies with equal importance and resonance in an ecological context, between human and biotic communities (Jennings and Gwiazdon 2021, p. 32).

Pananampalataya or faith. The spiritual aspect of the work of MaCEC is a crucial part of the organization's identity. *Pananampalataya*, or faith for MaCEC members, informs and motivates them to engage in their work as environmental stewards actively and sustains them in the protracted struggle to obtain justice from the Marcopper Mining Corporation. Rooted in their beginnings as a small Basic Ecclesial Community, MaCEC developed a more comprehensive program to share the Word of God to village chapters. The program, *Hangkaan at Bahaginan ng Pamayanang Kristiyano sa Salita ng Diyos* (Sharing of the Word of God among Christian Communities) helps spread the Word of God.

In the development of course modules, the knowledge of priests and pastoral workers, and seminarians of the diocese were pooled together, according to the members. The organization tapped local facilitators and resource persons to implement the integrated formation and skills development, including relevant modules in environmental justice and stewardship. Until recently, this combined formation is being applied and updated by the MACEC to cover timely issues. The ecological dimension of the program aims to develop environmental consciousness and values by eliciting actions from the members themselves that will encourage sustained commitment. Activities were about community organizing and holding a series and continuing education using modules such as understanding spiritual ecology and links to climate change, mining, health (as a response to the pandemic), and digital security related to the proliferation of misinformation and "fake news" in social media.

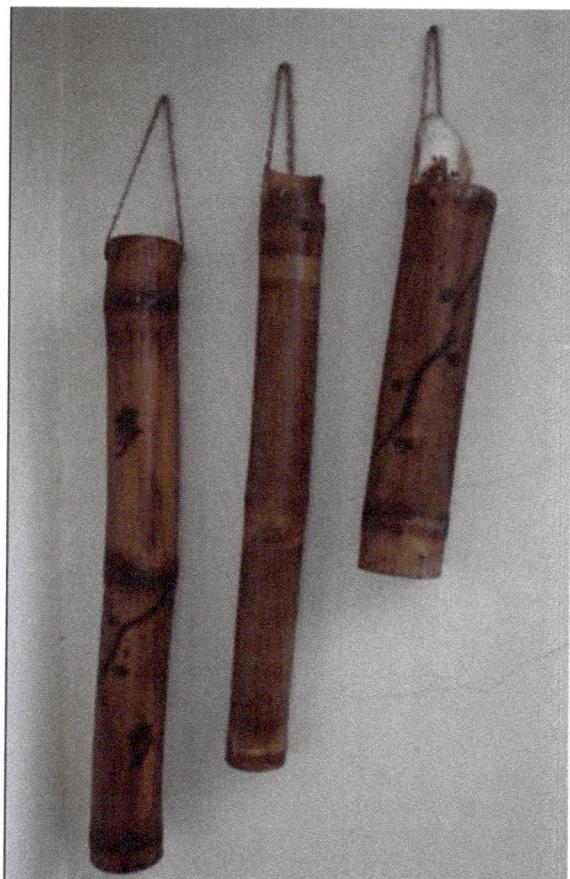

Figure 4. A sample of the bamboo raft used by families. Photo by the author.

Hand and Crowe (2012, p. 11) observe that in the US, greater exposure to church culture (through attendance), greater commitment to personal piety (through prayer), and a greater commitment to one's denominational identity does not generally increase pro-environmental beliefs and behavior. For Ramon Echica (2010, pp. 44–45), the devotional practices heavily promoted by the Catholic Church in the Philippines tend to focus on the "other-worldly" concerns and are apolitical. Both studies suggest that without widespread support from the public, including local government, non-government organizations, and other citizen-driven ecological movements, religiosity alone is not enough to elicit behavioral changes towards environmental action. MACEC has proved that faith and religiosity must intertwine with culture and environmentalism to effect meaningful and sustainable social transformation.

4.3. Greening the Moriones Festival

Marinduque is known for its Holy Week event, the *Moriones* festival. The original ritual would have male volunteers from the poorest *barrios* in Marinduque wear the costume of Roman soldiers and put on elaborate masks for one week to depict the *morions* who chased the Roman soldier, Longinus. In the Lenten rituals, Longinus was the first Roman soldier who converted to Christianity when he witnessed the death of Jesus on the cross

(Peterson 2007). According to Peterson, the men chose to enact *moriones* as a response to a *panata* (vow) to purge their sins. The *morion* mask, a symbol of repentance during the Holy Week, becomes a symbol for the MaCEC and its members. It reminds them of the challenges of being faithful to God (Peterson 2007, p. 311).

The Boac river, a victim of the mine tailings disaster, silently witnesses the Holy Week events as they unfold beside it. The presence, and the symbolic participation of the river, added to the lamentation of the members of MaCEC. Nonetheless, they managed to make the river into an active participant. According to the members, the *Moriones* Festival becomes a venue for commemorating the mine tailings spills on 24 March 1996 through Earth Day celebration, tree planting, Lenten recollection, and other environmental advocacy activities. Reflections of the members focus on the responsibility, rooted in faith, to be stewards of the environment, nature, and creation.

5. Conclusions: Ecological Care beyond Anthropocentrism

The heart-shaped island province of Marinduque is home to the members of MaCEC. In Filipino, the word *tahanan* refers to home. Its root word is *tahan* (hush). It evokes a mother rocking her fussy, crying baby to calm down and sleep. It pulls forth the original meaning of ecology, *Oikos*, a Greek word for home. Many Filipinos regard the home as the safest place as it evokes the warm embrace of a mother. Filipino psychologists have attempted to seek what they call cognitive and affective dimensions of biodiversity, which, according to them, have been lacking in many social and scientific studies on biodiversity conservation (Tan Siy 2008). In a study involving Filipino farmers and fisherfolks living on the banks of ecologically vulnerable Taal Lake in the southern part of Manila, Tan Siy claims that those who lived by the banks of the lake were more open and receptive to its rehabilitation and care. The results of this study highlighted the significant role people's affective bonds placed on the conservation and the protection of the lake. Moreover, the quality of respondents' answers was a function of their proximity to and dependence on the lake (Tan Siy 2008, p. 98).

Similarly, the members of MaCEC are deeply committed to their environmentalism, living as they do in a disaster-prone area and having experienced environmental disasters brought about by natural hazards and extractive industries. Their environmentalism developed into a community consciousness that regards members as thoroughly embedded in their ecological communities. Such is akin to Eckersley's (1992) ecocentric approach to environmentalism that views creations as formed by ecological interrelatedness.

Ecological care's dimensions of *pagtutulungan* (service to one another), *pakikiisa* (solidarity), and *pananampalataya* (faith) demonstrate its breadth and depth that includes "a recognition of systemic interdependence that means recognizing that self is deeply related to other, not just other human selves, but the natural world (water, air, other species) that impact our lives and whose lives and actions profoundly impact processes" (Bradbury 2003, p. 211).

Reflecting on the notion of ecological care of the members of MaCEC, we can appreciate this view of care as Christian praxis. Praxis refers to reflecting and acting upon and within the world to transform it. McFague (1997) challenges Christians to extend the Christian praxis to nature. Christian praxis is grounded in what Leonardo Boff calls "social ecology, the ways that human social and economic systems interact with the natural ecosystems" (Boff 1995, p. 88). This ecology underscores that whatever onslaught to the poor affects the natural world and vice versa.

Through the various stages of development, faith-based communities of environmental stewards actively participate in determining their role in ecological care and stewardship and transforming structures that cause inequalities. As MaCEC members subscribe to service to *Simbahan ng mga dukha* (Church of the Poor) and *likas-kayang pag-unlad* (sustainable development), the organization exemplifies a practical application of the ecological liberation theology, as advanced in Holden et al. (2017).

While the praxis of MaCEC members echoes that of liberation theology, it arises from their self-understanding of faith intertwining with service. According to the MaCEC members, the extended hands of Jesus on the cross signify service and solidarity; the hands of Jesus are reaching out to help. According to the organization and its members, the cross symbolizes the Christian faith in which all actions on ecological care are rooted. The organization's vision aptly reflects the values of service, solidarity, and faith ingrained in the local culture. In turn, these values contribute to the discourse McCarroll (2020) raises towards a re-imagining of ecological care that extends beyond anthropocentrism without losing the focus on social and environmental justice. Ecological care beyond anthropocentrism encompasses human activities that attend to the needs of the ecological community, promote its wellbeing and health, and work for the flourishing of all members of the ecological community. Those who extend ecological care beyond anthropocentrism recognize that ecosystems thrive and flourish when suitable conditions are present for everyone, including humans to be healthy. The research supports the continuing discussions on the many ways religion's commitment to ecological care reveals its promising potential, primarily the pro-environmental actions of faith-based communities.

Author Contributions: Conceptualization, J.C.P.; methodology, R.B.M.Q.; formal analysis, J.C.P. and R.B.M.Q.; investigation, J.C.P. and R.B.M.Q.; resources, J.C.P. and R.B.M.Q.; data curation, writing—original draft preparation, J.C.P.; writing—review and editing, R.B.M.Q. All authors have read and agreed to the published version of the manuscript.

Funding: This research received no external funding.

Institutional Review Board Statement: Not applicable.

Informed Consent Statement: Written informed consent has been obtained from all subjects involved in this study.

Acknowledgments: The authors acknowledge the support of the Institute for the Advanced Study of Asian Cultures and Theologies (IASACT) Program of the United Board for Christian Higher Education (UBCHEA) and the Chung Chi Divinity College, The Chinese University of Hong Kong. We acknowledge the support of the leaders and members of Marinduque Council for Environmental Concerns (MaCEC). We are grateful to our anonymous peer reviewers for their insightful and constructive comments that made the manuscript better and richer.

Conflicts of Interest: The authors declare no conflict of interest.

References

Beever, Jonathan. 2018. Anthropocentrism in the Anthropocene. In *Encyclopedia of the Anthropocene*. Edited by Dominick A. Dellasala and Michael I. Goldstein. Amsterdam: Elsevier, pp. 39–44. [CrossRef]

Boff, Leonardo. 1995. *Ecology and Liberation: A New Paradigm*. Maryknoll: Orbis Books.

Bradbury, Hillary. 2003. Sustaining the Heart of Action Research(ers): An Interview with Joanna Macy. *Action Research* 1: 208–23. [CrossRef]

Canceran, Delfo. 2018. Climate Justice: The Cry of the Earth, the Cry of the Poor (The Case of the Yolanda/Hayain Tragedy in the Philippines). *Solidarity: The Journal of Catholic Social Thought and Secular Ethics* 8: 1.

Catholic Bishops Conference of the Philippines (CBCP). 2019. An Urgent Call for Ecological Conversion, Hope in the Face of Climate Emergency. July 16. Available online: https://cbcponline.net/an-urgent-call-for-ecological-conversion-hope-in-the-face-of-climate-emergency/ (accessed on 4 December 2021).

CCS, MaCEC, and SAC-Northern Quezon. 2011. *Voyage to Disaster Resilience in Small Islands: A Guide for Local Leaders*; Quezon City: Christian Aid. Available online: https://www.dilg.gov.ph/PDF_File/reports_resources/DILG-Resources-2012112-2a91abbcac.pdf (accessed on 4 December 2021).

Cruz, John Kenneth, Jaime Baquiran Jr., John Kenneth Suan, and Imee Bren Villalba. 2020. Project Daluyan: Water quality, hydrology, and hydraulic analyses of Boac River, Marinduque. In *University of the Philippines College of Engineering Technical Bulletin: Professorial Chair and Teaching and Research Grant Award Book of Abstracts*. Available online: https://anyflip.com/aaerp/imee/basic (accessed on 8 December 2021).

Dagmang, Ferdinand. 2015. From Vatican II to PCP II to BEC Too: Progressive Localization of a New State of Mind to the New State of Affairs. In *Revisiting Vatican II 50 Years of Renewal Volume II: Selected Papers of the DVK International Conference on Vatican II (31 January–3 February 2013*. Edited by Shaji George Kochuthara. Bangalore: Dharmaram Publications, pp. 308–26.

Department of Natural Resources (DENR). 2020. Cimatu Vows to Restore Marinduque Rivers Hit by Marcopper Disaster. March 2. Available online: https://denr.gov.ph/index.php/news-events/press-releases/1467-cimatu-vows-to-restore-marinduque-rivers-hit-by-marcopper-disaster (accessed on 24 November 2020).

Dizon, Nikko. 2019. *The Marcopper Disaster: A Tragedy that Continues in People's Veins*. April 3, Available online: https://verafiles.org/articles/marcopper-disaster-tragedy-continues-peoples-veins (accessed on 29 November 2021).

Eade, Pauline, and Yvonne Su. 2018. Post-Disaster Social Capital: Trust, Equity, and Typhoon Yolanda. *Disaster Prevention and Management* 27: 334–45. [CrossRef]

Eballo, Arvin. 2018. Contextualizing Laudato Si' through People's Organization Engagement: A Kalawakan Experience. *Solidarity: The Journal of Catholic Social Thought and Secular Ethics* 8: 2.

Echica, Ramon. 2010. The Political Context of the Infancy Narratives and the Apolitical Devotion to Santo Nino. *Hapag* 7: 37–51. [CrossRef]

Eckersley, Robyn. 1992. *Environmentalism and Political Theory: Toward an Ecocentric Approach*. New York: SUNY.

Formilleza, Sammie P. 2010. Reflections on Building Disaster-Resilient Communities Case Study in Marinduque. In *Building-Disaster-Resilient Communities: Stories and Lessons from The Philippines*. Edited by Lenore Polotan-Dela Cruz, Elmer Ferrer and Maureen Pagaduan. Quezon City: CSWCD-UP, pp. 91–95.

Francis, Pope. 2015. *Laudato Si: Encyclical Letter of the Holy Father Francis on Care for our Common Home*. Pasay City: Paulines Publishing House.

Gaspar, Karl. 2010. The Story Behind the Indigenous Peoples' Sunday. *MindaNews*. Available online: https://www.mindanews.com/around-mindanao/2010/10/the-story-behind-the-indigenous-peoples-sunday/ (accessed on 27 December 2021).

Hand, Carl M., and Jessica Crowe. 2012. Examining the Impact of Religion on Environmentalism 1993–2010: Has the Religious Environmental Movement Made a Difference? *Electronic Green Journal* 1: 1–15. [CrossRef]

Holden, William. 2012. Ecclesial Opposition to Large-Scale Mining on Samar: Neoliberalism Meets the Church of the Poor in a Wounded Land. *Religions* 3: 833–61. [CrossRef]

Holden, William, Kathleen Nadeau, and Emma Porio. 2017. *Ecological Liberation Theology: Faith-Based Approaches to Poverty and Climate Change in the Philippines*. Cham: Springer.

Jennings, Bruce. 2015. Ecological Solidarity. *Minding Nature* 8: 4–10.

Jennings, Bruce, and Kathryn Gwiazdon. 2021. Water and Ecological Ethics in the Anthropocene. In *Ethical Water Stewardship, Water Security in a New World*. Edited by Ingrid L. Stefanovic and Zafar Adeel. Cham: Springer Nature, pp. 23–41. [CrossRef]

Jocson, Rosanne, and Rosario Ceballo. 2020. Resilience in Low-Income Filipino Mothers Exposed to Community Violence: Religiosity and Familism as Protective Factors. *Psychology Violence* 10: 8–17. [CrossRef]

Magalang, Miguel R. 2010. Mainstreaming Disaster Risk Reduction and Climate Change Adaptation in Mandatory Planning and Budgeting Processes of Barangays: A Case Study on Building Disaster-Resilient Communities in Marinduque. In *Building-Disaster-Resilient Communities: Stories and Lessons from The Philippines*. Edited by Lenore Polotan-Dela Cruz, Elmer Ferrer and Maureen Pagaduan. Quezon City: CSWCD-UP.

Malmstrom, Carolyn. 2010. Ecologists Study the Interactions of Organisms and Their Environment. *Nature Education Knowledge* 3: 88.

Maphill. 2011. Location Map of Marinduque, Philippines. Available online: http://www.maphill.com/philippines/region-4/marinduque/location-maps/physical-map/ (accessed on 27 December 2021).

Marinduque Council for Environmental Concerns (MaCEC). 2021. MaCEC Press Release: Pananawagan at Panindigan ng mga Marindukueno sa ika-25 taong Anibersaryo. Available online: https://www.alyansatigilmina.net/single-post/macec-press-release-pananawagan-at-panindigan-ng-mga-marindukueno-sa-ika-25-taong-anibersaryo (accessed on 3 December 2021).

McCarroll, Pamela R. 2020. Listening for the Cries of the Earth: Practical Theology in the Anthropocene. *International Journal of Practical Theology* 24: 29–46. [CrossRef]

McFague, Sally. 1997. *Super, Natural Christians: How We Should Love Nature*. Philadelphia: Fortress Press.

Ofreneo, Rosalinda Pineda, and Mylene D. Hega. 2016. Women's Solidarity Economy Initiatives to Strengthen Food Security in Response to Disasters: Insights from Two Philippine Case Studies. *Disaster Prevention and Management* 25: 168–82. [CrossRef]

Peracullo, Jeane. 2020. The Virgin of the Vulnerable Lake: Catholic Engagement with Climate Change in the Philippines. *Religions* 11: 203. [CrossRef]

Peterson, William. 2007. Holy Week in the "Heart of the Philippines": Spirituality, Theatre, and Community in Marinduque's Moriones Festival. *Asian Theatre Journal* 24: 309–38. [CrossRef]

Philippine Statistics Authority (PSA). 2020. *Updated Full Year 2018 Official Poverty Statistics of the Philippines*. Quezon City: PSA.

Picardal, Armado. 2013. Conversation with the Catholic Bishops of the Philippines during the Seminar on Spirituality of Stewardship, 22 January 2013. Available online: http://amadopicardal.blogspot.com/2013/01/seminar-on-spirituality-of-stewardship.html (accessed on 3 December 2021).

Province of Marinduque. 2011. *Provincial Disaster Risk Reduction and Management Plan 2011–19*. Marinduque: The Provincial Government of Marinduque.

Quindoza, Rosa Bella. 2015. Making Local Voices Heard: Collective Advocacy and Action in Local Disaster Management. Paper presented at The International Conference on Researches on Disasters in Asia, Tagbilaran, Bohol, January 20–21.

Sachs, Wolfgang. 2017. The Sustainable Development Goals and Laudato Si': Varieties of Post-Development? *Third World Quarterly* 38: 2573–87. [CrossRef]

Salvacion, Arnold R., and Damasa B. Magcale-Macandog. 2015. Spatial Analysis of Human Population Distribution and Growth in Marinduque Island, Philippines. *Journal of Marine and Island Cultures* 4: 27–33. [CrossRef]

Soriano, Cheryll Ruth, Earvin Charles Cabalquinto, and Joy Hannah Panaligan. 2021. Performing "Digital Labor Bayanihan": Strategies of Influence and Survival in the Platform Economy. *Sociologias* 23: 84–111. [CrossRef]

Tan Siy, Sherilyn. 2008. Cognitive and Affective Dimensions of Biodiversity Conservation. *Philippine Journal of Psychology* 41: 79–101.

Thompson, John D., Raphaël Mathevet, Olivia Delanoë, Chantal Gil-Fourrier, Marie Bonnin, and Marc Cheylan. 2011. Ecological solidarity as a Conceptual Tool for Rethinking Ecological and Social Interdependence in Conservation Policy for Protected Areas and their Surrounding Landscape. *Comptes Rendus Biologies* 334: 412–19. [CrossRef]

Tuazon, Rolando. 2018. Becoming Stewards of Creation: Ecological Virtue Ethics from the Perspective of Otherness. In *Fragile World: Ecology and the Church*. Edited by William Cavanaugh Eugene. Oregon: Cascade Books, pp. 192–209.

United Nations General Assembly (UNGA). 2017. Report of the Open-Ended Intergovernmental Expert Working Group on Indicators and Terminology Relating to Disaster Risk Reduction. Available online: https://www.preventionweb.net/files/50683_oiewgreportenglish.pdf (accessed on 14 August 2021).

United Nations International Strategy for Disaster Reduction (UNISDR). 2009. *Terminology on Disaster Risk Reduction*. Geneva: UNISDR, Available online: http://www.unisdr.org/files/7817_UNISDRTerminologyEnglish.pdf (accessed on 14 August 2021).

United Nations International Strategy for Disaster Reduction (UNISDR). 2017. UNISDR Strategic Framework 2016–2021. Available online: https://www.undrr.org/publication/unisdr-strategic-framework-2016-2021 (accessed on 3 December 2021).

UP Planning and Development Research Foundation (UP PLANADES). 1999. *Boac Rehabilitation Options: Cost-Benefit Analysis*. Quezon City: UP PLANADES.

White, Lynn. 1967. The Historical Roots of the Environmental Crisis. *Science* 155: 1203–7. [CrossRef] [PubMed]

Wickman, Matthew, and Jacob Sherman. 2020. Introduction: Faith after the Anthropocene. *Religions* 11: 378. [CrossRef]

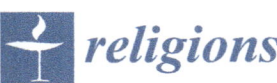

Article

Who Is My Neighbor? Developing a Pedagogical Tool for Teaching Environmental Preaching and Ethics in Online and Hybrid Courses

Leah D. Schade

Lexington Theological Seminary, Lexington, KY 40503, USA; lschade@lextheo.edu

Abstract: As theological education has moved increasingly to online and hybrid settings (both by choice and by pandemic necessity), practical theologians committed to teaching ecological theological education must navigate a paradox. How do we teach about interconnectivity and interdependence between the human and other-than-human inhabitants of a particular place when our classrooms are in disembodied digital spaces? This article examines a case study of a pedagogical tool developed by the author called the "Who Is My Neighbor" Mapping Exercise that enables students to explore and articulate how they conceptualize themselves and their faith communities embedded within their larger ecological contexts. This paper assesses the use of the mapping exercise in four different course contexts: three online and one hybrid online–immersion course. The author provides an overview of each of the four course contexts in which the tool was used, includes descriptions of how students engaged the tool, and assesses its effectiveness. The author uses three types of criteria for assessment of the pedagogical exercise: student feedback, level of competence demonstrated in student assignments (sermons, worship services, teaching events), and personal observations, particularly around the differences between online and onsite contexts. The author suggests that the mapping exercise is a tool that can be used by others teaching practical theology to help students understand their relationships within Creation and their communities, critically engage environmental justice issues, and apply what they learn to their ministry contexts.

Keywords: ecological theology; environmental ethics; environmental justice; homiletics; preaching; online teaching; pedagogy; practical theology

Citation: Schade, Leah D.. 2022. Who Is My Neighbor? Developing a Pedagogical Tool for Teaching Environmental Preaching and Ethics in Online and Hybrid Courses. *Religions* 13: 322. https://doi.org/10.3390/rel13040322

Academic Editors: Pamela R. McCarroll and HyeRan Kim-Cragg

Received: 18 February 2022
Accepted: 29 March 2022
Published: 3 April 2022

Publisher's Note: MDPI stays neutral with regard to jurisdictional claims in published maps and institutional affiliations.

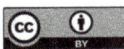

Copyright: © 2022 by the author. Licensee MDPI, Basel, Switzerland. This article is an open access article distributed under the terms and conditions of the Creative Commons Attribution (CC BY) license (https://creativecommons.org/licenses/by/4.0/).

1. Introduction

As a mainline Protestant homiletician with a passion for environmental issues, I have dedicated a great deal of my teaching, preaching, and writing to equip clergy for "greening" their preaching. A main tenet of my book, *Creation-Crisis Preaching*, is that preachers have a key role to play in helping congregations understand environmental issues as a matter of faith and moral/ethical obligation. However, in my research studying clergy attitudes and opinions around social issues and preaching, I have learned that pastors are sometimes hesitant to address issues such as climate change or species extinction in their sermons. For example, in a 2017 survey of mainline Protestant clergy in the U.S., I learned that environmental issues ranked among the lowest priorities for preachers to address. Only 30% of the 838 respondents said that they had mentioned environmental issues in their sermons in the previous twelve months (Schade 2017). Fortunately, that number rose to 47% when my team and I conducted the second survey wave with 2099 respondents in 2021 (Schade et al. 2021). Nevertheless, this still means that, by their own admission, more than half of the U.S. clergy who responded to this survey are not speaking about climate or environmental issues.

Given the acceleration and intensity of the numerous climate and environmental crises that are devastating communities, one might think that clergy would be willing to bring a prophetic and pastoral word about these issues to their congregations. As Fletcher Harper, executive director of GreenFaith, has written, "The world needs religious voices that clearly name the causes of this dire crisis, articulate a moral vision, and catalyze courageous action to meet the suffering that lies ahead while bending history's arc towards justice" (Harper 2021). Yet, a number of factors have contributed to the relative silence on environmental issues from the pulpit, including the politicization of topics such as climate change and fossil fuel extraction, as well as the negative pushback that clergy receive for being a "political" preacher when they address such issues.[1]

However, I have also found that many preachers and seminarians simply do not know *how* to bring biblical and theological language to environmental topics and to do so in a way that does not alienate or anger their congregations. Therefore, I have tried to design seminary courses that help students develop an environmentally literate approach to preaching, worship, and faith formation. Yet, as a professor whose courses are either online or hybrid, I recognize that there are challenges to this work when our classrooms are in disembodied digital spaces. So, I have experimented with pedagogical approaches to help students grasp the concepts of interconnectivity and interdependence between the human and other-than-human world.

To that end, this article examines a case study about the use of a pedagogical tool I developed called the "Who Is My Neighbor" Mapping Exercise. This tool is designed to help students explore and articulate how they conceptualize themselves and their congregations embedded within their larger ecological contexts and to share their insights through preaching, leading worship, or teaching in their faith community. I will provide an overview of each of the four course contexts in which I used the tool, include descriptions of how students engaged the tool, and assess its effectiveness. I will use three types of criteria for assessment of the pedagogical exercise: student feedback, level of competence demonstrated in student assignments, and my own observations, particularly around the differences between online and onsite contexts. I suggest that the "Who Is My Neighbor" Mapping Exercise is a tool that can be used by others teaching practical theology courses to help students understand their relationships within Creation and their communities, critically engage environmental justice issues, and apply what they learn to their ministry contexts.

2. The Need for Place-Based Ecological Education in Theological Studies

Taylor Tollison has noted that interest in "place-based" education is growing within academia (referencing Ark et al. 2020; Knapp 2014; Morris 2014; Sobel 2004). "In conjunction with this emphasis on place, many institutions are now highlighting not only the ways in which we should learn *from* or *about* a place, but also the ways in which we should learn *for* a place" (Tollison 2021, p. 3). How students and institutions are "embedded" within their communities and ecological contexts has implications not just for the institutions in which they learn, but for their formation as ministers or religious leaders in whatever contexts they serve. How might students "learn *from* the places in which they are embedded in order to learn *for* the places they are embedded?" (Ibid, p. 7).

These are questions I asked when I first began teaching environmental ethics in onsite classrooms. In those settings, I had the opportunity to take students outside to think about their embeddedness and interconnectedness with nature. I used an exercise described by Mark Wallace in his book, *Finding God in the Singing River*, called the Council of All Beings. In this activity, he takes students to a natural area and invites them to seek a connection with one of the lifeforms there. After spending significant time observing, listening, and communing with this lifeform, the group comes back together and shares what they learned by speaking as the lifeform itself. "The purpose of a Council," he explains, "is to foster compassion for all life-forms and heal the ugly splits that separate human beings from the natural world (Wallace 2005, p. 138).

Such imaginative speaking "for" and "with" other-than-human beings can have intriguing implications for preaching, leading worship, and faith formation from an ecological perspective. I have used this exercise for retreats and onsite classes, and it has yielded insights for participants to integrate into their sermons and their personal relationship with Creation. However, for students in an online classroom, there is no option to be together in one place in nature at the same time. Moreover, unless the Council of All Beings is conducted in the place where a student is engaged in ministry, the exercise is removed from their own context.

So, I wanted to develop a tool to help students root themselves in their own context and create a presentation that they could share both with the class and with their congregation. This would allow students in the digital course to articulate a "theology of place" (Inge 2003) rather than being relegated to a sterile classroom removed from their context. I envisioned an exercise that would enable both instructor and students to traverse digital and local spaces with an eye toward identifying ecojustice issues to address with their congregations. Ideally, such a tool would create a means by which students engaged in distance learning could experience embeddedness and a theology of place within their ecological contexts and then share that through sermons, worship services, and teaching events. I call this tool the "Who Is My Neighbor" Mapping Exercise.

3. Developing the "Who Is My Neighbor" Mapping Exercise

I originally developed the "Who Is My Neighbor" Mapping Exercise for preachers to use in their sermon preparation and in ministry with congregants to help them expand the notion of "neighbor" to include other-than-human beings. The goal was to enlarge a preacher's and congregation's circle of care to include other-than-human "persons" who suffer and languish because of environmental injustice. I wanted to give them a tool to survey their landscapes and expand the concept of neighbor to include our Earth-kin so that they could determine what issues need to be addressed in their congregations and communities. I also wanted draw on a biblical story to help frame this work as part of Jesus's mandate to care for those on the margins of our human society, regardless of barriers we might initially put in place.

I chose Luke 10: 25–37 (NRSV) which includes a lawyer's question to Jesus that prompts the parable known as "The Good Samaritan." The lawyer asks what he must do to inherit eternal life. Jesus answers with a question, "What is written in the law? What do you read there?" The lawyer replies by quoting the Torah: Love the Lord your God with all your heart, soul, strength, and mind; and love your neighbor as yourself. But after Jesus affirms his answer, the lawyer follows with a rejoinder: "And who is my neighbor?" Jesus responds with a parable about a Samaritan taking care of a beaten man when two others had ignored him. Jesus then asks, "Which of these three, do you think, was a neighbor to the man who fell into the hands of the robbers?" The lawyer replies, "The one who showed him mercy." The passage ends with Jesus instructing the man to "Go and do likewise."

As I explain in *Creation-Crisis Preaching*, "It is not the qualifications of the one who suffers that determine who should be considered 'neighbor.' It is the one who chooses to care who makes herself or himself a neighbor. In other words, 'neighborness' is not initiated by the one in need of care. It is determined by the one choosing to act in a caring way toward another" (Schade 2015, p. 63). Put another way, the lawyer's question could be restated as, "Who is worthy of my moral consideration? Who qualifies? And who can I justifiably and reasonably exclude?" Jesus turns the question around: "Who will you choose to care about?" In other words, neighborness is not determined by the receiver of compassion, but by the giver. From the Samaritan's perspective, the only qualification for neighborness was the suffering and need of the beaten man. All other lines, walls, hierarchies, and divisions fell away.

Using an ecohermeneutical lens[2] to interpret this passage, I make the case that we must think expansively about the concept of "neighbor" to include our other-than-human kin who, in a sense, lie beaten and bleeding on the side of the road by the "robbers" that have attacked all aspects of Creation. In class discussions, we talk about how we might reconsider this parable about moral obligations within the biotic realm and environmental justice issues. Are animals our neighbors? How about mountains? Ecosystems? The empty lot down the street filled with trash? The microscopic organisms in the stream killed by fracking waste-water? How far down the food chain and how far afield should we go?

This line of questioning spurs them to think about their own context. Who are the ecological neighbors of our congregation that need our attention and a Samaritan's care? How are people, plants, animals, land, and air suffering from human activity right in our own community? And in what ways might a congregation tend to their wounds with the compassion, attention, and the generosity of the Samaritan?

4. Criteria for Determining Eco-Ethical Obligation and Action

Invariably, students raise the thorny question that accompanies all environmental ethics about whether human beings should be prioritized over other lifeforms when it comes to determining moral obligations. As Cynthia Moe Lobeda describes the dilemma:

> Moral consciousness expanded to include the other-than-human is fraught with complexity. To illustrate: ... On what grounds do specific moral values and obligations apply differently to humans than to other-than-humans? What moral constraints ought be placed on human beings in light of our sameness with and dependence upon otherkind? (Moe-Lobeda 2013, p. 125)

In summarizing John Cobb's critique of deep ecology, Mark Wallace puts it this way: "If all beings—everything from megafauna such as human beings and blue whales to microflora such as mold spores and green algae—are sacred, if everything is equal in value and worth, then on what basis can decisions be made about what should be saved and protected and what can be used and destroyed?" (Wallace 2005, p. 150). In other words, without some sort of hierarchy of values, there would be no way to engage in eco-ethical decision making because value would collapse into sameness.

Wallace's approach to determining how we should make decisions about environmental ethics, which I offer to the students, is to ensure "the health and dynamism of the life cycle rather than protect the interests of added-value beings (such as human beings) whose inner life is more complex than other beings. Thus, green spirituality is able to make highly nuanced and sophisticated practical judgments about use and value, but it does so in biocentric rather than anthropocentric terms" (Wallace 2005, p. 151). He adds that judgments about value "should be based on keeping open the living channels of energy that make life possible ... [P]ractical decisions about resource allocations and the like should focus on ensuring the dynamism and vitality of the energy cycle, not on the particular needs of individual participants within the cycle, including the needs of individual human participants" (Ibid, pp. 152–53).

Building on Wallace's holistic focus on the life cycle, I suggest to the students that a key for determining ethical action is to apply the criteria of "the least of these", using the term from Matthew 25: 31–46, Jesus' parable of the "sheep and the goats". The "least of these" refers to those most vulnerable who are in need and have little to no voice or agency in their self-preservation. So, for example, on the human level, pregnant women and children are biologically and historically among the most vulnerable of human beings. Their needs would be prioritized when making environmental decisions about pesticides, mercury emissions from coal-fired power plants, and the use of plastics, for example. Applying the criteria to the biotic cycle, the most basic building blocks of life on a cellular and microbiotic level must be considered, and any activity that threatens them should be avoided. For instance, since fracking for methane gas involves the use of chemicals that kill microscopic life and poison the food chain at its most basic level, it should not be allowed.

Thus, rather than determining the rightness of a human activity from the top down (i.e., those in power protecting and promoting their immediate self-interest, gratification, and profit), we would gauge it from the bottom up. In other words, if it is not good for the children, the fish in the sea, or the microbes in the soil, an inverted pyramid of care dictates that it should not be done. Stated in a positive way, the "least of these" are what Jesus has said we are to protect, so whatever promotes their health and well-being fulfills the divine command of caring for them.[3]

5. "Who Is My Neighbor" Mapping Exercise: Description and Use in the Classroom

In Chapter 3 of *Creation-Crisis Preaching*, I offer practical suggestions and questions for mapping the ecological, social, cultural, and political location of a particular congregation to help preachers better contextualize their sermons. As I developed the tool, I chose activities that would help participants experience themselves and their congregations embodied within a particular ecological context while also seeing ecological issues related to the larger context of other justice issues. The activities and accompanying questions are designed to help participants think in an interconnected way about the ecological, social, cultural, and political location of a particular congregation in order to better contextualize their ministry.

For the course assignment, I ask students to pick six options from numbers 1–12, and then complete number 13 for their project. I encourage them to do this work in collaboration with a group of parishioners if possible so that the student can incorporate more voices and perspectives. Here are the options (Schade 2015, pp. 73–75):

1. **Walk**. Walk the grounds around the church building. Consider your surroundings, which include the land, the plants near you, the air you are breathing, and other living creatures perceptible to your senses. Who are your biotic neighbors? Also consider the houses, buildings, businesses, factories, and other human-made "neighbors." Reflect on the interactions that are occurring between you and these multi-faceted surroundings. Are they harmful? Beneficial? Neutral? How do your natural surroundings affect your physical or spiritual existence? Your feelings? Your values?

2. **Sit**. Choose a location where you can sit and quietly observe and reflect on the interactions that are occurring between you and your multi-faceted surroundings. Allow all of your senses to be engaged as you listen, sniff, and feel the world around you. Where do you perceive harm or pain? What interrelations are beneficial? How do your natural surroundings affect your physical or spiritual existence? Your emotions? Your values?

3. **Look at a topographical map of where the congregation is located.** Google Maps, Google Earth, or other online mapping services are free and can reveal a bird's eye view of your setting. Notice the local waterways and landscape features (mountains, desert, beach, green spaces, etc.). How are they disrupted, connected to, or otherwise intersecting with human civilization?

4. **Look at a map that shows the location of major businesses, industries, landfills, waste processing, etc.** Do some research of the basic demographics of the area (census data, income data, sociological data). In what ways do the major "players" interact and have an impact on each other and the biotic community?

5. **Talk with members of your congregation** to get a sense of "who" (in the expanded ecological sense) their neighbors are, and who has been beaten and lies along side of the road. Who are "the least of these" (Matthew 25: 40) in need of attention and care?

6. **Talk with other clergy** to learn the history of "neighbor-relations" in the community. What stories do they tell about neighbors helping each other (or not)? Do any of them have shared interest in environmental issues so that you may collaborate on preaching ideas?

7. **Talk with community members** to hear their stories about environmental issues that are part of the community's history. Were there any grassroots efforts to clean up blighted areas? Protest pollution? Confront toxic dumping? What was successful? What work remains to be done?

8. **Talk with local health care workers** such as doctors and nurses to find out what the key public health issues affect the community. There are often environmental connections to health concerns. Asthma, obesity, cancer, and depression, for example, are all exacerbated by deleterious environmental conditions such as air pollution, radioactive waste, waste incineration, etc.

9. **Meet with local chapters of environmental groups** such as Sierra Club, Clean Air Council, Interfaith Power and Light, and grassroots activist groups to find out what

environmental issues they are addressing in your community. Ask how local houses of worship can be helpful to their work.
10. **Talk with local naturalists, master gardeners, those who fish, hunters, farmers, beekeepers, or others whose work involves the natural elements**. Ask what changes they have observed in animal, plant, insect, fish, or other biotic communities in the last few decades. What would they like to see happen in terms of protecting or sustaining the health of the local ecosystems?
11. **Search for clean-energy businesses in your community** such as wind farms, solar farms, geothermal companies, etc. Inquire as to how they see their work in relation to the community and the planet.
12. **Meet with your elected officials.** Ask them who they consider "the least of these," those most vulnerable among their constituents. What are their main environmental concerns regarding their watersheds, land, forests, and biotic communities within their jurisdictions? What legislation or policies have they supported or opposed for environmental protection?
13. **Create a "map" of your findings.** This can take the form of an actual map with key features noted, a hand-drawn representation, a collage of photos or images, a video, PowerPoint, or some other kind of visual display of the "neighbors" surrounding your congregation. This can be a collaborative project with youth and adults.

Typically, I give students at least a week to complete the steps they choose from numbers 1–12 and then report on their initial findings through an online discussion board. I instruct students to share two to three insights or "a-ha" moments that came from completing the steps and to name the environmental issue they are considering as the topic for their sermon, worship service, or educational event. For the peer responses, I prompt them to ask questions of each other, give feedback as to what they'd like to learn more about, and to seek clarity about the topic their peer plans to address.

For the final project, I have experimented with requiring simple PowerPoint slides, to allowing a variety of formats such as photos of a visual display, videos, or narrated PowerPoints. Students are also required to write a 500–700-word paper in which they reflect on what was most meaningful for them in this exercise as well as their plan for sharing the project with their congregation. As I will describe in the examples that follow, some students presented their "maps" at educational forums, others wrote and preached a sermon, and still others designed a worship service around the theme from their mapping project.

6. Assessment 1: Lancaster Theological Seminary, Creation-Crisis Preaching Course

The first time I used the "Who Is My Neighbor" Mapping Exercise in an online course was in the fall of 2018 when I taught Creation-Crisis Preaching for Lancaster Theological Seminary as an adjunct instructor. Seven students registered for the five-week course which was online and asynchronous except for one Zoom meeting at the beginning. After completing readings which introduced them to environmental, theological, and biblical foundations for environmental preaching, the students completed the "Who Is My Neighbor" Mapping Exercise as a step toward their final sermon. The sermon was to be based on Luke 10: 25–37 and needed to connect to a local environmental issue of their choice in their community or region. For some students, this was the first time they were challenged to think about environmental issues at all, much less address one in a sermon. So, I provided a list of twenty-six possible topics ranging from air pollution to waste disposal with the option of identifying a different topic in consultation with me.

While each student completed the mapping assignment, most included just a few slides and only completed four or five of the options in the exercise. One student only submitted a topographical map with some scribbled notes. The sermons were average to above average in content and delivery. I shall highlight two examples.

One student was a White female whose church was situated in a small town in central Pennsylvania. In her mapping exercise, she walked around the church and streets of the town, sat to watch the environmental processes happening around her, talked with church members, and learned about a new initiative to restore streams and the health of the local water system. These activities were documented in the PowerPoint she created for the mapping assignment. In her sermon on the parable of the Good Samaritan, she began by talking about the idea of neighbors in a general way while referencing the South African concept of *ubuntu*, meaning "I am, because you are." Then she moved to expand the concept of neighbor to include God's Creation, noting that human beings can only exist because the rest of nature exists. This brought her to the "neighbor" suffering in their own community—the streams that run through their town and surrounding countryside that have been deteriorating due to nitrogen and chemicals from agricultural and yard runoff as well as silt accumulation. She made the case that the example of the Samaritan's extravagant service toward his neighbor urges us to be extravagant in the care we give our water system. She encouraged that care to be collective, systemic, and engaging local policy. However, she did not go as far as encouraging them to attend local meetings and express their support for water restoration projects or to engage in the projects themselves. So, in my feedback to her, I suggested that she offer those next steps to them in future conversations and sermons.

In contrast, another student, who was a Black female, served a church that was located in an urban area of Baltimore, Md. Through her mapping exercise as documented by her PowerPoint, she walked around the neighborhood and took pictures of deteriorating buildings, looked at city maps, talked with local residents and clergy, and educated herself about the effects of lead-based paint on the health of children. Building on the work her church was already doing to address the need for affordable, safe housing for local families, she drew three key points from the Lukan passage on the Good Samaritan: (1) stop (do not be a passerby), (2) do what you can, and (3) invite others to help. In my feedback, I recommended that she be even more specific and invitational by encouraging the congregation to become more involved in local efforts to clean up the neighborhood and support healthy homes for their friends and neighbors. I suggested that she identify projects that are happening in the community and invite the congregation to join in what she called "God's Samaritan work" in a tangible, concrete way.

Overall, while I received positive feedback from students about the mapping exercise, I felt that I had not clearly articulated my expectations for the final projects. This resulted in less than stellar submissions. So, I knew I needed to be more specific with the instructions when I used the tool in the future.

7. Assessment 2: Lexington Theological Seminary, Witness and Testimony in Appalachia Course

The second time I used the mapping exercise was for the course, Witness and Testimony in Appalachia, in the summer of 2019 at Lexington Theological Seminary where I serve as Associate Professor of Preaching and Worship.[4] I received a grant from the Appalachian Ministries Educational Resource Center (AMERC) to provide scholarships and funding for the course which covered transportation, lodging, and meals for twelve students.[5] The course was a hybrid of online and onsite learning elements. Before arriving for the immersion trip, students engaged online readings, videos, podcasts, and completed a short research paper about the coal region of eastern Kentucky. The four-day trip then provided the opportunity for students to learn first-hand about the complex ways in which geography, class, culture, race/ethnicity, and sexual orientation impact the conjoining challenges of environmental, socioeconomic, and public health issues in the region.

The students were assigned to create the "Who Is My Neighbor" Map to reflect the people we met (such as coal miners, high school students, clergy and their congregations, and local community organizers), and places and environmental "neighbors" we visited, including an historic coal mine, an old growth forest protected by Kentucky Natural Lands Trust, and mountains and waterways destroyed by mining. This time, I had the students consider guiding questions when thinking about their mapping assignments: what is it like to be you in this place? What would it be like if you could envision a positive future?

Whose stories do we tell? Who gets to tell these stories and how will those stories be told? These questions enabled students to engage in deep, pastoral listening to a variety of voices (including other-than-human neighbors in God's Creation), and to discern how they can preach the gospel in the midst of contentious community issues.

Unlike the first time I used the exercise where most students submitted a few PowerPoint slides, this time I received many different types of maps, including collages of labeled photographs, images overlayed across a map of the region, a radial chart, and a poster with the image of a web in the background to indicate the web of life. I intended the mapping exercise to help them organize their ideas for preaching a sermon when they returned to their home congregations. The sermon was to highlight what they learned in the Appalachian immersion experience and to demonstrate that they had thought critically about how one tells the story of a people and culture. Two of the more intriguing sermons were preached by students whose countries of origin were outside the U.S.

One was a male student who was a native of Ghana and served an African-native congregation in Louisville, Ky. He drew parallels between the way the environment is exploited for coal in Appalachia and how the rivers of his own country are polluted because of mining. He used the story of the Woman at the Well in John 4:4-14 to encourage his congregation to advocate for "living water".

Another student was a female native of Haiti serving a Haitian congregation in New York City. She noted that both the residents of Appalachia and the residents of Haiti are like the man in the parable of the good Samaritan in Luke—beaten, robbed, and left to die on the side of the mountain. She also connected the "neighbor" thread from the drug addicts in their neighborhood, to the mother who does not have enough money to feed her children, to the trees cut down in their homeland, to the sea crying out from being suffocated with trash. She encouraged her congregation to be a "Good Samaritan church" by teaching the youth to love God's Creation and by joining with their interfaith neighbors to clean up abandoned lots in their community.

I was much more pleased with the mapping assignment submissions the second time around. Not only were students creative and detailed in their maps, they also expressed appreciation for having a tangible reminder of the trip. Many of the submissions were so impressive that I decided to use them as examples to show students in the future when using this tool.

8. Assessment 3: Hartford Seminary, Environmental Ethics Course

In the third iteration of the "Who Is My Neighbor" Mapping Exercise, the course was not about preaching and worship but environmental ethics. I taught the online, asynchronous, semester-long course for Hartford Seminary in the spring of 2020. Unlike the first two Christian seminaries where I used the exercise, this was an interfaith seminary which meant that I had sixteen students from Christian, Muslim, Unitarian, non-denominational, and secular contexts. This made for a rich learning environment for the students and for myself.

Instead of using the mapping exercise as a lead-in for preaching or designing worship, I made it a stand-alone assignment and had the students present their mapping exercise to their faith community as an educational event. Because this course coincided with the emergence of the coronavirus pandemic that was causing houses of worship to close, I allowed the students to create narrated PowerPoints which could be shown during an online education event or accessed by congregation members asynchronously.

One student was a Muslim male in Houston, Tx, who began his presentation by comparing the parable of the good Samaritan with a teaching from An-Nisaa 4:36 about caring for "neighbors who are near, neighbors who are strangers, the companion by your side, the wayfarer (ye meet)." His PowerPoint then showed the wilderness of concrete and pavement around their masjid from the street view and from a Google Earth view. He zeroed in on one underdeveloped area of green space and encouraged his fellow congregants to join an effort to revitalize a local plan for parks, recreation, and open space in Harris County.

Another student was a White female faculty member at a co-educational boarding and day school for high school students in Connecticut. She used the mapping assignment to highlight not just the community and environmental neighbors, but to incorporate the voices of Indigenous Peoples. As she wrote in her reflection paper, "This project has inspired me to bring a proposal for land acknowledgement, education, and professional development to school leadership. I've been working with another colleague, and we've actually been making some great progress! We secured the funding to bring in a speaker from a Native community here in Connecticut." Her PowerPoint consisted of twenty-six well-designed and informative slides that incorporated nearly all of the twelve options from the mapping exercise and concluded with concrete "next steps", including a presentation the following month called "Dialogues on Difference" for the community.

Other student projects included preserving green spaces and partnering with local environmental groups in the church's community, water conservation for congregation members as well as the church's building and grounds, protecting a community against wildfires, and becoming a "zero waste" congregation. One student even created a live-action video about the lifecycle of a single-use plastic bottle. The video showed the interrelatedness of "neighbors" ranging from the oil that is used to produce the bottle, to the recycling facility, to the places where "recycled plastic" actually ends up—oceans, underdeveloped nations, and in the stomachs of fish and sea birds.[6]

This time around, the students were able to see models of the mapping exercise that I had collected from the previous course, and I believe this made a difference in the quality of their assignments. In all, the mapping exercise for this course provided a way for students to develop critical skills for theological analysis of and creative engagement with environmental challenges that their faith communities could address. The exercise also empowered them to provide education and, for some students, leadership on the issue they chose to address.

9. Assessment 4: Lexington Theological Seminary, Creation-Crisis Preaching Course

The fourth time I utilized the mapping exercise was in May 2021 at Lexington Theological Seminary. Twenty-two students registered for the four-week online course, sixteen of whom were part of a continuing education certificate program, "The Church and Creation", and were not required to submit assignments. This course was about incorporating environmental issues into both preaching and worship, so in addition to the sermon assignment, students were also required to design a Creation-centered worship service complete with prayers, hymns, readings, and a communion liturgy.[7] The "Who Is My Neighbor" Mapping Exercise, then, was intended to situate their worship design and sermon within the political, cultural, and biotic setting of the church.[8]

One White male student served a congregation in the Cumberland Plateau of Tennessee and focused on the "neighbors" of the East Fork of the Obed River and Dale Hollow Lake. He made it a point to speak with beekeepers, farmers, hunters, those who fish, winemakers, and others who work in natural elements. He referenced two biblical texts in his sermon. He used Isaiah 24: 4–5 ("The earth dries up and withers") to describe the pollution and neglect that the river suffers by the hands of humans. However, he also lifted up a vision of hope in Matt. 6: 25–33 ("Look at the birds of the air"). "Jesus' words serve as an example of looking to nature, so that we might learn from those other-than-human life forms; learn how-to live-in harmony with our biotic neighbors," he said in the sermon. He encouraged the congregation to care for "the least of these" through supporting local environmental and recreational groups, scout troops, and community organizations that are already working to revitalize the river and lake. He framed this as "environmental healing ministry" at the conclusion of the sermon. The student also designed a worship service with a theme of "taking care of God's *oikos* (household)", with hymns and prayers for Creation in general and rivers and water in particular.

Two time zones away, another student created her mapping assignment for her desert-dwelling congregation in Arizona. This White female student created a video highlighting the native plants, trees and birds, the local senior living facility, an elementary school, a food bank, and a community farm demonstrating desert food production and ecological restoration. She even showed pictures of the very edge of the church's property where a homeless encampment had left remnants of their stay that day. She stressed that all of these were the church's neighbors and that she intended to focus on the "circular, cyclical, self-balancing design of Creation" as symbolized by the church's large outdoor labyrinth. She preached her sermon outside standing in front of the labyrinth and drew parallels between the "deserted place" where Jesus fed the multitudes in Mark 6: 30–44, and the "deserted place" there in the Sonoran Desert, which had thrived ecologically before European colonization. She encouraged the congregation to listen to the teaching of Creation and of Jesus Christ to see the "hidden abundance" all around them. She concluded, "Jesus bids us to offer what we have, then sit down with all of Creation and be fed." She, too, designed a worship service complete with Creation-centered hymns, prayers, and other liturgical elements.

In this course, I noticed a marked improvement in the mapping exercises and sermons compared to those submitted the first time I taught the course in 2018. For instance, most of the PowerPoints in 2018 had 5–10 slides. For this course in 2021, however, the number of slides ranged from 10–24, included much more text and graphics, and showed evidence of completing six or more of the steps in the exercise. I think one of the reasons for the improved quality of the assignments was due to the fact that I provided examples of mapping exercises completed by students in the Appalachia immersion course and the Hartford course so that students could get ideas for their own projects. I found that the students engaged with much more depth, detail, and diligence in the project than the first time I assigned the exercise three years prior.

10. Possibilities for Future Research and Use in Teaching Contexts

While students have expressed unanimous appreciation for the "Who Is My Neighbor" Mapping Exercise, I do not know how their congregations responded or what long-term effects the projects had on the students' ministries. In the future, one way to gauge the effectiveness of this exercise would be to conduct a before-and-after survey of the congregation. Prior to the project, the congregation would receive a questionnaire asking about their attitudes toward religion and ecology as well as their knowledge about the topic the student would be addressing in their mapping exercise. Then, after the student completes the project, a second survey would be distributed asking the same questions as well as additional questions about how they felt moved to respond or put their faith into action in light of the student's sermon, worship service, or educational presentation. In this way, the comparative data would provide feedback not only about the student's individual project, but about the overall effectiveness of using the mapping exercise.

There is also the potential to develop a version of the exercise that guides students and members of a congregation to envision ways they can address environmental issues more fully as a community of faith. Working with a team in their congregation, the student could choose just one or two of the steps in the exercise as learning activities to be done with their congregants that would then inform the student's map-making. I would also welcome the opportunity to see others adapt the "Who Is My Neighbor" Mapping Exercise for Roman Catholic and Orthodox contexts within Christianity, as well as in other faith traditions such as Judaism or Islam.

11. Conclusions

In whatever ways students in theological education choose to address environmental issues in their ministries, I remind them that this work does make a difference. Research has shown that homilies and sermons can enhance the effectiveness of the message to embrace green Christianity. For example, the 2014 PRRI/AAR survey on religion, values, and climate change found that "Americans who say their clergy leader speaks at least occasionally about climate change are more likely to be climate change Believers than Americans who tend not to hear about climate change in church (49% and 36%, respectively)" (Jones et al. 2014, p. 4). In other words, people in the pews are listening to what their ministers have to say about climate and other environmental issues. Simply making the case that Creation-care is part of our responsibility as Christians is a vital message that clergy and faith leaders can and should convey.

As I reflect on the use of the "Who Is My Neighbor" Mapping Exercise for these four courses over the span of three years, I have come to see that the tool was a source of spiritual formation for many students. I encouraged them to prayerfully consider how the process of reading scripture, interpreting faith through an ecological lens, and attending to the suffering of their human neighbors as well as Earth kin could inform and shape their own faith and relationship with the Divine. In turn, they critically engaged matters of faith and ecological justice in local and global contexts.

The mapping exercise is also a useful reference point as I invite students to consider what concrete actions they might take on environmental issues beyond the conclusion of the course. Especially as they move beyond an individualistic framework (What should *I* do?) toward a more congregationally and community-based framework (What should *we* do?), the mapping exercise is a way for students to engage people in their houses of worship and local community on these questions.

As the examples above demonstrate, the mapping exercise also encouraged students to learn about the ways in which race, socioeconomics, culture, religion, and local context relate to and with environmental issues. Therefore, I suggest that this exercise could be used in any number of teaching contexts, courses, and disciplines to help inculcate a "theology of place" and emphasize the importance of learning *"from* the places in which they are embedded in order to learn *for* the places they are embedded" (Tollison 2021). For example, this mapping exercise could be used in courses on food and faith, climate ethics, God and nature, environmental law and policy, biodiversity and nature's rights, ecological racism, and climate migration and the church, to name just a few. The "Who Is My Neighbor" Mapping Exercise is a project that can enable students to develop an expansive and holistic understanding of environmental issues while making the case that Jesus' teaching about showing mercy extends to our biotic neighbors as well. "Go and do likewise."

Funding: This research was partially supported by a grant from the Appalachian Ministries Educational Resource Center which provided funding for students in the course, Witness and Testimony in Appalachia, Lexington Theological Seminary, June 2019.

Institutional Review Board Statement: Not applicable.

Informed Consent Statement: Not applicable.

Conflicts of Interest: The author declares no conflict of interest.

Notes

[1] In both the 2017 and 2021 survey, half of respondents said they received negative pushback in the form of angry emails, letters, or direct confrontation when preaching about social issues.

[2] Norman C. Habel suggests six guiding ecojustice principles: the principle of intrinsic worth, the principle of interconnectedness, the principle of voice, the principle of purpose, the principle of mutual custodianship, and the principle of resistance (Habel 2000, p. 2).

[3] According to Paul W. Taylor, "William Frakena delineated eight types of ethical theories which could generate moral rules and/or judgments concerning how rational agents should act with regard to the natural environment. The eight types are differentiated by their conceptions of moral subjects or patients. Each has its own view of the class of entities with respect to which moral agents can have duties and responsibilities. The eight types may be briefly delineated as follows: 1. Only what benefits or harms the agent himself is morally relevant to how anything else in existence should be treated. (Egoism.) 2. Only humans (or those humans who are also persons) are proper moral patients. How we ought to act with respect to the environment is determined ultimately by the effects of our actions on humans or on persons. 3. All conscious (or sentient) beings are proper moral patients. Conduct with regard to the environment is right if it alleviates the suffering or increases the pleasure of beings that can suffer or

[4] experience pleasure. 4. All living beings, conscious or not, are proper moral patients. Our moral concern should extend beyond humans to all animals and plants. 5. Everything in existence (other than God), whether taken distributively or collectively, is to be considered as that toward which we may have duties and responsibilities. 6. God is the only ultimate moral subject as far as human action is concerned. We owe duties only to God, and we should treat the natural world in such a way as to fulfill our duties to God. 7. Combinations of any two or more of the above. 8. Nature itself is a moral patient. We should either follow the ways of nature or let the ways of nature take their course without our intervention." (Taylor 1981). My assessment is that Wallace prioritizes #5. The "Who Is My Neighbor" Mapping Exercise utilizes a combination of #4, #5, and #6.

[4] Appalachia is a region of the United States spanning thirteen states across the Appalachian Mountains from southern New York to Mississippi. While blessed with beautiful mountains, valleys, forests, rivers, lakes, and abundant natural resources, some areas have suffered from environmental devastation, poverty, and public health issues (such as lung disease and addictions). In addition, harmful classist and cultural stereotypes, as well as tensions around race, ethnicity, and sexual orientation further complicate attitudes within and about the people of Appalachia.

[5] The mission of AMERC is to promote contextual, cross-cultural education for theological students, faculties, and other Christian leaders. Working primarily through an ecumenical consortium of theological schools, regional colleges or universities, oversight agencies of the church, and supporting organizations, AMERC supports experiential learning about the theological, spiritual, social, economic, and environmental aspects of Appalachian culture, especially for ministry in rural and small-town settings.

[6] The video can be accessed on Youtube: https://www.youtube.com/watch?v=NT4IJBiO7ws (accessed on 28 March 2022).

[7] In addition to *Creation-Crisis Preaching*, two other required texts were: *Liturgies from Below: Praying with People at the Ends of the World* by Cláudio Carvalhaes (Nashville, T, Abingdon Press, 2020), and *A Watered Garden: Christian Worship and Earth's Ecology* by Benjamin Stewart (Minneapolis, MN: Augsburg Fortress, 2011). A recommended text was *The Season of Creation: A Preaching Commentary* edited by Norman C. Habel,, David M. Rhoads, and H. Paul Santmire (Minneapolis, MN: Fortress Press, 2011).

[8] I also provided several website resources to the students to give them ideas for designing their worship service and preaching their sermon, including: Creation Justice Ministries resources for Earth Day. http://www.creationjustice.org/urgency.html (accessed on 28 March 2022); Let All Creation Praise, http://www.letallcreationpraise.org/ (accessed on 28 March 2022); EcoAmerica, https://ecoamerica.org/ (accessed on 28 March 2022); Blessed Tomorrow, https://blessedtomorrow.org/ (accessed on 28 March 2022; Climate Health, https://ecoamerica.org/health/ (accessed on 28 March 2022); Lutherans Restoring Creation, http://www.lutheransrestoringcreation.org/ (accessed on 28 March 2022); and Emerging Earth Community, http://www.emergingearthcommunity.org (accessed on 28 March 2022).

References

Ark, Tom Vander, Emily Liebtag, and Nate McClennen. 2020. *The Power of Place: Authentic Learning through Place-Based Education*. Alexandria: ASCD.
Habel, Norman. 2000. Readings from the Perspective of Earth. In *The Earth Bible*. Cleveland: Pilgrim Press.
Harper, Fletcher. 2021. Stop Preaching about Being Good Stewards of the Earth. *Sojourners*. Available online: https://sojo.net/articles/stop-preaching-about-being-good-stewards-earth (accessed on 28 January 2022).
Inge, John. 2003. *A Christian Theology of Place*. Explorations in Practical, Pastoral, and Empirical Theology. Edited by Leslie J. Francis and Jeff Astley. New York: Routledge.
Jones, Robert P., Daniel Cox, and Juhem Navarro-Rivera. 2014. *Believers, Sympathizers, and Skeptics: Why Americans are Conflicted about Climate Change, Environmental Policy, and Science: Findings from the PRRI/AAR Religion, Values, and Climate Change Survey*. Washington, DC: Public Religion Research Institute and American Academy of Religion. Available online: https://www.prri.org/research/believers-sympathizers-skeptics-americans-conflicted-climate-change-environmental-policy-science/ (accessed on 28 January 2022).
Knapp, Clifford E. 2014. Place-Based Curricular and Pedagogical Models. In *Place-Based Education in the Global Age: Local Diversity*. Edited by David A. Gruenewald and Gregory A. Smith. London: Routledge, pp. 5–27.
Moe-Lobeda, Cynthia D. 2013. *Resisting Structural Evil: Love as Ecological-Economic Vocation*. Minneapolis: Augsburg Fortress.
Morris, Michael Malahy. 2014. Place in Leadership Formation. In *Place-Based Education in the Global Age: Local Diversity*. Edited by David A. Gruenewald and Gregory A. Smith. London: Routledge, pp. 225–53.
Schade, Leah D. 2015. *Creation-Crisis Preaching: Ecology, Theology, and the Pulpit*. St. Louis: Chalice Press.
Schade, Leah D. 2017. "Preaching About Controversial Issues.". Unpublished survey data.
Schade, Leah D., Amanda Wilson Harper, Wayne Thompson, and Katie Day. 2021. Ministry, Preaching, and Social Issues. Unpublished survey data.
Sobel, David. 2004. *Place-Based Education: Connecting Classrooms & Communities*. Great Barrington: Orion Society.
Taylor, Paul W. 1981. Frankena On Environmental Ethics. *The Monist* 64: 313–24. [CrossRef]
Tollison, Wm Taylor. 2021. An Ecological Pedagogy of Embeddedness: Theological Education for Human Flourishing. Unpublished Paper. Available online: https://www.academia.edu/56599087/An_Ecological_Pedagogy_of_Embeddedness_Theological_Education_for_Human_Flourishing (accessed on 18 February 2022).
Wallace, Mark I. 2005. *Finding God in the Singing River: Christianity, Spirit, Nature*. Philadelphia: Fortress.

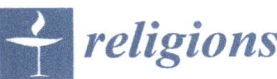

Article

Preaching Addressing Environmental Crises through the Use of Scripture: An Exploration of a Practical Theological Methodology

HyeRan Kim-Cragg

Emmanuel College of Victoria University, University of Toronto, Toronto, ON M5S 1K7, Canada; hyeran.kimcragg@utoronto.ca

Abstract: This article considers the critical roles of preaching in addressing the environmental crises by way of engaging with Paul Ballard's work as a particular practical theological methodology, namely the use of Scripture. This methodological consideration is followed by highlighting the work of the Earth Bible Team, which compliments Ballard's work. Both works are used as an example of a homiletical practice as well as a learning exercise, demonstrating how Scripture can be used as a homiletical resource of and hermeneutical source for doing practical theology with an eye to address environmental crises.

Keywords: environmental crises; preaching; homiletics; practical theological method; use of scripture; Earth Bible Team

Citation: Kim-Cragg, HyeRan. 2022. Preaching Addressing Environmental Crises through the Use of Scripture: An Exploration of a Practical Theological Methodology. *Religions* 13: 226. https://doi.org/10.3390/rel13030226

Academic Editor: Simon S. M. Kwan

Received: 13 January 2022
Accepted: 1 March 2022
Published: 7 March 2022

Publisher's Note: MDPI stays neutral with regard to jurisdictional claims in published maps and institutional affiliations.

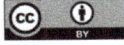

Copyright: © 2022 by the author. Licensee MDPI, Basel, Switzerland. This article is an open access article distributed under the terms and conditions of the Creative Commons Attribution (CC BY) license (https://creativecommons.org/licenses/by/4.0/).

1. Introduction

In the world of the COVID-19 pandemic, we often hear the phrase: "We are all in this together." However, not everyone is equally impacted by this problem. In a world experiencing the impacts of global warming, or a climate crisis, we hear a similar phrase: "we are all part of the problem, and we are also part of the solution." However, some individuals have suffered and will suffer more than others. Whether we are an individual, a corporation, or a nation, some people have contributed to the cause of the ecological problem more than others, and thus ought to grapple with this unequal injustice. I am saying these things as someone living in a nation that has been more of a cause to the ecological problem than its solution. I am also speaking as a Christian. I am taking a confessional posture regarding my own privileged social location. I am also taking a repentant stance acknowledging that in some Christian groups, the alarm of climate change and global warming is treated as fake news. I join with many Christians who are deeply dismayed by modern millennialists and creationists who believe that it is God's will to "burn up" this world. Facing climate-change-denying Christians, those concerned about climate change are reminded of Lynn White Jr.'s question: "Is Christianity the most anthropocentric religion that the world has ever known?" (White 1967).

In 1992, feminist homiletician Christine Smith defined preaching as weeping, confessing, and resisting in order to respond to structural evil. She was primarily concerned with six systematic injustices, namely, ableism, ageism, sexism, heterosexism, White racism, and classism (Smith 1992). While her work was prophetic and ahead of its time, ecological injustice was not presented on her list. This is not surprising; as John Cobb observed at the American Academy of Religion in the same year, Christian biblical and theological discourse proceeds as if there is no environmental crisis, sometimes as if there is no natural world at all (Cobb 1992, pp. 22, 38). Such omissions continue more than two decades later in recent publications, including *The Wiley Blackwell Companion to Practical Theology*, in which the volume lists racism, sexism, heterosexism, colonialism, postcolonialism, globalization, classism, ableism, and Christian-centrism as the issues, contexts, and perspectives of practical theology, but notably omits environmentalism (Miller-McLemore 2014).

The lack of, one, the keen awareness of and, two, the adequate attention to environmental crises[1] in practical theology and homiletics has contributed to re-inscribing oppressive and colonizing relationships among humans, and has also further isolated humans from the natural world. This article considers the critical roles of preaching in addressing the environmental crises by way of engaging with Paul Ballard's work as a particular practical theological methodology, namely the use of Scripture. This methodological consideration is followed by highlighting the work of the Earth Bible Team, which compliments Ballard's work. Considering both works enables an analysis of a sermon. This sermon is used as an example of homiletical practice as well as a learning exercise, demonstrating how Scripture can be used as a homiletical resource of and for conducting practical theology with an eye to address environmental crises.

Before delving into the use of Scripture as a practical theological method, let us consider the intersectional positionality of the environmental crises as a subject matter of practical theology. Practical theologians, including homileticians, need to take into account the ways in which different forms of oppressions converge. Ecofeminist theologians have already shown how patriarchy and anthropocentrism are interlocking forms of oppression (McFague 1993; Gebara 1999; Eaton 2005; Grey 2004; Kim-Cragg 2018). They point out that when nature is associated with women, and both are subordinated to the human male, accumulative injustice and collateral suffering often occurs. Making this intersectional stance visible is critical, as part of the challenge of addressing environmental crises in preaching exposes its invisibility and the resultant indifference of Christians towards it. Despite the wildfires, floods, and droughts occurring all over the world, it is still somehow difficult to display environmental crises as the central issue in Christian preaching practice. This is not just a Christians problem. The authors of *Eco Bible*, Rabbi Yonatan Neril and Rabbi Leo Dee, also note that most "Hebrew Bible study, teaching, and preaching occur without addressing the ecological crisis" in Jewish faith communities.[2] Many Christian and Jewish preachers do not seem to feel the rising global temperature, so to speak. That is why it is both urgent and imperative to make the issues of environmental crises explicit by using evocative language and tapping into the imagination in preaching. In this vein, Philosopher Wendy Lynn Lee's naming of fracking as a form of environmental rape is exemplary. Such naming is a visceral example of an intersectional analysis of how the forces of the oil and mining industry, capitalism, colonialism, and a sexist view of nature converge (Lee 2011).

2. Reasons for the Use of Scripture Addressing Environmental Crises in Preaching

It may be useful to delineate three reasons why the use of Scripture is a helpful research method for tackling these crises in homiletics. Despite the centrality of Scripture in Christian communities (and arguably in other Abrahamic religious communities as well), the use of Scripture in contemporary practical theologies seems weak (Ballard 2011). However, this is not the case for preachers who deny global warming and climate change. Scripture is extensively used to justify such denial. For example, John MacArthur preached a sermon titled "Cal Tech and the Global Warming Hoax," citing Revelation: "God intended us to use this planet, to fill this planet for the benefit of man. Never was it intended to be a permanent planet. It is a disposable planet. Christians ought to know that."[3] MacArthur is an influential preacher and the author of *Study Bible* (MacArthur 2013), which has sold almost 2 million copies. In the same sermon mentioned above, he apprehends the creation story in Genesis 1 literally and that God created the world in six days, dismissing the scientific evidence of evolution. This is the first reason why preachers should engage the use of Scripture. It is an important tool to adequately and critically counter Christian naysayers. An adequate and critical engagement requires preachers to go beyond interpreting the Bible literally. Yet, most adult Christians have a low level of biblical understanding. This is a problem Edward Farley bemoaned in pointing out the challenges of theological education in the 1980s (Farley 1983, pp. 152–53; 1988). A 2014 study shows that Christians feel that they need some help interpreting the Bible (Goff et al. 2014). This need is a call to practical theologians, such as preachers, to provide an informed biblical understanding for those in the pew and outside the church who may be otherwise easily misguided by an ideological interpretation coded in popular culture and social media (Beavis and Kim-Cragg 2017, p. xi).

Another reason why it may be instructive to maximize the use of Scripture is simply the fact that the Bible can offer robust arguments for why we should stop environmental destruction. Under the influence of hermeneutics, chiefly the work of Paul Ricoeur, the focus on biblical studies shifted from a focus on what lies "behind" the text to a focus on what is "before" or "in front of" the text.[4] Such a shift has introduced the importance of the context as a site for interpreting Scripture. This context provides a situated knowing and allows practical theology to make use of the life conditions of people as raw material in their theologizing (Fulkerson 2007, p. 7). The environmental crisis calls for practical theologians to interpret the Bible in ways that respond to the situated ecological conditions and complex suffering realities that result from ecological injustices.

The other reason why the use of Scripture is helpful in addressing the environmental crisis has to do with its capacity to influence the imagination. This is connected to the ability to observe the past and behold the future in a non-linear way. Postcolonial biblical scholar Tat-siong Benny Liew talks about having "yin and yang eyes", when one interprets the Bible (Benny Liew 2008, pp. 2, 19). Scripture is an ancient text. It comes from the past and captures a particular wisdom of ancestors regarding faith, their resilience, struggles, and failures as well as their faithfulness. Scripture, in this regard, is the written record of the past. However, this past is not unrelated to the present and the future. In fact, when we read the Scripture closely, guided by the Holy Spirit, we see that the issues that people in the Bible grappled with are not so foreign from what we, the people in the 21st century, are dealing with. However, to hear the voices from the past loud and clear, one needs to exercise the imagination. My point here is circular. We need the imagination to understand Scripture and we need Scripture to develop the imagination. The use of Scripture helps to cultivate the imagination (Kim-Cragg 2021, see chapter 2 on imagination, pp. 29–76). In a similar vein, to adequately and steadily address the environmental crises today, we need to behave as if the future is already here. We must be able to listen to the future heirs of planet Earth. To be able to see and hear the future generations of our descendants also requires the power of the imagination. The use of Scripture has the power to tap into people's imagination in such a way as to release this potential. With imagination, as the prophet Isaiah proclaimed, we will be able to hear the mountains and hills burst into song, and the trees of the field will clap their hands (Isaiah 55: 12).

3. The Use of Scripture: A Practical Theological Methodology

Paul Ballard proposes four different modes of the use of Scripture in practical theology. These modes emerged from collaborative research that was published under the title, "the Bible in Pastoral Practice Project" (2000–2005) (Ballard and Holmes 2006). The four modes of the use of Scripture include (1) the Bible as resource, (2) Bible in worship and spirituality, (3) Bible as wisdom for theological reflection, and (4) Bible as a source of empirical research (Ballard 2011, pp. 165–71). A brief examination of these modes is helpful here as I employ them, respectively, in the analysis of the sermon in the next section.

The first mode views Scripture as a resource for performing practical theology. The term "resource" has multi-layered meanings. For Ballard, using Scripture as a resource means that it can provide a normative framework for practical theology in general and pastoral counseling in particular. The notion of Scripture as a resource assumes that Scripture is a living text, which invites readers to correlate it to a present reality. Scripture is also used as a resource for performing contextual analysis, for examining the sociocultural and economic realities, both then and now. This is a mode that is often taken up by liberation theologians. In summary, the mode of Scripture as a resource identifies it as a reservoir into which practical theologians can tap. Scripture contains many different, albeit partial, stories and events that can shed light on current issues and present-day situations, while illuminating how God is at work in those situations.

The second mode of the use of Scripture is found in liturgy or worship settings. It is in the corporate and consistent practice of worshipping together as a gathered body of Christ that Scripture is most prevalently used, directly cited in the case of preaching or during sacraments, praise and prayers. In this regard, the use of Scripture is closely related to congregational studies as it compliments liturgical theology where the concern is not only what the Bible says, but how it has been used, enacted and re-membered as the work of the people of God in a setting in relation to worship.

The third mode of the use of Scripture is hermeneutics. This interpretive mode helps readers to discern where God is at work in the Bible and today. It supports and enhances a spiral praxis model of performing theological reflection, starting from the current reality, through the critical analysis, and moving on to action, a spiral that is especially important for a participatory action approach to practical theology. Theological reflection may also begin from the reality in the Bible, which relates to the contemporary context or a reality that informs a pastoral prophetic response from a correlational theological perspective.

The fourth mode is to view the Bible as an object of practical theological research. As a topic of the research in practical theology, the following questions can be asked of it: how has a scriptural text been received in the church (i.e., the congregational and/or denominational study), how has the Bible been used as content and a process (i.e., Christian education and faith formation), how is the Bible read and understood by the laity or clergy, and how has the Bible been portrayed or distorted (i.e., in or by popular culture and media studies or socio-cultural studies).

Ballard's approach brings the Bible into critical conversation with the work of practical theology. Yet, a more substantial and sustained attempt to engage with the Bible is required in order to address environmental crises. One such attempt is found in the work of the Earth Bible project, which was first developed by a team of biblical researchers from Adelaide, South Australia.[5] The project grew as a collaboration of scholars from around the world who use specific eco-justice principles to foreground their reading and analysis of biblical texts.

The Earth Bible Team underscores the agency of the natural world as they suggest six ecojustice principles for developing a hermeneutic method to read the Bible. These principles, developed over several years, are chosen to facilitate a dialogue with biologists, ecologists, and other religious leaders beyond the Christian Church. These principles state that (1) the Earth has intrinsic worth (the Earth is valuable in itself and not just in a utilitarian sense as a means to an human end), (2) all life is interconnected (the earth and human life are interdependent), (3) the Earth has a voice (and its own language), (4) the Earth has purpose (which can be found in the cycle of life), (5) the Earth is subject to mutual custodianship (the Earth and humans have co-responsibility for the household, oikumene), and (6) the Earth is an agent of resistance (the Earth has the power to survive and revive) (The Earth Bible Team 2000). These principles provide a helpful way to pose questions of the biblical text by using a hermeneutic of both suspicion and retrieval. Readers, including preachers, should suspect that the Bible was written by privileged men and that the work of interpretation calls for a retrieval of the Earth community that has been suppressed or hidden.

In the present work, a specific sermon is analyzed by highlighting the work of Ballard and the Earth Bible Team's six principles to demonstrate how the use of Scripture in preaching as a particular method of conducting practical theology can be employed in relation to the environmental crises, and how it can inform necessary actions. It should be noted that not all four modes of Ballard's work and not all six principles are fully reflected in the analysis of the sermon.

4. Sermon as an Example of the Use of Scripture for Addressing Environmental Crises

Sermon Title: The Pruning God[6]

Scripture Passages: John 15: 1–2

"I am the true vine, and my Father is the vine grower. 2 He [sic] removes every branch in me that bears no fruit. Every branch that bears fruit he [sic] prunes to make it bear more fruit." (NRSV)

One sunny afternoon many years ago, my partner and I were in my old stomping grounds in Toronto's Koreatown near Christie on Bloor. We had stopped to admire a concrete planter full of flowers sitting at the edge of a grocery store parking lot. A woman entering her house just beyond noticed us standing there. She told us she had planted these flowers. They were not on her property, but since the big planters had been left unattended, she had taken it upon herself to see that there were flowers in them, a wonderful act of service to the neighbourhood. After a very short visit with this lovely lady, she surprised us further by inviting us into her backyard to show us her own private little vineyard! She enjoyed telling us how the grapes grew and how she made wine from them. She told us that she had to prune and tend to the vines, a 10 min lesson in grape growing. It was a remarkable and joyful encounter.

Some years passed and my family moved to Saskatoon. A church friend in Saskatoon invited my family to visit their home one summer day. Our friends are gardeners and had all kinds of plants in their backyard but we were particularly taken by their grape vine. We tasted the grapes. They tasted heavenly. Our friends encouraged us to grow our own vine and gave us a few plants to get started. We found the sunniest and warmest spot in our garden and put them in a row. Every day, we faithfully checked the plants, watered them, put supports in so that the vines could grow and weave.

In the Gospel of John, God is the vine grower and Jesus is the true vine and we are his branches. As a good gardener, God removes every branch that bears no fruit. God does a bit of pruning. God is the pruning God.

Vineyards were familiar to Jesus' disciples and also to the Jewish Christian community within which the Gospel of John was written. Jesus' followers and the earliest Christians would pass vineyards as they walked from place to place every day. Some likely had their own vineyard or worked in a vineyard. They were able to discern fruitful branches from those that would drain the vine's energy and yield no fruit in return. They would learn how to trim branches, all the while feeling good about the surgical purpose of their work. Pruning might seem cruel, but it renews the vine's vitality. Useless branches drain the plant's strength to leave them in place serves no purpose and reduces the value of the vineyard. The vine growers need to cut away unfruitful branches and burn them to get rid of them.

Crisis events often require us to prune our lives. We learn to prioritize things that really matter, not just as individuals but for the community collectively. COVID 19 pruned us. It cut some aspects of our lives down to the bare necessities. It also showed us where branches of our community tree need tending. This pandemic revealed poverty, racism, sexism, ageism, ableism, ecological danger and violence. It revealed things in society, branches of human-centric anthropocentrism, that should not be there, branches of our culture that need pruning.

Though there are signs that the vaccines are helping us move out of the pandemic, we will not be able to return to the ways things were before COVID 19. There are areas of life that have been changed and will not come back. But there are also new shoots pushing out to replace what was lost. We have to keep a careful watch, as followers of the Pruning God. Has there been damage to the vine that needs tending to? Are old unfruitful branches in danger of springing back?

Crises are one thing that will prune our lives. Moving is another. And if that move means traveling thousands of kilometers and adjusting to a new language and culture, that will require even more. This past year I have been working on a book project to write about preaching in the United Church of Canada, anticipating a centennial anniversary of our Church in 2025. My colleague from St. Andrew's College, Prof. Don Schweitzer and I have collected sermons from a variety of UCC preachers going back 110 years! We have sermons from well-known preachers such as George Pidgeon, Lois Wilson, Cliff Elliott, and Stan Lucyk. We also included sermons from lesser known preachers such one preached in a Japanese internment camp during the Second World War and two short Christmas sermons preached to French congregations in Quebec. In order to behold the future, we need to look back on the past. Reading through these sermons from the past has been comforting and assuring because I have found many of them so insightful, visionary, and bold, grappling with their own issues of the day, which are mysteriously not so different from our own issues today. I felt God's presence in these sermons.

One sermon speaks very powerfully to me and shares a similar message that we have heard from the Gospel of John today. It is the sermon of the Right Rev. Dr. Sang Chul Lee, the former moderator of the United Church of Canada and the former Chancellor of Victoria University in the University of Toronto. This is Rev. Lee's inaugural sermon which he preached on the very first Sunday at Toronto Korean United Church in 1969. The Rt. Rev. Sang Chul Lee served that church for more than 20 years and, of course, went on to be the moderator of the UCC in 1988. Keep in mind, however when you hear his words today, that in 1969 he was relatively new to Canada and that he was preaching to a group of immigrants. Most of the congregation members would have arrived in Canada no earlier than 1966, the year Canada's immigration policy changed allowing more racialized people to settle in the country. Therefore, most of the congregation would have been in Canada no more than three years when Rev. Lee preached this sermon to them. That is at the heart of Rev. Lee's message. Let me translate his words for you:

The new world developing before us is amazing and bright. But those things that we have become psychologically attached to in the past still call out to us and create a kind of hesitation and anxiety. We have not been practicing the new way of life. Still we have to spur ourselves on and try to throw ourselves into this new world. For this is the life we have been given. This is the duty that needs our secret stores of courage. It is a task of great value.

Those old things that we need to get rid of are the things our bodies have become used to and things we have become familiar with and so throwing them away will cause sorrow. But in order to learn new things we have to clear those things out . . . . It requires us to cut away a long-accrued part of our life and this is a task which is marked with pain. This cutting requires vulnerability. It is a work of completely exposing our weakness and ignorance. That is why it is not something we can do without suffering and passion. But there is a reward of being open to newness. It is like having the innocent heart of a child.

The Rt. Rev. Lee invited his congregation to cut away the old way of life. For Lee, allowing God to prune and teach results in a renewed life.

The Greek word for "pruning" in the Gospel of John is kathaírō (κατχάιρο)—which means to make clean by purging (removing undesirable elements); eliminating what is fruitless by purifying. The word, pruning, kathairo means to cleanse and purify. The pruning God is a decisive God. God engages a decisive action to cut things off and remove things that are taxing the life of the vine and preventing the fruit of new life to come forward. Humans need to confess a pruning and purifying God and join God's work today more than ever.

Take environmental crises seriously, for example.

Dear people of faith,

This is an issue that I feel, more than any other, requires our attention today. "The UN Report on Climate Change" in August 2021 is startling. God is calling us to make decisions and prune our life in ways that will allow human life to continue to thrive on the planet. We need to follow God who engages decisive actions that will stop global warming. God is urging us to cut food waste, cut garbage, and cut the use of energy for heating and cooling, cut buildings that are inefficient and energy burning houses in the suburbs and cities, cut out our private car use, and much more besides!

This old Greek wisdom on pruning is so instructive to those of us living in the current climate crisis and ecological devastation.

Mark Carney, the former governor of both the bank of Canada and the bank of England, now a UN special envoy on Climate and Finance, gave the 2020 BBC Reith Lecture based on his book, Values: Building a Better World for All (Carney 2021). He identified three crises facing the world today, each starting with the letter "C": COVID-19, Credit, and Climate. The recovery from COVID-19 and the recovery of the economy are closely related to the restoration of the damaged planet earth. He said that the ultimate test of a fair economy will be how it addresses the growing climate crisis. What is valued is not always the same as what is profitable. In fact, we painfully learned during the pandemic that financial values have to be replaced with communal and social values. I would add that market values are not greater than the divine values, what God favors. And I say again, market values are not greater than the divine values.)

When the ecosystem is on the verge of collapse, many economic considerations need to be cut away. The sooner we act, the less costly it will be. Speed and scale will be critical. The goal of achieving net zero carbon emissions must be our priority. The good news is that 140 big countries have committed to achieve this goal and the numbers of the countries are increasing. The manufacture of certain cars that pollute the air will be pruned in Europe in 2030. The Canadian government also pledged that the sale of gas running cars will be purged by 2035. Cutting out the use of coal as fuel has yet to happen. There is lots to do, still.

Dear branches of the True Vine,

I invite you to look at your home, your workplace, and your congregation! What needs to be pruned in order to tackle the climate crisis? What decisive action do you as a community of faith need to make to allow life on earth to flourish? What pruning can you think of as a spiritual discipline to cut down waste and eliminate overconsumption? How shall we contribute to saving the earth as a daily Christian practice?

Let me suggest how we can join God in the work of pruning every day of the week individually and collectively.

Monday for Meditation. Think about, read about, learn about our planet and what we need to do to keep it healthy. Monday for Meditation includes simply delighting in the beauty of the life around you in creation while walking and biking or doing nothing else.

Tuesday for Turning off machines and lights. Try not to use cars or airplanes and look out for lights left on.

Wednesday for Waste free. Try not to make unnecessary waste, whether it is food, water or other waste.

Thursday for Thrift. Don't throw things out that can be used later or by others. Spend less. Borrow or lend something rather than buying something new.

Friday for Future. This motto is not my original idea but the international movement of young people that started by Greta Thunberg, August 2018, exactly 3 years ago. Millions of young people from over 150 countries are doing a prophetic act, demonstrating on Friday to demand action from political leaders to take action to prevent climate change and for the fossil fuel industry to transition to renewable energy.

Saturday for Sabbath. This is an ancient Jewish practice of resting. Resting can be good for you and I. It is also good for the Earth! We join this Jewish practice as a way of pruning our life and saving the earth, even if as Christian we celebrate Sunday as our sabbath.

Sunday for Sharing. As we gather as a congregation, let's find ways to share the work we have done to prune our lives for a thriving planet! Be with people that you love and who need your love. Encourage one another!

Monday for Meditation, Tuesday for Turning Off, Wednesday for Waste Free, Thursday for Thrift, Friday for the Future, Saturday for Sabbath and Sunday for Sharing. I will look forward to hearing how you have been doing regarding this matter next time when we meet in person.

These are some tips for pruning. The guiding principle of all these actions is to prune branches of despair and apathy so that branches of hope and renewal can flourish. Pruning is holy work. May God, the chief gardener, bless your gardening this day and always.

What happened to the vine we grew in Saskatoon? Well, let's just say we did not leave that house with a vineyard in the backyard! We did our best, but God is the real gardener. And sometimes God saves and gives life by pruning. God in Jesus can give you life–life abundant and free. A life that grows, a life that bears fruit, a life that takes root even in these troubled times. If we do our part, the divine gardener will do the gardener's part. And not only will the dead flowerpots on the street corner come back to life but the dead dreams, dead relationships, dead careers, and even this dying, nearly dead world will come back to life.

Amen and thanks be to God.

5. Sermon Analysis: A Critical Reflection

The main idea of the sermon is to invite the congregation to observe God as the pruning God, while drawing our attention to environmental crises. While we must admit that God as Father is still androcentric and anthropocentric, thus, a hermeneutic of suspicion is warranted as the Earth Bible Team pointed out (Habel 2000, p. 39), it is God in Jesus as the True Vine who embodies a community of interconnectedness, which is the second principle suggested by the Earth Bible Team. In embracing both an androcentric and plant-centered theology, the sermon focuses on John 15:2, and highlights the verb, *prune*. Here, this verse containing the particular verb serves as a resource of practicing theology that addresses the environmental crises, resonating with Ballard's first mode of Scripture. This verb is active, involving a human agency inviting a costly and vulnerable act, affirming the work of the Earth Bible Team. It further develops the idea of the original Greek word for pruning, *kathaírō*, which means purging and purifying, to address the current reality of the COVID-19 pandemic and urge concrete actions. The sermon taps into the ancient text in order to relate to the current context that calls for action addressing environmental crises, which is the third mode suggested by Ballard. Hermeneutically speaking, to name God as the pruning God is to interpret the biblical text by unearthing a divine activity that is not obvious. One may argue that not only is the agency of the Earth community is hidden, but also that of God is overlooked in our theological understanding. This draws on the insight of the Earth Bible Team regarding the retrieval of hidden traditions.

Preaching takes place in worship and contributes to the strengthening of the spirituality of the people in the pew as well as of the preacher. As a central piece in the sermon, it can easily demonstrate Ballard's second mode of the use of Scripture for enhancing worship and spirituality. The sermon was preached during a Sunday in summer, intentionally celebrating the liturgical season of the creation. Congregations were invited to deeply encounter the natural world in this season, while hearing about the U.N. report on climate change and that of the COP 26 Conference was being organized in October 2021. Ballard's third mode of the use of Scripture, viewing the Bible as hermeneutical wisdom for theological reflection, is employed in this sermon. Following the Earth Bible Team's third principle, the scripture allows us to hear the cries of the creation (Habel 2000, pp. 46–48). Instead of allowing itself to be co-opted by a dominant reading, a reading that silences the language of the Earth, we are also able to hear the voice of the Earth, groaning and resisting, through the agony of God as a gardener who must cut the branch off and unroot the plant that is not going to bear fruit. Using the words of the Earth Bible Team's fourth principle, the Earth has a purpose, which is to sustain life in all its diversity and beauty. Hence, the use of Scripture in this sermon helps preachers proclaim God who attends to the condition of the creation and invites humans to join in this work.

The writer of the Gospel of John uses the theological metaphor of chief gardener and True Vine. The sermon highlights this theological metaphor by evoking the congregation's capacity to imagine Jesus in a non-androcentric and non-anthropocentric way. This promotes ecological consciousness and interdependent perspectives. The very agenda of practical theology is found in the use of the theological metaphor. Bonnie Miller-McLemore proposed that the future of practical theology lies in the shift of the guiding metaphor from "living human document" to "living human web", with the recognition of interdependence between personal, political and public well-being (Miller-McLemore 1993). Yet, a decade later, she admitted that this shift did not observe the presence of the "non-human" natural world and noted the absent theme for pastoral theologians (Miller-McLemore 2020). The sermon, in this regard, reveals the interdependence of and inseparability between the Triune God, humans and non-human lives for the sake of addressing compounded by environmental crises.

The sermon presented here, entitled "The Pruning God," compels us to grapple with human greed to confess, expose, and resist our exploitation of nature in ways that reorient our priority to make decisive actions by pruning our life with a view to the Earth's purpose. The sermon has a confessional posture. This confessional posture meets the resistance of the Earth. The resistance of the Earth is what reveals sin and judgement in a way that is similar to how Hebrew Scripture relays God's judgements and calls to repentance (Jer. 12: 4, 7–11, Hos. 4:1–3). Canadian ecofeminist theologian Heather Eaton, commenting on the Earth Bible Team's principles, notes that the last principle, resistance, "requires imagining the Earth not only as a subject capable of agency, but one that has a sensitivity toward justice for the Earth and to the human community." (Eaton 2000, p. 69). The sermon shares the preacher's personal experience. It indirectly communicates the Earth's intrinsic agency and purpose. Yet, the sermon equally calls for an interdependent stance vis– vis human, creation, and Creator.

The sermon proclaims God's desire to mend the broken relationship between the non-human creation and that of humans, even if this mending requires pruning, a costly and uneasy reorientation, a radically different way of life. In this regard, the sermon moves to invite people to participate in concrete (and manageable) actions, highlighting the value of mutual custodianship as the fifth principle laid out by the Earth Bible Team. To follow and believe in the pruning God requires repentance involving a change of heart and habits. Repentance as truth-telling requires honesty. Repentance requires vulnerability. Repentance requires courage. It is hard work. That is why we need to seek the help of our ancestors in faith who have traveled the way of confession and repentance ahead of us. Tapping into the wisdom of the ancestors is similar to imagining that they are tapping on our shoulders, by encouraging us to see that we are not alone in performing the hard work of repentance. That is why repentance as an essential practice of Christianity is related to remembering the past. Confession as a part of repentance in this regard involves naming our own mistakes, complacency, and complicity and actively drawing wisdom from our ancestors guided by the work of the Holy Spirit, so that we can turn to God, a re-orientation toward the Earth and the Divine mystery, as a source of life.

Drawing wisdom from our ancestors in faith through the Book of Revelation, John Holbert argues that this particular biblical text exposes the horror of the economic and social monster of the Roman Empire in the first century, and that it can help us to repent of our complicity in similarly monstrous empires in the twenty-first century (Holbert 2011, p. 86). The same point can be made in the Gospel of John, the text for the sermon, because, arguably, it is the same author, John, or the community to which John belonged who wrote both the Gospel and Revelation. It is also important to note that the author, John, did not write the books specifically for us with our context in mind. Yet, we "overhear" what was written and "tell" it to our own people in a confessional manner (Craddock 2002). This overhearing and telling is what it means to proclaim the Gospel in an age of environmental crises. This is the preaching act. It is about bearing public witness to the exposure of a sinful act, by owning our own complicity and complacency and inviting the hearers to take necessary action. Confession and repentance, in a homiletical sense, are not doctrinal but performative. John of Patmos himself, writing the book of Revelation, performed a funeral liturgy and delivered a sermon exposing the ugly face of the Roman Empire (Rev. 18). John the homilist helped his hearers envision the end of the world of the imperial economic system. We overhear his homily and it is our task to tell it to our people by addressing today's Empire (Keller 2005, p. 2), which threatens the ecosystem of the Earth.

6. Conclusions

The article has attempted to showcase how the use of Scripture as a methodology of practical theology, following Ballard's four modes, and the Earth Bible Team's six ecojustice principles, can be effective in addressing environmental crises through preaching. It suggests that Scripture can be used as a resource for and of conducting practical theology. In particular, the preaching ministry unveils sins by way of truth-telling as confession, and invites congregations to practice repentance, turning to God who is at work healing the ecological wounds and reorienting the human mind and spirits towards a concern for the wellbeing of the planet.

Funding: This research received no external funding.

Conflicts of Interest: The author declares no conflict of interest.

Notes

[1] The term "environmental crises" is mainly used to encompass various and inter-locking problems of climate change, global warming, environmental racism, and forced migration. The use of this term is also conducive to the Special Issue of this journal theme.

[2] See (Neril and Dee 2020, p. xvi). It is published through The Interfaith Center for Sustainable Development, found at www.interfaithsustain.com.

[3] https://www.youtube.com/watch?v=ZTlYl8E_B14&t=1s, accessed on 3 March 2022; see the critical review of his sermon, John MacArthur on Cal Tech and the Global Warming Hoax, https://theconversation.com/god-intended-it-as-a-disposable-planet-meet-the-us-pastor-preaching-climate-change-denial-147712, accessed on 18 February 2022.

[4] *Semeia* 4: Paul Ricoeur on Biblical Hermeneutics (1975). Additionally, Ricoeur's work on hermeneutics is found in 1980. *Essays on Biblical Interpretation.* Edited by Lewis S. Mudge. Philadelphia: Fortress. Available online: https://www.religion-online.org/book/essays-on-biblical-interpretation (accessed on 3 March 2022).

[5] The Earth Bible Project. Available online: http://www.webofcreation.org/Earthbible/ebteam.html (accessed on 3 March 2022).

[6] This sermon was preached in August, 2021, at a local United Church Congregation in Toronto.

References

Ballard, Paul. 2011. The Use of Scripture. In *The Wiley Blackwell Companion to Practical Theology*. Edited by Bonnie J. Miller-McLemore. Hoboken: Blackwell Publishing Limited, vol. 63, pp. 163–72.

Ballard, Paul, and Stephen Holmes, eds. 2006. *The Bible in Pastoral Practice: Readings in the Place and Function of Scripture in the Church.* Grand Rapids: Eerdmans.

Beavis, Mary Ann, and HyeRan Kim-Cragg. 2017. *What Does the Bible Say? A Critical Conversation with Popular Culture in a Biblically Literate World*. Eugene: Cascade.

Benny Liew, Tat-Siong. 2008. *What Is Asian American Biblical Hermeneutics? Reading the New Testament*. Honolulu: University of Hawai's Press.

Carney, Mark. 2021. *Values: Building a Better World for All*. New York: Public Affair.

Cobb, John. 1992. Postmodern Christianity and Eco-Justice. In *After Nature's Revolt: Eco-Justice and Theology*. Edited by Dieter T. Hessel. Minneapolis: Augsburg.

Craddock, Fred. 2002. *Overhearing the Gospel*. Revised and Expanded Version. St. Louis: Chalice.

Eaton, Heather. 2000. Ecofeminist contributions to an Ecojustice Hermeneutics. In *Readings from the Perspective of Earth*. Sheffield: Sheffield Academic Press, p. 69.

Eaton, Heather. 2005. *Introducing Ecofeminist Theologies*. New York: Bloomsbury.

Farley, Edward. 1983. *Theologia: The Fragmentation and Unity of Theological Education*. Minneapolis: Augsburg.

Farley, Edward. 1988. *The Fragility of Knowledge: Theological Education in the Church and University*. Minneapolis: Fortress.
Fulkerson, Mary McClintock. 2007. *The Place of Redemption: Theology for a Worldly Church*. Oxford: Oxford University Press.
Gebara, Ivone. 1999. *Longing for Running Water: Ecofeminism and Liberation*. Minneapolis: Fortress.
Goff, Phillip, Arthur Farnsley, and Peter Thuesen. 2014. *The Bible in American Life: A National Study by the Center for the Study of Religion and American Culture*. Indianapolis: Indianapolis University-Purdue University.
Grey, Mary. 2004. *Sacred Longings: The Ecological Spirit and Global*. London: SCM.
Habel, Norman C., ed. 2000. *Readings from the Perspective of Earth*. Sheffield: Sheffield Academic Press.
Holbert, John C. 2011. *Preaching Creation: The Environment and the Pulpit*. Eugene: Cascade.
Keller, Catherine. 2005. *Apocalypse Now and Then: A Feminist Guide to the End of the World*. Minneapolis: Fortress.
Kim-Cragg, HyeRan. 2018. *Interdependence: A Postcolonial Feminist Practical Theology*. Eugene: Pickwick.
Kim-Cragg, HyeRan. 2021. *Postcolonial Preaching: Creating a Ripple Effect*. Lanham: Lexington.
Lee, Wendy Lynn. 2011. Fracking Is a Variety of Environmental Rape Abetted by the Law: Governor Corbett's Pennsylvania, Inc. Raging Chicken Press. December 15. Available online: https://ragingchickenpress.org/2011/12/15/fracking-is-a-variety-of-environmental-rape-abetted-by-the-law-governor-corbetts-pennsylvania-inc/ (accessed on 7 November 2021).
MacArthur, John. 2013. *Study Bible*. Nashville: Thomson Nelson.
McFague, Sallie. 1993. *The Body of God: An Ecological Theology*. Minneapolis: Augsburg Fortress.
Miller-McLemore, Bonnie. 1993. The Human Web: Reflections on the State of Pastoral Theology. *Christian Century* 367: 366–69.
Miller-McLemore, Bonnie. 2014. *The Wiley Blackwell Companion to Practical Theology*. Chichester: Blackwell.
Miller-McLemore, Bonnie. 2020. Trees and the 'Unthought Known': The Wisdom of the Nonhuman (or Do Humans "Have Shit for Brains"?). *Pastoral Psychology* 69: 424. [CrossRef]
Neril, Yonatan, and Leo Dee. 2020. *Eco Bible: An Ecological Commentary on Genesis and Exodus*. Jerusalem: Interfaith Center for Sustainable Development.
Smith, Christine. 1992. *Preaching as Weeping, Confessing, and Resistance: Radical Responses to Radical Evil*. Louisville: Westminster John Knox.
The Earth Bible Team. 2000. Guiding Ecojustice Principles. In *Readings from the Perspective of Earth*. Edited by Norman C. Habel. Sheffield: Sheffield Academic Press, pp. 38–53.
White, Lynn, Jr. 1967. The Historical Roots of Our Ecological Crisis. *Science* 10: 1203–207. [CrossRef] [PubMed]

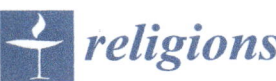

Article

Eco-Anxiety and Pastoral Care: Theoretical Considerations and Practical Suggestions

Panu Pihkala

Faculty of Theology, HELSUS Sustainability Science Institute, University of Helsinki, P.O. Box 4, 00014 Helsinki, Finland; panu.pihkala@helsinki.fi

Abstract: The environmental crisis is producing an increasing number of both physical and psychological impacts. This article studies the challenge of eco-anxiety for pastoral care, drawing from both interdisciplinary research and ecological theology. The aim is to help both practitioners and researchers to encounter eco-anxiety more constructively. The rapidly growing research about eco-anxiety and therapy is discussed in relation to pastoral care. The various forms of eco-anxiety are briefly analyzed. The role of the caregivers is discussed by using sources that study the challenges of therapists in relation to eco-anxiety. The existential depths of eco-anxiety are probed in the light of recent research and older existentialist theory. It is pointed out that the political character of ecological issues, especially climate change issues, causes many kinds of challenges for pastoral care. As the constructive conclusion of the article, various possibilities and resources for encountering eco-anxiety in pastoral care are discussed, along with the connections with wider pastoral theology. It is argued that pastoral care providers should engage in self-reflection about their own attitudes and emotions related to ecological issues, preferably with the support of trusted peers or mentors. Various organizational developments are also needed to support caregivers. Dialectical thinking is one tool that can help to navigate the complex dynamics related to environmental responsibility, eco-emotions, and questions of hope or hopelessness.

Keywords: eco-anxiety; pastoral care; climate anxiety; pastoral theology; spiritual care; psychology; existentialism; eco-theology; ecological grief; therapy

Citation: Pihkala, Panu. 2022. Eco-Anxiety and Pastoral Care: Theoretical Considerations and Practical Suggestions. *Religions* 13: 192. https://doi.org/10.3390/rel13030192

Academic Editors: Pamela R. McCarroll and HyeRan Kim-Cragg

Received: 31 January 2022
Accepted: 18 February 2022
Published: 23 February 2022

Publisher's Note: MDPI stays neutral with regard to jurisdictional claims in published maps and institutional affiliations.

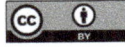

Copyright: © 2022 by the author. Licensee MDPI, Basel, Switzerland. This article is an open access article distributed under the terms and conditions of the Creative Commons Attribution (CC BY) license (https://creativecommons.org/licenses/by/4.0/).

1. Introduction

"It's in those bleak, liminal times before dawn that the eco-anxiety hits hardest. I lie in bed praying, desiring with all my heart that there be a future; that I might have again that taken-for-granted confidence that I'll live to see grandchildren, great-grandchildren. Now young people are deciding not to have children at all" (Personal reflections by Anglican theologian Frances Ward; Ward 2020, p. 141).

The concept "eco-anxiety" refers to a variety of difficult emotions and mental states that are significantly related to environmental problems, while "climate anxiety" refers to the climate-change-related forms of eco-anxiety (for discussion about terminology, see Pihkala 2020a; Wardell 2020). Some people felt eco-anxiety already decades ago (Clinebell 1996, pp. 13–14, 31–32), but it is currently an increasingly widespread phenomenon. For example, a recent global survey about climate change among 10,000 children and youth in 10 countries revealed that 56% of them thought that "humanity is doomed", while 75% felt the climate future to be frightening; 42% reported having felt at least some hesitation in having children because of the climate crisis (Hickman et al. 2021).

Even amidst the COVID-19 pandemic, climate concerns and worries are very high (Pew Research Center 2021). Worry and anxiety can be separated technically from each other, but in relation to climate change and other ecological problems, these mental phenomena are deeply connected (Ojala et al. 2021). People may feel climate-related fear, anxiety, and worry because of many kinds of things, for example, the uncertainty of the future, the damage that has already been done to ecosystems and social systems, changes in identities and lifestyles, and the loss of hope and dreams (for various kinds of climate-related loss, see Tschakert et al. 2019). Some people recognize these feelings as related at least partly to the climate crisis, while some people try to avoid making that link for various reasons such as group pressure or internal psychological anguish (for climate denial as a coping mechanism, see Haltinner and Sarathchandra 2018). Thus, there is both explicit and implicit climate anxiety (cf. Weintrobe 2021; LaMothe 2021a).

Eco-anxiety and climate anxiety have received growing attention in public discussions and research. There are disputes about what terms would be the best and about the framing of these phenomena, but even more fundamentally, there is a growing concern about the resilience of people amidst the growing ecological damage (see, e.g., Cunsolo et al. 2020). It seems evident that varieties of eco-anxiety will increasingly feature in the lives of people who seek pastoral care support or, more widely, spiritual care. This provides many challenges and possibilities. How will providers of pastoral care frame eco-anxiety—as mainly a mental health issue or as a broad phenomenon that also includes action tendencies and moral emotions? Will providers of pastoral care show care and recognition to people who feel eco-anxiety? What kind of methods will they use, and what ways forward will they offer people?

In this article, the challenges and potentials of pastoral care in relation to eco-anxiety are studied from an interdisciplinary perspective. Theological reflection is included, but a major focus in the article is the application of the contemporary interdisciplinary research about eco-anxiety and eco-emotions into pastoral care. Recent research and discussion from related fields are briefly introduced, and needs for further research and discussion are pondered. A special emphasis is given to the application of the emerging literature about therapy and eco-anxiety into pastoral care. While some scholars, including the author of this article, have made observations about eco-anxiety in the context of pastoral theology and pastoral care, as a whole, this subject has received relatively little attention (see Calder and Morgan 2016; Clinebell 1996; Pihkala 2016a, 2020b; LaMothe 2019, 2020, 2021a; McCarroll 2020; Helsel 2018; LaMothe 2016, 2021b, 2021c).

The structure of the article is as follows. First, the multifaceted character of eco-anxiety is briefly analyzed by using interdisciplinary research sources. It is argued that caregivers should be able to recognize that there may be various manifestations of eco-anxiety, both paralyzing and adaptive. Second, three major challenges and potentials for pastoral care in relation to eco-anxiety are delineated: the role of the caregivers, the existential depth of the issue, and the political dimensions of the issue.

It is pointed out that research about therapists shows the difficulty of caregivers to respond constructively to eco-anxiety: inner work and social support are needed to build resources for encounters and to enable a personal process to move forward, which will support efforts to help others.

The existential depth of eco-anxiety provides both challenges and possibilities for pastoral care: people are grappling with issues related to the meaning of life, finitude, and responsibility. Belief systems can help to provide existential resilience, but this requires an approach that takes the existential questions seriously and does not offer too-easy hope or too-easy redemption.

The political character of climate issues challenges caregivers and pastoral theologians to engage with their own attitude towards political participation. Pastoral theologians who are sensitive to eco-anxiety, such as Ryan LaMothe, Pamela McCarroll, and Storm Swain, have argued that pastoral theologians have a vocation to address the sources of suffering, which means engaging with politics and climate action. Furthermore, pastoral care providers need sensitivities to analyze the socio-political factors which affect people's eco-emotions. Intersectional justice issues also affect eco-anxiety.

In the final part of the article, many possibilities and resources for pastoral care in relation to eco-anxiety are discussed. These include the role of emotional skills and the possibility to draw from various kinds of therapies and psychologies. Special attention is given to eco-psychology and dialectical thinking, which can help to navigate the complex dynamics related to the topic, such as the relationship between individual environmental responsibility and structural issues or the relationship between hope and hopelessness. The connections between wider pastoral theology and ecological theology bring out the possibilities to encounter eco-anxiety constructively in education, environmental action, and ritual or spiritual practices. Various organizational developments are also needed to support caregivers, such as the inclusion of teaching related to eco-anxiety in theological seminaries and universities. A table is provided about the key results of the article: the various possibilities and learning goals in relation to eco-anxiety and pastoral care.

2. Eco-Anxiety: Practical, Paralyzing, and Existential

The term anxiety is notoriously wide-ranging (Barlow 2004; LeDoux 2016). Many health professionals use it in the connotation of anxiety disorders. Philosophers and theologians tend to use the term in the connotation of existential angst: anxiety about the human condition, and yet further, emotion researchers point out that anxiety is also an emotion that arises in relation to potential threats, which include some kind of problematic uncertainty from the point of view of the individual (Kurth 2018).

When interdisciplinary research about anxiety and the ecological crisis is evaluated, it can be discerned that the word anxiety is used in all of these connotations in relation to eco-anxiety (Pihkala 2020a). Eco-anxiety can manifest as strong anxiety, and it can be paralyzing (e.g., Clayton 2020; Taylor 2020); sometimes, the philosopher Glenn Albrecht's (Albrecht 2011) concept of "eco-paralysis" is used to refer to the paralyzing form (see also Albrecht 2019). Existential psychologists, philosophers, and theologians have increasingly written about the dimensions of eco-anxiety that have the characteristics of existential anxiety: people are grappling, for example, with questions of freedom and guilt, and meaning and meaninglessness, in relation to the vast ecological crisis (e.g., Budziszewska and Jonsson 2021; Pihkala 2018a), and in interdisciplinary research, it has been increasingly noticed that eco-anxiety does include the motivational dimension. Using anxiety philosopher Charlie Kurth's terminology about practical anxiety, Pihkala (2020a, 2020c) has called this dimension "practical eco-anxiety". It is practical and adaptive because it stems from the perception of real problems that need attention. Challenges arise because these socio-ecological problems are so difficult to solve and they require international cooperation; individuals and even groups can easily feel relatively powerless, which easily increases the feelings of uncontrollability which intensify anxiety (for these anxiety dynamics, see Grupe and Nitschke 2013).

Eco-anxiety research is currently growing rapidly, but so far, this research has mainly concentrated on the more paralyzing forms of eco-anxiety. This can easily strengthen the view of eco-anxiety as something at least nearly pathological, but scholars increasingly oppose this kind of emphasis, pointing out the adaptive fundamental character of eco-anxiety (Hickman et al. 2021; see also, e.g., Wullenkord et al. 2021; Verplanken et al. 2020). Among pastoral theologians, LaMothe (2020) has observed the various possibilities of eco-anxiety, both the paralyzing and the motivating ones (see also LaMothe 2021a).

Eco-anxiety is related to numerous phenomena and factors because it is connected with reacting to the ecological crisis and all the related social complexity (Crandon et al. 2022). There are many psychological phenomena that share at least some aspects with eco-anxiety, such as ecological trauma or climate trauma (Pihkala 2020d; Woodbury 2019), coping and adapting to the ecological crisis (e.g., Bradley and Reser 2017; Doherty and Clayton 2011), and various emotions and feelings related to these processes (e.g., Pihkala 2022a; Hamilton 2020; Albrecht 2019). Among the emotions and feelings, some have received special attention, such as grief or sadness (e.g., Comtesse et al. 2021; Cunsolo Willox and Landman 2017), guilt and/or shame (e.g., Jensen 2019; Fredericks 2021), and anger and/or rage (e.g., Antadze 2020). Because of the complex social dynamics related to these issues, scholars have argued that a psychosocial view would be highly necessary (e.g., Andrews and Hoggett 2019; see also the social psychology approaches in, e.g., Clayton and Manning 2018).

In a recent article, the theological and spiritual literature related to eco-anxiety prior to 2020 is briefly reviewed (Pihkala 2020b). New writings on related topics appear regularly, and many of these are cited below (e.g., Malcolm 2020a, 2020b; Ward 2020; Joyce 2020; see also the reflections about ecological trauma and pastoral theology in Swain 2020). Most of the sources discussing spiritual care and eco-anxiety have focused on Christianity, but there is an article about Hindu spiritual care and climate trauma (Patel 2020).

Pastoral care providers need support and information so that they can see the various dimensions of eco-anxiety and not just one or two of them. Seeing the fundamental role of eco-anxiety as practical anxiety helps to avoid pathologization and over-therapization, and seeing the possibilities of eco-anxiety to turn into a paralyzing condition helps to understand the importance of providing enough psychosocial and spiritual support for people.

3. The Role of the Caregivers

A crucial challenge is the resilience and attitudes of the caregivers (in this case, the pastoral care providers). In relation to caregivers in general, it has been increasingly noted that the ecological crisis is a psychologically demanding topic for them, too. The sheer weight and intensity of the crisis are difficult to bear (if proof is needed, the natural sciences offer plenty of data and predictions; see, e.g., Steffen et al. 2015). The issue is made more difficult by the fact that everyone is implicated in the crisis: the topic challenges people's behavioral habits, their values, their identities, their beliefs, and their dreams about the future. Furthermore, people may already have so many other difficulties in their lives that it is challenging to give any resources to the ecological issues. As a result of all this complexity, people have been noticed to be prone to distancing reactions, in other words, to disavowal and various other forms of denial. These dynamics can also be analyzed as forms of maladaptive or adaptive coping or as either healthy or problematic defense mechanisms. (The research literature on these topics is very large. For popular introductions, see Stoknes 2015; Marshall 2015. For an academic overview, see Jylhä 2017).

For a long time, the people who felt eco-anxiety had strong difficulties in finding caregivers or therapists who could resonate with their experiences and support them on an emotional level. There are many reminiscences of encounters with therapists who simply have disavowed the reality of the issue and suggested that some inter- or intrapersonal matters are the real cause of the person's feelings (see already Macy 1995; and, e.g., Stoknes 2015). While the inter- and intrapersonal matters may indeed shape people's experiences, there is a large and rapidly growing research evidence showing that eco-anxiety can simply result from knowing and feeling about environmental issues (see Section 2 above).

Currently, there is a growing research literature about the difficulties of therapists in facing ecological issues and especially the climate crisis. Haseley (2019) discusses the relationship between other mental health issues and climate anxiety and observes that the therapists' own disavowal or denial can be a challenging obstacle. Seaman (2016) surveyed how therapists see the role of climate issues and noted that younger therapists recognized climate issues more often in their work, which resulted in the hypothesis that these younger therapists were better able to resonate with their clients' issues related to the climate crisis. Since the time of that study, the climate issues have become even more pressing, and it is probable that they feature also even more in therapy.

In recent research, Silva and Coburn (2022) analyze these dynamics on the basis of eight in-depth interviews of Australian therapists. They make highly useful categorizations of the various difficulties that therapists experience. Topics that are discussed include the challenges for the self-identity and psychological well-being of the therapist, the existential and socio-political challenges included in climate issues, the therapists' experiences of how clients increasingly bring these matters into therapeutic encounters, and many professional challenges and uncertainties that the therapists experience.

The personal actions and attitudes of the therapist in relation to climate action may be evoked in many ways in therapeutic encounters. Clients may expect from the therapist or caregiver a certain kind of attitude towards climate issues, either a positive or a negative one. For example, those in disavowal or denial may expect their caregiver to manifest a similar attitude and offer them psychosocial support in their own stance, and others may expect a commitment to climate action manifested by the caregiver.

Furthermore, the therapist or caregiver may himself/herself wrestle with inner conflicts related to climate action, as has been noted in research (Silva and Coburn 2022; cf. Orange 2017). Therapists may feel anxiety because their own lifestyle contributes to climate emissions and because they feel either inner or outer pressure to make changes. This distress may cause many kinds of results: some therapists or caregivers may try to avoid the distressing topic altogether, while others may try to solve the problem by engaging in various kinds of behavior and emotion regulation.

It is to be expected that similar difficulties occur with pastoral care providers. There are some discussions of this dynamic in literature (Pihkala 2016a; McCarroll 2020; LaMothe 2019, 2020, p. 143), but the author is not aware of wider empirical research about eco-anxious people's experiences with pastoral care providers. The fact that so little research and other literature has been published about pastoral care and eco-anxiety—with various terms—points to the probability that many pastoral care providers are struggling to integrate eco-anxiety sensitivity into their work. Many authors have emphasized that much self-compassion is needed because the situation is indeed difficult (Davenport 2017; Ray 2020; see also Brach 2019).

Pastoral care providers thus need both individual work and social support in order to encounter eco-anxiety constructively. Intention and determination are important (Greenspan 2004), but the contexts of people are very different, and support from others is crucial, too. Below, in Section 6, the possibilities of a dialectical approach are discussed (drawing especially from Lewis et al. 2020), and in Section 7, certain organizational means for support are listed. However, the existential weight of eco-anxiety makes things more difficult and also more pressing, and this theme is discussed next.

4. The Existential Depth of Eco-Anxiety

The wording "existential crisis" can be used in two connotations in relation to the climate crisis. First, the term is sometimes used to refer simply to the life-threatening character of this global crisis. For many people, the climate crisis is an existential threat to their very survival or their well-being. Second, the term can be used in the sense of existentialism, referring to the difficult questions and feelings related to being human in a vast universe.

Pioneering scholars and therapists have long since noticed the existential character of eco-anxiety, even while the concept of eco-anxiety was not yet used. The influential therapist Clinebell (1996) discussed the phenomenon with the term angst and observed already in the 1990s many of the emotions which can be connected with it, such as guilt and sadness. Clinebell also noticed the connections between death anxiety and eco-anxiety, although he did not develop this theme fully.

The author has in his studies pointed out that the existential theologian Paul Tillich had much ecotheological content in his works and also briefly discussed some aspects of eco-anxiety, especially the shame and horror which can be related to realizing how strongly humankind has damaged the more-than-human world (see Pihkala 2018a, 2018b; Pihkala 2020b; Tillich 1963). The author also pointed out that the three major aspects of Tillich's view of existential anxiety all apply strongly to eco-anxiety. There is eco-anxiety related to fate and death, to emptiness and meaninglessness, and to guilt and condemnation (Pihkala 2018a; Tillich 1952; see also generally Scott and Weems 2013).

Currently, scholarship is deepening the understanding of the existential character of eco-anxiety. For example, existential psychologists Budziszewska and Jonsson (2021) studied the climate anxiety of 10 Swedish therapy clients and applied the existential theories of Tillich, Irvin Yalom, and Ernesto Spinelli. These researchers observed that people may experience existential isolation in the midst of the climate crisis, and they raise up important aspects related to authenticity, freedom, and responsibility.[1] The existential depth of eco-anxiety has also been noted by many other scholars (e.g., Pienaar 2011; Passmore and Howell 2014; Silva and Coburn 2022).

The dynamics of these existential aspects are wider and more complex than what can be discussed here. Deep down, they seem to be related to the challenge of finding meaning amidst suffering and practicing responsibility without burning out (cf. Pihkala 2018a; Jamail 2019; Clinebell 1996; see also the similar reflections in eco-anxiety books that do not operate with the concept of meaning, such as Gillespie 2020; Ray 2020; Weber 2020). In the following, some aspects of the existential dimensions are discussed in order to provide examples of what kind of issues may be related to pastoral care encounters of eco-anxiety.

As noted above, guilt has been found to be one of the common emotions related to climate issues because so many things in the lifestyles of industrialized countries contribute to global warming. Climate guilt can be so severe that it has an existential dimension: it becomes related to the way in which the person exists in the universe. Climate guilt may also have elements of what existential psychologists such as Rollo May and Irvin Yalom have called existential guilt: people may feel that they are not fulfilling their potential as beings. This feeling of not being what one should or could be comes close to shame, which is another prominent climate emotion (Jensen 2019; Fredericks 2021; Orange 2017). Scholars have noted that there exists "species shame": some people feel shame as members of the human species, which has so profoundly damaged the ecosystems.

These feelings are closely related to many other notions discussed in existentialism, such as freedom and authenticity. They may also be connected with feelings of isolation, another major existentialist theme (Yalom 1980; for climate anxiety and isolation, see Budziszewska and Jonsson 2021). People may feel isolated and lonely in relation to climate issues because of many reasons. One possible reason is guilt and/or shame. Another is that their climate grief is not recognized by others and it turns into disenfranchised grief (Cunsolo Willox and Ellis 2018; Kretz 2017). Yet another reason is simply the experience that others in one's vicinity do not take climate issues seriously, as they practice denial or disavowal (Budziszewska and Jonsson 2021; Weintrobe 2021). "Climate isolation" as a feeling may eventually have elements of existential isolation, the feeling that one cannot find the connection between oneself and the world.

Authenticity is an existentialist concept that has been used in various connotations: it refers to being true to one's being (for a review of various views about it, see Mkono 2020). Here, it is only pointed out that issues of authenticity feature in people's experiences of the climate crisis: the crisis provokes many people to ponder their deepest values and their life choices, and the practical situations amidst the crisis may cause conflicts related to authenticity (see also the brief reflections in Budziszewska and Jonsson 2021). As an example of these, tourism scholar Mkono has analyzed the experiences of authenticity and inauthenticity related to "eco-conscious" travelers and their choices. Often these travelers fail to live up to the moral standards which they espouse, which can raise accusations of hypocrisy. Mkono insightfully points out that these kinds of issues are both social debates and potentially existential distresses: feelings of inauthenticity may reach an existential level of not being true to what one thinks and believes one should be.

In the next section, the problems related to the issue of individual ecological actions are discussed, and the need for a socio-political critique of many power structures is emphasized. There are profound structural problems and ethical problems related to the ways in which the division of responsibility between individuals and collectives is often presented or felt. Now, a final dimension of existential aspects is discussed here: the one related to death and finitude.

One of the big challenges related to both existential anxiety in general and to eco-anxiety in particular is the connection with death anxiety. It seems evident that this dark background is activated in people's minds in relation to ecological threats, and this often causes distancing reactions, as for example, the research in terror management theory has shown (for an insightful discussion, see Adams 2016, pp. 109–28). The author has himself written about the connections between ecotheology, death, and eco-anxiety (Pihkala 2018b).

However, death is in itself a very tough topic to engage with, and the task of engaging with both death and eco-anxiety seems to be too much for most people, even though these topics are actually interconnected. As scholars Affifi and Christie (2018) note in their insightful study on environmental education and pedagogy of death, "Very rare is the soul who can dwell in existential angst by day and not watch Netflix at night" (p. 11).

This discussion of the existential depth of eco-anxiety is bound to be disturbing also for pastoral theologians, but it is regrettably a very necessary disturbance in the current global circumstances. The crucial thing is to understand how deep an existential crisis the ecological crisis can be for contemporary people (see also Pienaar 2011; Hickman 2020; Malcolm 2020a; for reflections by a person of color, see Heglar 2020). Pastoral care providers need to think about both the psychosocial factors that affect the people they encounter and also the possible existential dimensions of people's experiences. For example, climate guilt can be both a social, a political, a psychological, and an existential issue. Many of these existential issues can also be issues for the caregiver himself/herself, perhaps already recognized, perhaps not yet. For religious people, these existential concerns may be linked with deep spiritual and religious crises. As many texts show, people are grappling with questions about how their religion, for example, Christianity, functions in such circumstances (e.g., Malcolm 2020a; Ward 2020; McIntosh 2008). Eco-anxiety raises deep issues related to the meaning of life and the meaning in life.

However, pastoral care providers have many resources that they can develop and utilize to respond to the existential issues related to eco-anxiety. This can be conceptualized, for example, as existential resilience: the ability to withstand the existential questions arising from changing circumstances (see Foster 2015; Pihkala 2018a). The possible resources is discussed more below after the important political dimension is discussed.

5. The Political Dimension and Justice Issues

Eco-anxiety is furthermore complicated by the strong political character of ecological and climate issues. This character can cause hesitation in many therapists and pastoral care providers, who would not like to take political stances in their work (cf. LaMothe 2016). As for eco-anxiety itself, it is often made more difficult by social and political disputes. Anxiety is lessened if there is a feeling that the collectives around oneself are taking determined action to prepare and mitigate the threats which cause anxiety. However, unfortunately, the responses of collectives towards climate issues are often ambiguous, and sometimes, the leaders are in denial or disavowal (for a scathing critique of this, see the recent climate psychology book by Weintrobe 2021). For example, young people have often reported that their climate anxiety has grown worse because political leaders do not engage in ambitious climate politics (e.g., Hickman 2020; Jones and Davison 2021; cf. Hickman et al. 2021; Johnson and Wilkinson 2020).

Several pastoral theologians and ecotheologians have argued that Christians simply must accept the political dimension of the ecological crisis and act according to ethical values (for a wide argument about this, see LaMothe 2021c). This does not mean adhering to any one particular political party, but it does mean the demand to critically evaluate the environmental politics of various parties. The biosphere is degrading at a very alarming rate. A pioneering Lutheran ecotheologian, H. Paul Santmire, has proposed that the climate crisis and the wider ecological crisis actually form a "status confessionis": a situation where Christians simply cannot stay passive and silent because there are too dire violations of God's will (Santmire 2020, p. 130). The concept of status confessionis has a long and partly contested history in Christian theology, and it was famously applied, for example, by Lutherans in relation to the apartheid racism in South Africa in the 1970s and 1980s (for the history of the concept, see DeJonge 2017).

There are numerous kinds of justice issues in relation to eco-anxiety. There is a tendency in various parts of the world that the most vulnerable populations are also the most susceptible to various kinds of climate-related harm. In Christian theology, the calls for "climate justice" have found deep roots in the eco-justice tendencies of ecotheology, which have been strong since the 1960s (see already the research bibliography by Bakken et al. 1995). Many proponents of ecotheology have called for justice towards both humans and non-humans (this has been especially prominent in animal theology and in posthumanism-leaning ecotheology; see, e.g., Latour 2009). Local and regional inequalities are very strong in many countries, as is discussed, for example, by environmental ethicist and theologian Jenkins (2013). In the 2000s, the movements for climate justice have been growing, and these movements have started to raise the issue that also the paralyzing forms of climate anxiety are distributed unequally (for the wide challenge of climate change and climate justice for Christian ecotheology, see Conradie and Koster 2019; for climate justice more widely, see Jafry 2019).

There are also justice issues related to the connections between climate anxiety, gender, and the legacies of racism and colonialism. In many studies, women have self-reported much more eco-anxiety than men (e.g., Hickman et al. 2021; Searle and Gow 2010). In many societies and regions, there are strong inequalities related to political power, race, and gender, which also affect climate politics and climate emotions (see, e.g., O'Dell-Chaib 2019). From the point of view of indigenous peoples, the climate crisis can appear as just a new form of oppression and suffering wrought on them by industrialized countries (e.g., Whyte 2017).

For pastoral theologians and pastoral care providers, these connections with politics and justice issues are very important to note. Many such dynamics shape people's eco-anxiety and also their attitudes towards how these issues are framed (Ray 2021). For example, in their study about climate anxiety in South Africa, Barnwell and colleagues (2020) noticed psychological impacts of climate change but also observed that many people did not resonate with the wording climate anxiety, which for them sounded more related to other people in other kinds of circumstances. There needs to be sensitivity to the wordings that are used in different contexts: sometimes such wordings as chronic stress or distress may function better than climate anxiety or eco-anxiety, and sensitivity to justice issues helps to provide recognition.

There has been much discussion in general about the question of engaging with the sources of suffering as part of the work of the therapist or the slightly different work of the pastoral care provider. Pastoral and political theologian LaMothe endorses famous therapist and social thinker Franz Fanon's approach, where the aforementioned task is seen as a crucial part of the work (LaMothe 2020, 2021a). LaMothe (2020, pp. 146–47) argues: "To fail to make the connection [between political-economic realities and the experiences of the people in therapy] would not only be unethical, because it would collude with the powers and institutions that caused suffering; it would also not be therapeutic, because it would mystify patients' suffering". In these views, the therapeutic and the political become interconnected (see also Clinebell 1996, pp. 10–11).

6. Possibilities and Resources for Pastoral Care

Pastoral care providers, and pastoral theologians more broadly, have many possibilities to help people channel their eco-anxiety more constructively. By engaging with the topic, pastoral theologians are at the same time dealing with their own emotions about these issues. As discussed above, the role of the caregivers is both crucial and difficult: they need to be able to notice the ways in which their own attitudes and emotions affect the pastoral care situations. On the positive side, it is an ancient truth that one may be personally helped by helping others.

Many kinds of actions, practices, and ways of non-action can give pastoral theologians resources to encounter eco-anxiety (for a review of these kinds of methods in general, see Baudon and Jachens 2021, although their use of the word "treatment" is slightly problematic in the author's view since it underscores the pathological dimensions). First, there is a need for intention and determination to work with these issues (Greenspan 2004). Because the ecological issues may feel difficult both in relation to practice and emotional life, people need both intention and support. One way forward could be to engage in a spiritual journey in relation to learning more about eco-anxiety and its existential challenge. With the support of natural environments, spiritual practice, and preferably trusted peers or mentors, it becomes more bearable—and more probable—to engage with dark eco-emotions. Chase (2011a, 2011b) provides resources for nature-oriented spiritual practice in relation to these themes, and Ward (2020) offers a journey of theological and emotional reflection in her monograph. Reading Ward's eco-anxiety book together with others and staying with the biblical passages quoted in the text is one possibility. For more global perspectives, the article collection edited by Malcolm (2020a) provides stories of both climate grief and courage from Christians around the world. The ancient theological method of lamenting is one resource explored in the book, together with poetry and other textual forms (see also Malcolm 2020b; Saler 2016). Methods and resources for social support are currently being researched and implemented: for example, the British Christian environmental organization GreenChristian has set up a discussion group method of encountering eco-anxiety (see Deep Waters 2022).

Second, various kinds of emotional methodologies provide support. The pastoral theologian can educate himself/herself with these and perhaps then educate others to use similar skills. There is a wide range of useful approaches, such as emotion-focused therapy (EFT, see, e.g., Greenberg 2004), Karla McLaren's emotion work methodology (McLaren 2010; for anxiety, McLaren 2020), and explicitly eco-emotional methodologies such as Joanna Macy's "The Work That Reconnects" (Macy and Brown 2014; The Work That Reconnects Network 2022) or Doppelt's (2016) transformational resilience methodology (for discussion of various eco-emotional methodologies and research about their impacts, see Hamilton 2020). Generally, developing a positive attitude towards all kinds of emotions is highly important (Greenspan 2004; Lomas 2016).

Third, methods of eco-psychology and eco-therapy provide many resources. Pastoral care providers can think critically about their own "environmental identity" (Clinebell 1996; in general, see Clayton and Opotow 2003; Doherty 2018) and utilize literature that encourages therapists to work with their own nature relationship (Lassloffy and Davis 2018; Rust 2020; for pastoral theological reflections, see also Clinebell 1996; Helsel 2018). There are both outdoor and indoor eco-psychological activities that can help with various eco-emotions (for general literature, see Jordan and Hinds 2016; Rust and Totton 2012; Buzzell and Chalquist 2009). There are creative and partly radical methodologies available, such as Trebbe Johnson's method of engaging directly with "wounded places" in more-than-human nature (Johnson 2018; Johnson 2017; for theological reflections about wounded natural places, see Stewart 2016; Pihkala 2020e). This method encourages people to be open to all kinds of emotions that environmental damage and changes may engender. There is much discussion about sadness and grief, but also about the possibility that "radical joy" may emerge through full-bodied emotional engagement (Johnson 2018; cf. Pihkala 2017a; Erickson 2020). In general, spiritual practices may help to encounter ecological grief, which is often accompanied by anxiety (Christie 2013; Menning 2017).

A special part of a holistic eco-psychological approach is one's relation to one's own body, which is the physical connecting element with the more-than-human world. Among others, Clinebell (1996) argued that a healthy relationship to the larger environment requires developing a healthy appreciation of one's body. This theme of how one regards one's body links together eco-psychology, emotion research, and wider discussions about the role of the body in Christian theology (for that wider discussion, see, e.g., Brown 2007; Isherwood and Stuart 1998). In eco-anxiety literature, the importance of many kinds of embodied practices is emphasized as means to encounter difficult emotions (e.g., Davenport 2017; Weber 2020).

Fourth, it is possible to draw from various other therapies and clinical psychology. A therapeutic approach to eco-anxiety, which takes its paralyzing potential seriously but does not pathologize it, has been developed by experienced environmental psychologist Thomas Doherty (e.g., 2018). Together with colleagues, he has recently published an overview of clinical psychology and ecological, especially climate-related concerns (Doherty et al. 2021).

For example, acceptance and commitment therapy (ACT) can be applied to eco-anxiety (see also Feather and Williams 2022). Learning to tolerate uncertainty and ambivalence helps; this provides counter-resources to "intolerance of uncertainty", a psychological construct that is closely related to eco-anxiety (Pihkala 2020a).

In the wide literature about stronger anxiety, which often focuses on state anxiety and anxiety disorders, there are many tips and guidelines about practices that can help when such anxiety arises (for an overview of such research, see Cox and Olatunji 2019). These kinds of tips have been applied directly to eco-anxiety by some therapists and authors (see esp. Weber 2020, pp. 110–22; see also Grose 2020; Davenport 2017; Doppelt 2016).

Because of the existential dimensions of eco-anxiety, existential therapies and meaning-focused therapies can be especially helpful. Many of the authors who have written about eco-anxiety offer their versions of such approaches (see, e.g., Clinebell 1996; Doppelt 2016). The meaning-centered approach called logotherapy, developed originally by Victor Frankl, is one such approach, but meaning-focused therapies have also gained new interest and new forms in the 2000s (see, e.g., Batthyany and Russo-Netzer 2014; Hicks and Routledge 2013; Vos 2018). There is more work to do in applying the rich discussions about meaning in pastoral theology explicitly with eco-anxiety issues, and there is already some literature that applies the thoughts of classic philosophers of meaning such as Rollo May into the issues of our ecological era (e.g., Softas-Nall and Woody 2017).

Therapists Lewis et al. (2020) have recently applied dialectical thinking to the difficult questions related to eco-anxiety and ecological action, and this promising venture is given special attention here. These therapists emphasize the need to keep difficult issues dialectically open: for example, to appreciate individual actions and still emphasize the structural character of socio-ecological problems. The therapist and the client can together discuss and practice accepting ambivalence in relation to environmental responsibility: there is an ethical need to do better, but because structural problems limit the possibilities of individuals, there must be an emphasis on civil and political action towards structural change. Here, theologians may draw from various resources in Christian theology where both repentant action and acceptance of forgiveness and grace are emphasized (cf. Pihkala 2016a).

This kind of dialectical approach also enables one to explore hope while admitting that there are also feelings of despair and hopelessness. More-than-human nature can function both as a source of comfort and a source of threat; there are both certainties and uncertainties, and the social reality may be incongruent with climate reality (Lewis et al. 2020). Instead of both the listener and the client succumbing to binary thinking—which can be really tempting in the midst of anxiety—therapists and pastoral care providers should work to keep the dialectic open.

Their discussion of dialectical thinking brings reminds a theological reading of the influential "dialectical theology" in the 20th century (Karl Barth, Emil Brunner, and others). The influence of this dialectical theology extended beyond those theologians who were associated with this particular, albeit loose, school of theology. The theologians of the period between the 1910s and 1940s were hardened by the harsh reality of the two world wars, and many of the so-called "realist theologians" manifested influences from dialectical thought. Some of the theologians from these two broad schools of theology had already then environmental sensitivities (Pihkala 2017b; summary available in Pihkala 2016b). Perhaps now, when the industrialized world has had to return to the reality of suffering after a period of optimism and belief in progress since the Second World War, these earlier theologies will gain new interest and new applications in the context of eco-anxiety. There are many common tones in the therapeutic proposals by Lewis et al. (2020) and in the theologies of such figures as Daniel Day Williams, H. Richard Niebuhr, and Joseph Sittler. Naturally, these earlier theologians did not yet have climate awareness, and their thoughts also need to be augmented with more sensitivity to issues of race, gender, and postcolonialism (for the challenges of postcolonialism to spiritual care in general, see Lartey and Moon 2020). However, these theologians produced profound discussions of hope and tragedy.

Currently, the public discussion abounds with implicit and explicit talk about the various forms of hope, despair, and hopelessness in relation to the ecological crisis and the climate crisis (for discussion of this in popular books, see, e.g., Sherrell 2021). There are naturally many stances on these issues. Some advocate for "realistic" hope, which is empathetic towards the suffering (e.g., Kelsey 2020), while others in a rather similar vein emphasize "radical hope", hoping even while there cannot be knowledge about what exactly could save the situation (this approach was championed by philosopher Jonathan Lear; see, e.g., Williston 2012). Some are more pessimistic: there are notable social movements, albeit countercultural, which base their action on the firm belief that there will be major socio-ecological collapses in the near future. Additionally, theological reflections of this vein have started to emerge (e.g., Bradford 2020; see also Robinson 2020). The members of these movements sometimes accuse other people of practicing "hopium", an addictive belief that there is still hope in the form of optimism. However, the author here joins the eco-anxiety writer Weber (2020) in his critique of both "hopium" and "reverse hopium": the latter term pointing to another form of binary thinking where it is held evident that there can be no hope.

It seems that the way forward could indeed be a dialectical one: a kind of pilgrimage that takes place between hope and hopelessness or through fluctuations of them. LaMothe, who has written in depth about the issues of hope and hopelessness amidst the ecological and political crises, champions a roughly similar view (the widest discussion of this is in LaMothe 2021c, Chp. 6). Discussing the striking book by theologian Miguel de la Torre, *Theology of Hopelessness*, LaMothe argues that courageous care should be the main emphasis, not hope. Drawing from philosopher Agamben's notion of inoperativity, LaMothe argues that hope could be seen as inoperative: it would not be the frame in which issues are interpreted, but rather people should practice care nevertheless. The author's own earlier emphasis on "tragic hope" (Pihkala 2017a, 2018a) and the centrality of the concept of meaning have many similarities with LaMothe's view. Quoting Kaur, LaMothe summarizes his view: "This is our defiance—to practice love even in hopelessness" (LaMothe 2021c, end of chp. 1 (LaMothe)).

Table 1 summarizes the possibilities and learning goals related to eco-anxiety, which have been explored in this article via interdisciplinary and theological research.

Table 1. Possibilities and learning goals related to eco-anxiety for pastoral theologians.

Possibilities and Learning Goals Related to Eco-Anxiety (Themes and Subthemes)	Examples of Sources That Discuss This Issue
Studying the various **forms** of eco-anxiety	(Pihkala 2020a; Clayton 2020)
- Understanding that eco-anxiety can be both paralyzing and adaptive and learning about the empirical evidence	(Hickman et al. 2021; Wullenkord et al. 2021)
- Learning about various socio-ecological dynamics which shape people's eco-anxiety	(Crandon et al. 2022)
Learning about the challenges of **caregivers** in relation to eco-anxiety	(Silva and Coburn 2022; LaMothe 2019)
- Understanding dynamics related to identity, emotions, and psychosocial factors	(Silva and Coburn 2022)
- Engaging with the possible disavowal by the caregiver	(Haseley 2019)
- Practicing self-compassion	(Ray 2020; Brach 2019)
Becoming acquainted with the various **existential dimensions** that can be linked with eco-anxiety	(Budziszewska and Jonsson 2021)

Table 1. *Cont.*

Possibilities and Learning Goals Related to Eco-Anxiety (Themes and Subthemes)	Examples of Sources That Discuss This Issue
- Understanding the crucial role of responsibility and guilt in relation to ecological issues	(Jensen 2019; Fredericks 2021)
- Understanding how death anxiety may be linked with eco-anxiety	(Pihkala 2018b; Pienaar 2011)
- Understanding the prevalence of various forms of sadness in relation to ecological changes	(Cunsolo Willox and Landman 2017)
Thinking critically about the **political dimensions** of eco-anxiety and ecological issues	(LaMothe 2020, 2021a)
- Understanding the need to personally reflect on one's attitude towards ecological action and climate politics	(LaMothe 2016)
- Being able to analyze political and social dynamics that shape various people's experiences of eco-anxiety and their preferred language about it	(Barnwell et al. 2020; Ray 2021)
- Understanding how factors related to gender, race, and colonialism may shape people's eco-anxiety	(O'Dell-Chaib 2019; Whyte 2017)
Learning about various **possibilities and resources** for encountering eco-anxiety more constructively	(Clinebell 1996; Weber 2020; Baudon and Jachens 2021)
- Developing an emotion-positive attitude, seeking social support, and manifesting intention to work with eco-anxiety	(Greenspan 2004; McLaren 2010)
- Understanding how many therapeutic and psychological approaches can be utilized for eco-anxiety work	(Doherty et al. 2021; Davenport 2017)
- Learning about religious and Christian resources	(Pihkala 2018a; Christie 2013; Macy and Brown 2014)
- Learning about emotion-focused methods	(Hamilton 2020; Greenspan 2004; McLaren 2020)
- Learning about and utilizing eco-psychological methods and thinking about one's environmental identity	(Rust 2020; Clinebell 1996)
- Appreciating one's body as the connecting element with the more-than-human world and using various embodied activities to encounter eco-anxiety	(Clinebell 1996; Davenport 2017; Weber 2020)
- Applying dialectical thinking in relation to the difficult dynamics of the ecological crisis, such as the relationship between individual action and collective action for structural change	(Lewis et al. 2020)
- Understanding how issues of hope, despair, and hopelessness are connected with eco-anxiety	(LaMothe 2021c; Pihkala 2017a)
Understanding how eco-anxiety is connected with **wider pastoral theology and ecological theology**	(LaMothe 2021c; McCarroll 2020; Swain 2020)
- Realizing the connections between ecological action and eco-anxiety and the need to develop emotional resilience in environmental activism	(Ray 2020; Weber 2020)
- Understanding the ways in which rituals and spiritual practices may help in encountering eco-anxiety	(Chase 2011a; Malcolm 2020a, 2020b; Pihkala 2021)
- Encountering eco-anxiety in education and formation of pastoral care providers	(Calder and Morgan 2016; cf. Pihkala 2020b)
- Launching and supporting organizational developments such as the integration of eco-anxiety teaching in seminaries and universities	(Clinebell 1996)

7. In Conclusions: Pastoral Theology in the Era of Eco-Anxiety

This article has studied the challenges and possibilities related to eco-anxiety for pastoral care. Many observations have been made about therapeutic encounters in general, including various forms of spiritual care. The wider context related to pastoral theology as a whole has been much present and is given more attention in these final comments, together with its relation to eco-theology.

The recent efforts to integrate ecological theology and pastoral theology (see LaMothe 2016; McCarroll 2020; Swain 2020; cf. Clinebell 1996) are very relevant for the topic of this article. This article has focused on the emotional and psychosocial dimensions of ecological issues, but naturally, the wider spheres of action and various forms of pro-environmental behavior are interrelated with the psychological dimension. Action may help to channel eco-anxiety constructively, but if there is no space for emotion work, people may burn out (Ray 2020; Hoggett and Randall 2018; Nairn 2019). Indeed, some environmental organizations nowadays include eco-emotion workshops and support procedures in their work (see, e.g., the discussion in Weber 2020). There may thus be an element of pastoral care in the ecological activities of congregations and other collectives, and the explicit offering of such support is an important thing to consider.

In general, participating in various kinds of environmental action usually helps with various difficult eco-emotions, and there is a rich literature about various ways in which religious communities can participate in this (see, for example, the materials produced by ecumenical and denominational environmental movements, such as Laudato Si Movement 2022; A Rocha 2022; World Council of Churches 2022). The potential strengths and challenges for various denominations in encountering eco-anxiety is a topic for future research (for some reflections on certain denominations, see Pihkala 2016a; Ward 2020).

Various kinds of rituals can be organized in relation to eco-anxiety and other eco-emotions (Pihkala 2021), and sometimes, rituals related to ecological concerns have implicit dimensions related to the processing of eco-emotions (cf. Fredericks 2021). While these rituals are maybe not pastoral care per se, if the caregiver is aware of these kinds of methods, they can be recommended to people on suitable occasions. Engaging in spiritual practices can help both the caregiver and the "client" to process their eco-anxiety (cf. Malcolm 2020b). The author has written elsewhere of the need for religious leaders to work critically with eco-guilt, eco-anger, and ecological grief and sadness in spiritual care, rituals, and wider action (Pihkala 2022b). Case examples in English are available, for example, about ways to encounter ecological shame via creative Christian worship (Powell 2019) or ecological grief via outdoor spiritual practices (Hirschfeld and Blackmer 2021; see also many articles in Malcolm 2020a).

The education and formation of pastoral care providers is an area that needs attention in relation to eco-anxiety. First of all, many who undergo such training are young of age, and many of them feel eco-anxiety in some form. They require support from their teachers (cf. Pihkala 2020b). Second, students can be taught constructive ways to encounter eco-anxiety, as has been the aim in Calder and Morgan's pioneering approach (Calder and Morgan 2016). Teaching about eco-anxiety and eco-emotions should be included in theological seminaries and universities. Furthermore, pastors, counselors, and other providers of pastoral care may find it difficult to devote time to learn more about contemporary issues such as eco-anxiety in the midst of their daily life and work. One potential means to help in this is to organize workshops where various professionals focus on environmental issues, including their emotional dimension. Various frameworks have been applied to the process of transformation of identity and attitudes that the ecological crisis requires, such as the "ecological conversion" championed by Francis (2015) and the "affective transformation" delineated by environmental scholar Verlie (2022).

It is notable that anxiety researcher and philosopher Kurth (2018) discusses the positive sides of anxiety often through the examples of religious figures, such as John Woolman and Martin Luther King. Kurth points out that it was exactly anxiety that caused these people to act: they felt problematic uncertainty about moral issues, and this anxiety did not let them go. They were able to cultivate anxiety as a moral emotion and not to stifle it or run away from it. This dynamic can be the positive power of eco-anxiety: if it does not become too intense, it causes people to "stay with the trouble" (see Haraway 2016) and search for ways to practice morality and responsibility, even amidst ambiguous circumstances. Religions may offer people sources of existential resilience, which help to bear eco-anxiety, but this needs effort and intention since religion can also become a hiding place from the troubles of the world.

Funding: This research was supported by a personal grant from Finnish Cultural Foundation, granted in February 2019 (no grant number given).

Institutional Review Board Statement: Not applicable.

Informed Consent Statement: Not applicable.

Data Availability Statement: Not applicable.

Acknowledgments: The author expresses gratitude to the two anonymous peer reviewers for their feedback about how to improve the article.

Conflicts of Interest: The author declares no conflict of interest. The funders had no role in the design of the study; in the collection, analyses, or interpretation of data; in the writing of the manuscript, or in the decision to publish the results.

Notes

[1] There are several more research articles about eco-anxiety and existential issues currently either in press or in peer review. See, for example, the two forthcoming books edited by Douglas Vakoch and Sam Mickey, *Climate Psychology in a Pandemic: Environmental Health in Lockdown* and *Eco-Anxiety and Planetary Hope: The Experience of COVID-19 and the Climate Crisis*.

References

A Rocha International. 2022. Available online: https://www.arocha.org/en/ (accessed on 17 February 2022).
Adams, Matthew. 2016. *Ecological Crisis, Sustainability and the Psychosocial Subject: Beyond Behaviour Change*. London: Palgrave Macmillan.
Affifi, Ramsey, and Beth Christie. 2018. Facing Loss: Pedagogy of Death. *Environmental Education Research* 25: 1143–57. [CrossRef]
Albrecht, Glenn. 2011. Chronic Environmental Change: Emerging 'Psychoterratic' Syndromes. In *Climate Change and Human Well-Being: Global Challenges and Opportunities*. Edited by Inka Weissbecker. New York: Springer, pp. 43–56.
Albrecht, Glenn. 2019. *Earth Emotions: New Words for a New World*. Ithaca: Cornell University Press.
Andrews, Nadine, and Paul Hoggett. 2019. Facing up to Ecological Crisis: A Psychosocial Perspective from Climate Psychology. In *Facing Up to Climate Reality: Honesty, Disaster and Hope*. Edited by John Foster. London: Green House Publishing, pp. 155–71.
Antadze, Nino. 2020. Moral Outrage as the Emotional Response to Climate Injustice. *Environmental Justice* 13: 21–26. [CrossRef]
Bakken, Peter W., Joan Gibb Engel, and J. Ronald Engel. 1995. *Ecology, Justice, and Christian Faith: A Critical Guide to the Literature*. Westport: Greenwood Publishing Group.
Barlow, David H. 2004. *Anxiety and Its Disorders: The Nature and Treatment of Anxiety and Panic*, 2nd ed. New York: Guilford Press.
Barnwell, Garret, Louise Stroud, and Mark Watson. 2020. Critical Reflections from South Africa: Using the Power Threat Meaning Framework to Place Climate-Related Distress in Its Socio-Political Context. *Clinical Psychology Forum* 332: 7–15.
Batthyany, Alexander, and Pninit Russo-Netzer, eds. 2014. *Meaning in Positive and Existential Psychology*, 1st ed. New York: Springer. [CrossRef]
Baudon, Pauline, and Liza Jachens. 2021. A Scoping Review of Interventions for the Treatment of Eco-Anxiety. *International Journal of Environmental Research and Public Health* 18: 9636. [CrossRef]
Brach, Tara. 2019. *Radical Compassion: Learning to Love Yourself and Your World with the Practice of RAIN*. New York: Penguin Books.
Bradford, David T. 2020. *Spiritual Life on a Burning Planet: A Christian Response to Climate Change*. Eugene: Wipf and Stock.
Bradley, Graham L., and Joseph P. Reser. 2017. Adaptation Processes in the Context of Climate Change: A Social and Environmental Psychology Perspective. *Journal of Bioeconomics* 19: 29–51. [CrossRef]
Brown, David. 2007. *God and Grace of Body: Sacrament in Ordinary*. London: Oxford University Press.
Budziszewska, Magdalena, and Sofia Elisabet Jonsson. 2021. From Climate Anxiety to Climate Action: An Existential Perspective on Climate Change Concerns Within Psychotherapy. *The Journal of Humanistic Psychology* 61. [CrossRef]
Buzzell, Linda, and Craig Chalquist. 2009. *Ecotherapy: Healing with Nature in Mind*. San Francisco: Sierra Club Books.
Calder, Andy S., and Jan E. Morgan. 2016. 'Out of the Whirlwind': Clinical Pastoral Education and Climate Change. *Journal of Pastoral Care & Counseling* 70: 16–25. [CrossRef]
Chase, Steven. 2011a. *A Field Guide to Nature as Spiritual Practice*. Grand Rapids: W.B. Eerdmans Pub.

Chase, Steven. 2011b. *Nature as Spiritual Practice*. Grand Rapids: Eerdmans.
Christie, Douglas E. 2013. *The Blue Sapphire of the Mind: Notes for a Contemplative Ecology*. New York: Oxford University Press.
Clayton, Susan. 2020. Climate Anxiety: Psychological Responses to Climate Change. *Journal of Anxiety Disorders* 74: 102263. [CrossRef]
Clayton, Susan D., and Christie Manning, eds. 2018. *Psychology and Climate Change: Human Perceptions, Impacts, and Responses*. London: Academic Press (Elsevier).
Clayton, Susan, and Susan Opotow, eds. 2003. *Identity and the Natural Environment: The Psychological Significance of Nature*. Cambridge: MIT Press.
Clinebell, Howard John. 1996. *Ecotherapy: Healing Ourselves, Healing the Earth: A Guide to Ecologically Grounded Personality Theory, Spirituality, Therapy, and Education*. Minneapolis: Fortress Press.
Comtesse, Hannah, Verena Ertl, Sophie M. C. Hengst, Rita Rosner, and Geert E. Smid. 2021. Ecological Grief as a Response to Environmental Change: A Mental Health Risk or Functional Response? *International Journal of Environmental Research and Public Health* 18: 734. [CrossRef]
Conradie, Ernst M., and Hilda P. Koster, eds. 2019. *T&T Clark Handbook of Christian Theology and Climate Change*. London: Bloomsbury Publishing Plc.
Cox, Rebecca C., and Bunmi O. Olatunji. 2019. Anxiety and Related Disorders: An Introduction. In *The Cambridge Handbook of Anxiety and Related Disorders*. Edited by Bunmi O. Olatunji. Cambridge Handbooks in Psychology. Cambridge: Cambridge University Press, pp. 1–10. [CrossRef]
Crandon, Tara J., James G. Scott, Fiona J. Charlson, and Hannah J. Thomas. 2022. A Social–Ecological Perspective on Climate Anxiety in Children and Adolescents. *Nature Climate Change* 12: 123–31. [CrossRef]
Cunsolo, Ashlee, Sherilee L. Harper, Kelton Minor, Katie Hayes, Kimberly G. Williams, and Courtney Howard. 2020. Ecological Grief and Anxiety: The Start of a Healthy Response to Climate Change? *The Lancet Planetary Health* 4: e261–63. [CrossRef]
Cunsolo Willox, Ashlee, and Neville R. Ellis. 2018. Ecological Grief as a Mental Health Response to Climate Change-Related Loss. *Nature Climate Change* 8: 275–81. [CrossRef]
Cunsolo Willox, Ashlee, and Karen Landman, eds. 2017. *Mourning Nature: Hope at the Heart of Ecological Loss & Grief*. Montreal and Kingston: McGill-Queen's University Press.
Davenport, Leslie. 2017. *Emotional Resiliency in the Era of Climate Change: A Clinician's Guide*. London: Jessica Kingsley Publishers.
Deep Waters: A Project of Borrowed Time. 2022. Available online: https://greenchristian.org.uk/deep-waters-a-project-of-borrowed-time/ (accessed on 17 February 2022).
DeJonge, Michael P. 2017. Bonhoeffer, Status Confessionis, and the Lutheran Tradition. *Stellenbosch Theological Journal* 3: 41–60. [CrossRef]
Doherty, Thomas J. 2018. Individual Impacts and Resilience. In *Psychology and Climate Change: Human Perceptions, Impacts, and Responses*. Edited by Susan D. Clayton and Christie M. Manning. Amsterdam: Academic Press, pp. 245–66.
Doherty, Thomas J., and Susan Clayton. 2011. The Psychological Impacts of Global Climate Change. Edited by Susan Clayton. *American Psychologist* 66: 265–76. [CrossRef]
Doherty, Thomas J., Amy Lykins, Nancy A. Piotrowski, Zoey Rogers, Derrick D. Sebree, and Kristi E. White. 2021. Clinical Psychology Responses to the Climate Crisis. In *Reference Module in Neuroscience and Biobehavioral Psychology*. Amsterdam: Elsevier. [CrossRef]
Doppelt, Bob. 2016. *Transformational Resilience: How Building Human Resilience to Climate Disruption Can Safeguard Society and Increase Wellbeing*. Saltaire: Taylor & Francis.
Erickson, Jacob. 2020. Grief and New Creation: Theopoetics for a Pandemic. *Dialog: A Journal of Theology* 59: 73–74. [CrossRef]
Feather, Gabrielle, and Matt Williams. 2022. The Moderating Effects of Psychological Flexibility and Psychological Inflexibility on the Relationship between Climate Concern and Climate-Related Distress. *Journal of Contextual Behavioral Science* 23: 137–43. [CrossRef]
Foster, John. 2015. *After Sustainability: Denial, Hope, Retrieval*. London and New York: Routledge.
Francis, Pope. 2015. *Laudato Si': On Care for Our Common Home*. Vatican: Vatican Press.
Fredericks, Sarah E. 2021. *Environmental Guilt and Shame: Signals of Individual and Collective Responsibility and the Need for Ritual Responses*. London: Oxford University Press.
Gillespie, Sally. 2020. *Climate Crisis and Consciousness: Re-Imagining Our World and Ourselves*. London and New York: Routledge.
Greenberg, Leslie S. 2004. Emotion–Focused Therapy. *Clinical Psychology & Psychotherapy: An International Journal of Theory & Practice* 11: 3–16.
Greenspan, Miriam. 2004. *Healing through the Dark Emotions: The Wisdom of Grief, Fear, and Despair*. Boulder: Shambhala.
Grose, Anouchka. 2020. *A Guide to Eco-Anxiety: How to Protect the Planet and Your Mental Health*. London: Watkins.
Grupe, Dan W., and Jack B. Nitschke. 2013. Uncertainty and Anticipation in Anxiety: An Integrated Neurobiological and Psychological Perspective. *Nature Reviews Neuroscience* 14: 488–501. [CrossRef]
Haraway, Donna J. 2016. *Staying with the Trouble: Making Kin in the Chthulucene*. Experimental Futures. Durham: Duke University Press.
Haltinner, Kristin, and Dilshani Sarathchandra. 2018. Climate Change Skepticism as a Psychological Coping Strategy. *Sociology Compass* 12: e12586. [CrossRef]

Hamilton, Jo. 2020. Emotional Methodologies for Climate Change Engagement: Towards an Understanding of Emotion in Civil Society Organisation (CSO)-Public Engagements in the UK. Doctor of Philosophy dissertation, University of Reading, Reading, UK. Available online: http://centaur.reading.ac.uk/95647/3/23861657_Hamilton_Thesis_Redacted.pdf (accessed on 17 February 2022).

Haseley, Dennis. 2019. Climate Change: Clinical Considerations. *International Journal of Applied Psychoanalytic Studies* 16: 109–15. [CrossRef]

Heglar, Mary Annaïse. 2020. Climate Change Isn't the First Existential Threat. Medium. February 18. Available online: https://zora.medium.com/sorry-yall-but-climate-change-ain-t-the-first-existential-threat-b3c999267aa0 (accessed on 17 February 2022).

Helsel, Philip Browning. 2018. Loving The World: Place Attachment and Environment in Pastoral Theology. *Journal of Pastoral Theology* 28: 22–33. [CrossRef]

Hickman, Caroline. 2020. We Need to (Find a Way to) Talk about . . . Eco-Anxiety. *Journal of Social Work Practice* 34: 411–24. [CrossRef]

Hickman, Caroline, Elizabeth Marks, Panu Pihkala, Susan Clayton, R. Eric Lewandowski, Elouise E. Mayall, Britt Wray, Catriona Mellor, and Lise van Susteren. 2021. Climate Anxiety in Children and Young People and Their Beliefs about Government Responses to Climate Change: A Global Survey. *The Lancet Planetary Health* 5: e863–73. [CrossRef]

Hicks, Joshua A., and Clay Routledge, eds. 2013. *The Experience of Meaning in Life: Classical Perspectives, Emerging Themes, and Controversies*. Dordrecht: Springer.

Hirschfeld, A. Robert, and Stephen Blackmer. 2021. Beyond Acedia and Wrath: Life during the Climate Apocalypse. *Anglican Theological Review* 103: 196–207. [CrossRef]

Hoggett, Paul, and Rosemary Randall. 2018. Engaging with Climate Change: Comparing the Cultures of Science and Activism. *Environmental Values* 27: 223–43. [CrossRef]

Isherwood, Lisa, and Elizabeth Stuart. 1998. *Introducing Body Theology*. Introductions in Feminist Theology. Sheffield: Sheffield Academic Press.

Jafry, Tahseen, ed. 2019. *Routledge Handbook of Climate Justice*. London and New York: Routledge, Taylor & Francis Group.

Jamail, Dahr. 2019. *End of Ice: Bearing Witness and Finding Meaning in the Path of Climate Disruption*. New York: The New Press.

Jenkins, Willis. 2013. *The Future of Ethics: Sustainability, Social Justice, and Religious Creativity*. Washington, DC: Georgetown University Press.

Jensen, Tim. 2019. *Ecologies of Guilt in Environmental Rhetorics*. Palgrave Studies in Media and Environmental Communication. Cham: Palgrave Macmillan.

Johnson, Trebbe. 2017. *101 Ways to Make Guerrilla Beauty*. Radjoy Press.

Johnson, Trebbe. 2018. *Radical Joy for Hard Times: Finding Meaning and Makin Beauty in Earth's Broken Places*. Berkeley: North Atlantic Books.

Johnson, Ayana Elizabeth, and Katharine K. Wilkinson, eds. 2020. *All We Can Save: Truth, Courage, and Solutions for the Climate Crisis*. New York: One World.

Jones, Charlotte A., and Aidan Davison. 2021. Disempowering Emotions: The Role of Educational Experiences in Social Responses to Climate Change. *Geoforum* 118: 190–200. [CrossRef]

Jordan, Martin, and Joe Hinds, eds. 2016. *Ecotherapy: Theory, Research and Practice*. London: Palgrave.

Joyce, Cullan. 2020. Responses to Apocalypse: Early Christianity and Extinction Rebellion. *Religions* 11: 384. [CrossRef]

Jylhä, Kirsti M. 2017. Denial Versus Reality of Climate Change. In *Encyclopedia Of The Anthropocene*. Edited by Dominick A. DellaSala and Michael I. Goldstein. Amsterdam: Elsevier, pp. 487–92. [CrossRef]

Kelsey, Elin. 2020. *Hope Matters: Why Changing the Way We Think Is Critical to Solving the Environmental Crisis*. Vancouver and Berkeley: Greystone Books.

Kretz, Lisa. 2017. Emotional Solidarity: Ecological Emotional Outlaws Mourning Environmental Loss and Empowering Positive Change. In *Mourning Nature: Hope at the Heart of Ecological Loss & Grief*. Edited by Ashlee Cunsolo Willox and Karen Landman. Montreal and Kingston: McGill-Queen's University Press, pp. 258–91.

Kurth, Charlie. 2018. *The Anxious Mind: An Investigation into the Varieties and Virtues of Anxiety*. Cambridge: The MIT Press.

Laudato Si' Movement. 2022. Available online: https://laudatosimovement.org/ (accessed on 17 February 2022).

LaMothe, Ryan. 2016. This Changes Everything: The Sixth Extinction and Its Implications for Pastoral Theology. *Journal of Pastoral Theology* 26: 178–94. [CrossRef]

LaMothe, Ryan. 2019. Giving Counsel in a Neoliberal-Anthropocene Age. *Pastoral Psychology* 68: 421–36. [CrossRef]

LaMothe, Ryan. 2020. On Being at Home in the World: A Psychoanalytic-Political Perspective on Dwelling in the Anthropocene Era. *The Psychoanalytic Review* 107: 123–51. [CrossRef]

LaMothe, Ryan. 2021a. Illusions, Political Selves, and Responses to the Anthropocene Age: A Political-Psychoanalytic Perspective. *Free Associations* 84: 1–18. [CrossRef]

LaMothe, Ryan. 2021b. A Radical Pastoral Theology for the Anthropocene Era: Thinking and Being Otherwise. *Journal of Pastoral Theology* 31: 54–74. [CrossRef]

LaMothe, Ryan. 2021c. *Radical Political Theology for the Anthropocene Era*. Eugene: Wipf and Stock.

Lartey, Emmanuel Y., and Hellena Moon, eds. 2020. *Postcolonial Images of Spiritual Care*. Eugene: Wipf and Stock.

Lassloffy, Tracey A., and Sean D. Davis. 2018. Nurturing Nature: Exploring Ecological Self-of-the-Therapist Issues. *Journal of Marital and Family Therapy* 45: 176–85. [CrossRef] [PubMed]

Latour, Bruno. 2009. Will Non-Humans Be Saved? An Argument in Ecotheology. *Journal of the Royal Anthropological Institute* 15: 459–75. [CrossRef]

LeDoux, Joseph. 2016. *Anxious: Using the Brain to Understand and Treat Fear and Anxiety*. New York: Penguin Books.

Lewis, Janet, Elizabeth Haase, and Alexander Trope. 2020. Climate Dialectics in Psychotherapy: Holding Open the Space between Abyss and Advance. *Psychodynamic Psychiatry* 48: 271–94. [CrossRef] [PubMed]

Lomas, Tim. 2016. *The Positive Power of Negative Emotions: How Harnessing Your Darker Feelings Can Help You See a Brighter Dawn*. London: Piatkus.

Macy, Joanna. 1995. Working through Environmental Despair. In *Ecopsychology: Restoring the Earth, Healing the Mind*. Edited by Theodore Roszak, Mary E. Gomes and Allen D. Kanner. San Francisco: Sierra Club, pp. 240–69.

Macy, Joanna, and Molly Young Brown. 2014. *Coming Back to Life: The Updated Guide to the Work That Reconnects*. Gabriola Island: New Society Publishers.

Malcolm, Hannah, ed. 2020a. *Words for a Dying World: Stories of Grief and Courage from the Global Church*. London: SCM Press.

Malcolm, Hannah. 2020b. Grieving the Earth as Prayer. *The Ecumenical Review* 72: 581–95. [CrossRef]

Marshall, George. 2015. *Don't Even Think about It: Why Our Brains Are Wired to Ignore Climate Change*. New York: Bloomsbury Publishing USA.

McCarroll, Pamela R. 2020. Listening for the Cries of the Earth: Practical Theology in the Anthropocene. *International Journal of Practical Theology* 24: 29–46. [CrossRef]

McIntosh, Alastair. 2008. *Hell and High Water: Climate Change, Hope and the Human Condition*. Edinburgh: Birlinn.

McLaren, Karla. 2010. *The Language of Emotions: What Your Feelings Are Trying to Tell You*. Boulder: Sounds True.

McLaren, Karla. 2020. *Embracing Anxiety: How to Access the Genius inside This Vital Emotion*. Boulder: Sounds True.

Menning, Nancy. 2017. Environmental Mourning and the Religious Imagination. In *Mourning Nature: Hope at the Heart of Ecological Loss & Grief*. Edited by Ashlee Cunsolo Willox and Karen Landman. Montreal and Kingston: McGill-Queen's University Press, pp. 39–63.

Mkono, Mucha. 2020. Eco-Hypocrisy and Inauthenticity: Criticisms and Confessions of the Eco-Conscious Tourist/Traveller. *Annals of Tourism Research* 84: 102967. [CrossRef]

Nairn, Karen. 2019. Learning from Young People Engaged in Climate Activism: The Potential of Collectivizing Despair and Hope. *Young* 27: 435–50. [CrossRef]

O'Dell-Chaib, Courtney. 2019. Desiring Devastated Landscapes: Love After Ecological Collapse. Doctor of Philosophy in Religion dissertation, Syracuse University, New York, NY, USA. Available online: https://surface.syr.edu/etd/1045/ (accessed on 17 February 2022).

Ojala, Maria, Ashlee Cunsolo, Charles A. Ogunbode, and Jacqueline Middleton. 2021. Anxiety, Worry, and Grief in a Time of Environmental and Climate Crisis: A Narrative Review. *Annual Review of Environment and Resources* 46: 35–58. [CrossRef]

Orange, Donna. 2017. *Climate Change, Psychoanalysis, and Radical Ethics*. New York: Routledge.

Passmore, Holli-Anne, and Andrew J. Howell. 2014. Eco-Existential Positive Psychology: How Experiences in Nature Can Address Our Existential Anxieties and Contribute to Well-Being. *The Humanist Psychologist* 42: 370–88. [CrossRef]

Patel, Gopal D. 2020. Hindu Approaches to Climate Trauma. In *Hindu Approaches to Spiritual Care: Chaplaincy in Theory and Practice*. Edited by Vineet Chander and Lucinda Mosher. London: Jessica Kingsley Publishers, pp. 261–68.

Pew Research Center. 2021. Climate Change Concerns Make Many Around the World Willing to Alter How They Live and Work. *Pew Research Center's Global Attitudes Project*, September 14. Available online: https://www.pewresearch.org/global/2021/09/14/in-response-to-climate-change-citizens-in-advanced-economies-are-willing-to-alter-how-they-live-and-work/ (accessed on 17 February 2022).

Pienaar, Mariska. 2011. An Eco-Existential Understanding of Time and Psychological Defenses: Threats to the Environment and Implications for Psychotherapy. *Ecopsychology* 3: 25–39. [CrossRef]

Pihkala, Panu. 2016a. The Pastoral Challenge of the Eco-Reformation: Environmental Anxiety and Lutheran 'Eco-Reformation'. *Dialog: A Journal of Theology* 55: 131–40. [CrossRef]

Pihkala, Panu. 2016b. Rediscovery of Early Twentieth-Century Ecotheology. *Open Theology* 2: 268–85. [CrossRef]

Pihkala, Panu. 2017a. Environmental Education After Sustainability: Hope in the Midst of Tragedy. *Global Discourse* 7: 109–27. [CrossRef]

Pihkala, Panu. 2017b. *Early Ecotheology and Joseph Sittler*. Studies in Religion and the Environment. Zürich: LIT Verlag.

Pihkala, Panu. 2018a. Eco-anxiety, Tragedy, and Hope: Psychological and Spiritual Dimensions of Climate Change. *Zygon* 53: 545–69. [CrossRef]

Pihkala, Panu. 2018b. Death, the Environment, and Theology. *Dialog* 57: 287–94. [CrossRef]

Pihkala, Panu. 2020a. Anxiety and the Ecological Crisis: An Analysis of Eco-Anxiety and Climate Anxiety. *Sustainability* 12: 7836. [CrossRef]

Pihkala, Panu. 2020b. Theology of 'Eco-Anxiety' as Liberating Contextual Theology. In *Contextual Theology: Skills and Practices of Liberating Faith*. Edited by Sigurd Bergmann and Mika Vähäkangas. New York: Routledge, pp. 181–204.

Pihkala, Panu. 2020c. Eco-Anxiety and Environmental Education. *Sustainability* 12: 10149. [CrossRef]

Pihkala, Panu. 2020d. The Cost of Bearing Witness to the Environmental Crisis: Vicarious Traumatization and Dealing with Secondary Traumatic Stress among Environmental Researchers. *Social Epistemology: The Cost of Bearing Witness: Secondary Trauma and Self-Care in Fieldwork-Based Social Research; Guest Editors: Nena Močnik and Ahmad Ghouri* 34: 86–100. [CrossRef]

Pihkala, Panu. 2020e. Ritualizing Grief. In *Words for a Dying World: Stories of Grief and Courage from the Global Church*. Edited by Hannah Malcolm. London: SCM Press, pp. 167–72.

Pihkala, Panu. 2021. Ympäristöahdistus ja rituaalit: Analyysia ympäristötunteiden rituaalisesta käsittelystä [Eco-anxiety and Rituals: An analysis of methods for encountering eco-emotions ritually]. *Uskonnontutkija Religionsforskaren* 10. [CrossRef]

Pihkala, Panu. 2022a. Toward a Taxonomy of Climate Emotions. *Frontiers in Climate* 3: 199. [CrossRef]

Pihkala, Panu. 2022b. Religious Communities and Climate Emotions: Encountering Climate Grief, Guilt, and Anger. In *Brooding Over Creation: Affective Ecologies, Religion, and Theology*. Edited by Jacob Erickson. London: Bloomsbury, Forthcoming.

Powell, Russell C. 2019. Shame, Moral Motivation, and Climate Change. *Worldviews* 23: 230–53. [CrossRef]

Ray, Sarah Jacquette. 2020. *A Field Guide to Climate Anxiety: How to Keep Your Cool on a Warming Planet*. Oakland: University of California Press.

Ray, Sarah Jaquette. 2021. Who Feels Climate Anxiety? *The Cairo Review of Global Affairs*. No. 43 (Fall 2021). Available online: https://www.thecairoreview.com/home-page/who-feels-climate-anxiety/ (accessed on 17 February 2022).

Robinson, Timothy. 2020. Reimagining Christian Hope(Lessness) in the Anthropocene. *Religions* 11: 192. [CrossRef]

Rust, Mary-Jayne. 2020. *Towards an Ecopsychotherapy*. London: Confer Books.

Rust, Mary-Jayne, and Nick Totton, eds. 2012. *Vital Signs: Psychological Responses to Ecological Crisis*. London: Karnac.

Saler, Robert C. 2016. Pastoral Care and Ecological Devastation: Un-Interpreting the Silence. *Journal of Lutheran Ethics*. 16. Available online: https://elca.org/JLE/Articles/1140 (accessed on 17 February 2022).

Santmire, H. Paul. 2020. *Celebrating Nature by Faith: Studies in Reformation Theology in an Era of Global Emergency*. Eugene: Cascade.

Scott, Brandon G., and Carl F. Weems. 2013. Natural Disasters and Existential Concerns: A Test of Tillich's Theory of Existential Anxiety. *Journal of Humanistic Psychology* 53: 114–28. [CrossRef]

Seaman, Elizabeth B. 2016. *Climate Change on the Therapist's Couch: How Mental Health Clinicians Receive and Respond to Indirect Psychological Impacts of Climate Change in the Therapeutic Setting*. Theses, Dissertations, and Projects 1736. Northampton: Smith College for Social Work. Available online: https://scholarworks.smith.edu/theses/1736 (accessed on 17 February 2022).

Searle, Kristina, and Kathryn Gow. 2010. Do Concerns about Climate Change Lead to Distress? *International Journal of Climate Change Strategies and Management* 2: 362–79. [CrossRef]

Sherrell, Daniel. 2021. *Warmth: Coming of Age at the End of the World*. New York: Penguin Books.

Silva, Jules F. B., and Jennifer Coburn. 2022. Therapists' Experience of Climate Change: A Dialectic between Personal and Professional. *Counselling and Psychotherapy Research*. [CrossRef]

Softas-Nall, Sofia, and William Douglas Woody. 2017. The Loss of Human Connection to Nature: Revitalizing Selfhood and Meaning in Life through the Ideas of Rollo May. *Ecopsychology* 9: 241–52. [CrossRef]

Steffen, Will, Katherine Richardson, Johan Rockström, Sarah E. Cornell, Ingo Fetzer, Elena Bennett, Reinette Biggs, and de Vries Wim. 2015. Planetary Boundaries: Guiding Human Development on a Changing Planet. *Science* 347: 1259855. [CrossRef]

Stewart, Benjamin M. 2016. What's the Right Rite? Treating Environmental Degradation as Sickness or Sin. *Currents in Theology and Mission (Online)* 43: 3–8.

Stoknes, Per Espen. 2015. *What We Think About When We Try Not To Think About Global Warming: Toward a New Psychology of Climate Action*. White River Junction: Chelsea Green Publishing.

Swain, Storm. 2020. Climate Change and Pastoral Theology. In *T&T Clark Handbook of Christian Theology and Climate Change*. Edited by Ernst M. Conradie and Hilda P. Koster. London: T&T Clark, pp. 615–26.

Taylor, Steven. 2020. Anxiety Disorders, Climate Change, and the Challenges Ahead: Introduction to the Special Issue. *Journal of Anxiety Disorders* 76: 102313. [CrossRef]

The Work That Reconnects Network. 2022. Available online: https://workthatreconnects.org/ (accessed on 17 February 2022).

Tillich, Paul. 1952. *The Courage to Be*. New Haven: Yale University Press.

Tillich, Paul. 1963. Man and Earth. In *The Eternal Now: Sermons*. London: SCM Press, pp. 54–64.

Tschakert, Petra, Neville R. Ellis, C. Anderson, A. Kelly, and J. Obeng. 2019. One Thousand Ways to Experience Loss: A Systematic Analysis of Climate-Related Intangible Harm from around the World. *Global Environmental Change* 55: 58–72. [CrossRef]

Verlie, Blanche. 2022. *Learning to Live with Climate Change: From Anxiety to Transformation*. Routledge Focus. London: Routledge.

Verplanken, Bas, Elizabeth Marks, and Alexandru I. Dobromir. 2020. On the Nature of Eco-Anxiety: How Constructive or Unconstructive Is Habitual Worry about Global Warming? *Journal of Environmental Psychology* 72: 101528. [CrossRef]

Vos, Joel. 2018. *Meaning in Life: An Evidence-Based Handbook for Practitioners*. London: Bloomsbury.

Ward, Frances. 2020. *Like There's No Tomorrow: Climate Crisis, Eco-Anxiety and God*. Durham: Sacristy Press.

Wardell, Susan. 2020. Naming and Framing Ecological Distress. *Medicine Anthropology Theory* 7: 187–201. [CrossRef]

Weber, Jack Adam. 2020. *Climate Cure: Heal Yourself to Heal the Planet*. Woodbury: Llewellyn Publications.

Weintrobe, Sally. 2021. *Psychological Roots of the Climate Crisis: Neoliberal Exceptionalism and the Culture of Uncare*. New York: Bloomsbury.

Whyte, Kyle Powys. 2017. Is It Colonial Déjà vu? Indigenous Peoples and Climate Injustice. In *Humanities for the Environment: Integrating Knowledge, Forging New Constellations of Practice*. Edited by Joni Adamson and Michael Davis. London and New York: Routledge, pp. 88–104.

Williston, Byron. 2012. Climate Change and Radical Hope. *Ethics & the Environment* 17: 165–86.
Woodbury, Zhiva. 2019. Climate Trauma: Toward a New Taxonomy of Trauma. *Ecopsychology* 11: 1–8. [CrossRef]
World Council of Churches. 2022. Care for Creation and Climate Justice. Available online: https://www.oikoumene.org/what-we-do/care-for-creation-and-climate-justice (accessed on 17 February 2022).
Wullenkord, Marlis, Josephine Tröger, Karen Hamann, Laura Loy, and Gerhard Reese. 2021. Anxiety and Climate Change: A Validation of the Climate Anxiety Scale in a German-Speaking Quota Sample and an Investigation of Psychological Correlates. *Climatic Change* 168: 1–23. [CrossRef]
Yalom, Irvin D. 1980. *Existential Psychotherapy*. New York: Basic Books.

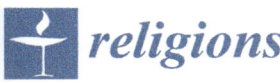

Article

Children and Climate Anxiety: An Ecofeminist Practical Theological Perspective

Joyce Ann Mercer

Yale University Divinity School, New Haven, CT 06511, USA; joyce.mercer@yale.edu

Abstract: As awareness grows of global warming and ecological degradation, words such as "climate anxiety", and "eco-anxiety" enter our vocabularies, describing the impact of climate change on human mental health and spiritual wellbeing. Distress over climate change disproportionately impacts children, who also are more susceptible to the broader health, economic, and social effects brought about by environmental harm. In this paper, I explore children's vulnerability to climate change and climate anxiety through the lens of ecofeminist practical theology. Ecofeminism brings the liberatory concerns of feminist theologies into engagement with those theologies focused on the life of the planet. Drawing on ecofeminism, practical theology must continue and deepen its own ecological conversion, and practical theologies of childhood must take seriously the work of making an ecological home, oikos, in which children are embedded as a part of the wider ecology that includes the more-than-human world. This requires foregrounding religious education with children toward the inhabitance of the earth in good and just ways. However, these theologies also must address children's lived realities of increased anxiety over planetary changes that endanger life through practices of spiritual care with children that engage and support them in their distress toward participatory empowerment for change.

Keywords: climate anxiety; children and eco-anxiety; ecotheology; practical theology; child theology; climate education; feminist theology

Citation: Mercer, Joyce Ann. 2022. Children and Climate Anxiety: An Ecofeminist Practical Theological Perspective. *Religions* 13: 302. https://doi.org/10.3390/rel13040302

Academic Editors: Pamela R. McCarroll and HyeRan Kim-Cragg

Received: 18 February 2022
Accepted: 29 March 2022
Published: 31 March 2022

Publisher's Note: MDPI stays neutral with regard to jurisdictional claims in published maps and institutional affiliations.

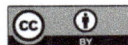

Copyright: © 2022 by the author. Licensee MDPI, Basel, Switzerland. This article is an open access article distributed under the terms and conditions of the Creative Commons Attribution (CC BY) license (https://creativecommons.org/licenses/by/4.0/).

1. Introduction

Children today know the earth and all its creatures are in trouble. They are born into life on a dying planet and increasingly demonstrate their awareness of this travesty through heightened levels of anxiety. Their "eco-anxiety" is a global phenomenon, not restricted to a single population of children, although intersectional identities and oppressions may amplify or blunt its effects among particular groups of children as well as its conscious articulation by them (Hickman et al. 2021, p. 106, ital. in original). This paper considers the phenomenon of children experiencing eco and climate anxiety through an ecofeminist practical theological lens. Recent attention to the differential effects of climate change on children calls for a recentering of ecological attention within theologies prioritizing the wellbeing of children.

Climate anxiety and eco-anxiety[1], as used here, refer not only to the self-conscious articulation of angst about the demise of the planet by children of affluence and privilege—children who are genuinely disturbed yet protected from many of the direct effects of climate change. Eco-anxiety also stands as a descriptive category for the lived experiences of precarity faced by children bearing the brunt of climate change in the here-and-now of their lives. Ecofeminist theology brings the liberatory concerns of feminist theologies into engagement with those focused on the life of the planet, meaning that advocacy for children and for planetary solidarity both fit within its purposes.

Feminist practical theologies of childhood must take seriously children's lived realities of increased anxiety and precarity amid ecological changes that endanger all life. Such theologies must bear witness to the particular suffering of children caused both by present-day ecological harms and by the erasure of a sustainable future for the earth caused by ecological degradation. My goals in this essay are modest: I first critique the absence of attention to the non-human creation in practical theologies of childhood. I then build on the work of two practical theologians, Jennifer Ayers and Annalet van Schalkwyk, to retrieve *oikos* as a particularly fruitful frame for ecological awareness and for addressing eco-anxiety in theological reflections concerned with the wellbeing of children. I then make a case for attending to children and eco-anxiety, first by identifying the particular vulnerabilities of children to the harmful effects of climate change and then by addressing a few common critiques. I conclude by calling upon practical theologians to take seriously children's experiences of eco-anxiety, and invite us to turn to the work of developing concrete, practical theological strategies to transform it in solidarity with the whole of God's creation.

2. Treating Children as Extra-Terrestrial Beings

Attention to the climate crisis and to children's lived realities of coping with it constitute critical elements for any contemporary theology of childhood. With some recent notable exceptions (see Hearlson 2021), a focus on children and climate change has been missing from many of these theological accounts, including my own (Mercer 2005a).[2] Collectively, those of us working at the intersections of childhood studies and Christian theology have confronted significant concerns in the lives of children, from violence against children to childhood poverty. We seem to have addressed these important matters, however, while inadvertently treating children as extra-terrestrial beings—creatures who reside in families and participate in faith communities that somehow stand outside of the realities impacting the wellbeing of the earth. As Bonnie Miller-McLemore exclaims about her changing consciousness, "Years ago, I argued for the 'living *human* web' as a better metaphor for pastoral theology's subject matter than the 'living *human* document'... But I seldom imagined its *nonhuman* extension. How did I miss this?"(Miller-McLemore 2020, p. 434, ital. in original).

To think theologically about childhood today requires recognition of this extended web. While I have argued elsewhere for theological anthropology formed around the "interrelatedness, interreliance, and contingency" of human beings with the non-human creation (Mercer 2017, p. 306), I have not brought these ecotheological interests into conversation with childhood. Pamela McCarroll (2020) critiques practical theology for its silence in the face of the climate crisis. She follows Panu Pihkala's (2020a) work on the dynamics of climate anxiety—which include denial and avoidance—to help explain this silence. In an effort to break through practical theological silence about children and the climate crisis, I first draw upon the work of Jennifer Ayres.

3. Making an *Oikos* for Children

Ayres, a religious educator, makes a compelling case for combatting climate despair through religious education toward what she terms inhabitance. "An inhabitant is a creature who lives well within the context and bounds of its habitation. ... An inhabitant desires and cultivates the wisdom necessary to live in God's world well" (Ayres 2019, pp. 2, 4). She notes that the root words for ecology, *oikos* (household, home, or habitation) and *logos* (logic or knowledge) render ecology as "the knowledge... of inhabiting" (Ayres 2019, p. 9). This "oikos" theme has been engaged by many in general discussions of ecotheology.[3] Inhabitance is a way of life conscious of human embeddedness within the non-human extension of the web proposed by Miller-McLemore. Ayres puts forward a vision of an "ecological theological anthropology" that understands the human vocation as "the work of inhabiting God's world well" (Ayres 2019, p. 9). Children have a "central role in awakening of the whole community to the gifts and responsibilities of inhabitance", writes Ayres (2019, pp. 120–21). Although she does not develop this point about children, her comment is a recognition that children can manifest ecological awareness inviting adult commitments that might otherwise be absent.

The *oikos* imaged by Ayres is one in which "together, human and nonhuman creatures are members of a household, a site of nurture and a site of obligation" (Ayres 2019, p. 8). Her description evokes constitutive notions of home—nurture and obligation (or responsibility)—that are central to children's lives. From an ecological standpoint, making a home for children situates them beyond what is generally understood to be a solely human web of connection, to recognize the presence and significance of those others making up the household—not only non-human creatures and plant life but also water, land, and air. These too participate in the nurture of children. Human household inhabitants (including children) have responsibilities to live well with the non-humans constituting their *oikos*. It is insufficient to view a child's development apart from this wider ecology. Accounting theologically for such expanded anthropology, then, requires adopting an "ecological faith [that] looks for patterns, relationships, and effects from the standpoint of an *embedded member* of the habitat" (Ayres 2019, p. 9).

I find Ayres' engagement of *oikos* and inhabitance as a theological description of an ecological way of life to be a helpful framework for thinking theologically about children. These guiding metaphors have special significance when brought to bear on childhood because of the power of "home" to so strongly define a child's world. Inhabitance makes clear that our ways of defining home have been too narrow, causing us to raise up children who think of home as an autonomously human habitation, unaware of their radical interdependence with non-human animals and the rest of the creation, and this ecology's role in constituting their very being.

Problematically, however, home- and household- metaphors contain historical, patriarchal associations with the subordination of women and children. Ecofeminism's theorizing of the connections between gender oppression and ecological harm is well known, analyzing the gendering of "nature" as feminine, with both women and nature treated as objects to be subdued and brought under control (Merchant 1980; Plumwood 1993). Under conditions of patriarchy, households become primarily consumer units ruled by the paterfamilias to whom other household members are subordinated. In the context of a discussion about ecology, household and home images risk reinscribing such oppressive meanings. Reimagining the *oikos* inhabited by children together with other non-human creatures thus necessitates a feminist retrieval of alternative meanings of *oikos* apart from such patriarchal and capitalist appropriations. In order to be of use in a liberatory ecological theology of childhood, the *oikos* must be reconfigured as an intentional connectional ecology that is life-giving for all.[4]

Feminist theologian Letty Russell pre-figured this contemporary ecological discussion more than three decades ago in an earlier work on feminist theology and authority in which she addressed the Greco-Roman *oikos*, "the arena of wives, slaves, and children ruled over by 'free' men" as "a household of bondage" (Russell 1987, p. 26). In place of such associations, Russell invokes "the biblical understanding of God's *oikonomia*, or householding of the whole earth" for which she uses the metaphor of a "household of freedom" as an "alternative translation of the phrase 'kingdom of God'" (Russell 1987, p. 26).[5] In the household of God, the logic of the *oikos* is not the logic of domination. An ecotheological perspective on childhood, drawn from this alternative, divine *oikonomia*, understands children and nurtures children's understanding of themselves as creatures situated within an *oikos*—part of a much larger ecology of God's making and delight. This *oikos tou Theou* as a "household of freedom" cannot be freedom for its human inhabitants alone. In fact, one lesson embodied in children's more obvious creaturely vulnerability is the embedded status of human beings within an ecology (both human and non-human) that is home. Embeddedness means the wellbeing of all oikos-dwellers is contingent upon one another's welfare. Harm or oppression of members of the *oikos* limits the freedom and flourishing of all who dwell therein.

South African ecofeminist theologian Annalet Van Schalkwyk (2012) also draws upon the relationship between oikos and ecology in her work, describing the earth as the *oikos* of God. Her "Oikos Cycle of Care" transposes the Deep Ecology cycle of Arne Naess (1990) onto the familiar "Pastoral Circle" of pastoral and practical theology

(Henriot 2000; Wijsen et al. 2005). In the pastoral circle (which can constitute both a template for action in ministry and for the reflective work of practical theology), one moves from experience to questioning, then to commitment, and finally to action. The Deep Ecology movement's cycle describes a process of conversion that "alters one's life orientation from anthropocentric to biocentric"(Van Schalkwyk 2012, p. 106).

Van Schalkwyk connects "experience" in the pastoral circle to the Deep Ecology cycle's initial step of immersion in nature, through which one can experience "God's creative love and God's revelation in and through nature", with the subsequent realization of "coming to understand nature and how humanity is a part of nature" (Van Schalkwyk 2012, p. 108) The immersive experience and the awareness it engenders leads to *ecophilia* (loving nature). Mapping the Deep Ecology Cycle onto the second moment in the pastoral circle, questioning, Van Schalkwyk sees this as a place from which one's *ecophilia* generates a critical interrogation of human disregard for the wider ecology, raising questions such as, "If the ecology works in this wonderful way, they why does humanity ignore it, disregard and exploit it, and live in unsustainable ways? What is wrong with our understanding of our faith, if this is the way in which we relate to the ecology? What can be the solutions to these destructive ways? What are the theological alternatives?" (Van Schalkwyk 2012, p. 108).

These two movements issue into a third one that van Schalkwyk names as a "deep commitment to protect and heal the ecology… This is also a deep commitment of faith, because one's understanding of the place of the ecology—of which humanity is part—transforms the way one believes in the creator-Saviour God" (Van Schalkwyk 2012, p. 108). Such commitments involve the formation of eco-values, and an "understanding the wisdom of nature", or *ecosophia*. Deep commitments ultimately lead to an ethic of care and eco-justice, "the willingness to change one's actions, and to act with care and justice, so as to alter the way in which humanity relates to the ecology and to the *oikos*. Thus, it leads to a transformation of values and ethics" (Van Schalkwyk 2012, p. 108). Together, then, the experience, wisdom, and questioning bring about a conversion: a profound commitment to the created world that becomes embodied in actions of love toward the earth.

Feminist interpretations of the earth as the *oikos tou theou* resonate with the priority that home has in the lives of children and the need to reconstruct how human adults and children understand their relationship to this *oikos*. Both Ayres and van Schalkwyk offer clues toward the kind of conversion needed from a household of human domination and disregard of the non-human ecology to one of aware embeddedness.[6] Children are not extra-planetary creatures. They "live and move, and have their being " (Acts 17:28) within a living web of relationships, human and non-human, held within the lands and waters of the earth.

4. Eco-Anxiety in Childhood

As awareness grows concerning the earth's perilous state, words such as "climate anxiety" also called "eco-anxiety" (Clayton et al. 2017), "solastalgia" (Albrecht 2005), "climate/environmental grief", and "psychoterratic syndromes" (Albrecht 2011) enter contemporary lexicons. Such terms seek to depict different dimensions of the impact of climate change on human mental and physical health and spiritual wellbeing. The American Psychological Association (APA) report on "Mental Health and Our Changing Climate" defines eco-anxiety as "chronic fear of environmental doom" (Clayton et al. 2017, p. 68). Within the growing body of psychological research attending to the mental health-related effects of climate change, the concept of eco-anxiety arose in response to the need to characterize the range of human emotional responses that include high levels of worry, fear, despair, sorrow, grief, depression, and existential anxiety felt in relation to ecological destruction and environmentally-related stressors (Ojala et al. 2021; Pihkala 2020a). Eco-anxiety may also include traumatic stress responses, particularly when ecological destruction is more directly experienced, as might be the case among children caught up in an extreme weather event or another climate-related disaster or those who must migrate from their homelands due to environmental factors.

I use eco-anxiety and climate anxiety as general terms to describe this range of bodily, spiritual, and psychological distress related to the effects of climate change. Eco-anxiety refers to emotions that have their origin in concern for the earth itself and for the suffering of non-human creatures. It also references feelings of anxiety generated by one's own experience of the impacts of climate change. In other words, a child might feel eco-anxiety in the form of worry over the ocean's sickness from plastic waste or worry for the Florida panther facing extinction. Another child's eco-anxiety might center more on the impact of climate change on people, such as the worry that their community will run out of fresh drinking water or that poor air quality is harmful to their friend who suffers from asthma. Still, another child, living as part of a household displaced by drought-driven famine, experiences climate anxiety as chronic, existential worry about the threat posed to their family's life and wellbeing by ecological degradation.

Eco-anxiety for children thus may include the "emotional response that can be seen even where there is no immediate physical evidence of impact of climate change on one's own life, a projected and anticipated anxiety into the future"(Hickman 2020, p. 414). The future-oriented aspects of eco-anxiety are characterized by worry, grief, and loss and sometimes by trauma, especially in situations of direct exposure to climate-related disaster events, climate migration, and displacement, in relation to which children may experience post-traumatic stress effects well beyond the event itself (Currie and Deschênes 2016; Garcia and Sheehan 2016; Gislason et al. 2021; Kousky 2016). All of this is to underscore the centrality of eco-anxiety's connection to time in the experience of children: ecological degradation brings harm in the present but is simultaneously tied to threatened harms and the after-effects of trauma extending in the future, creating uncertainty.[7] The future-related aspects of climate anxiety are born in part out of the stress of not knowing what takes place amid anticipation of catastrophe, alongside the long-term "chronicity" of eco-anxiety (Clayton 2020; Clayton et al. 2017).

5. Children as Especially Vulnerable to Climate Harms

Children are particularly subject to climate anxiety for a reason: climate scientists and mental health experts alike agree that children are among the most vulnerable to its negative effects (Burke et al. 2018; Clayton et al. 2017; Hickman et al. 2021; Sheffield and Landrigan 2011; Stanley et al. 2021). An overarching aspect of such vulnerability that cuts across physical, social, and mental health dimensions concerns the greater proportion of children's lives spent under the conditions of the climate crisis. That is, the young today live their entire lives under its sway. Because they have a longer life expectancy than do the adults coming before them, children risk longer exposure to "newly developing or worsening environmental hazards in the future" (Sheffield and Landrigan 2011, p. 292) in addition to the present-day impacts of such hazards.

Children also experience particular vulnerability to the effects of climate change due to their developmental status (Vergunst and Berry 2021), including their emotional capacities for dealing with stress and distress, which are still maturing. They, therefore, are more vulnerable to the effects of ongoing, chronic stress on the brain's structure, which Wu and colleagues consider a risk factor for mental illness: "As such, the stress of a climate crisis during a crucial developmental period, coupled with an increased likelihood of encountering repeated stressors related to climate change throughout life will conceivably increase the incidence of mental illness over the life course" (Wu et al. 2020, p. e435). Physically, children have "less effective heat adaptation capacity than do adults", and they experience higher exposure of air- and water-toxins per body weight in their still-developing systems (Sheffield and Landrigan 2011, p. 292).

The World Health Organization (WHO) maps what they call the "global burden of disease", a measure of the percentage of the overall morbidity and mortality carried by various population groups around the world. Looking at diseases and risk factors for disease attributable to climate change two decades ago, the WHO held that more than "88% of the existing burden of disease due to climate change occurs in children < 5 years of age in both developed and developing countries" (Zhang et al. 2007 in Sheffield and Landrigan 2011, p. 292). According to the WHO, 1.7 million children under the age of five died in 2012 from environmentally-related causes, and 2021 WHO information shows that 25% of the "disease burden" in children under five can be accounted for by environmental risks.[8] This means children as a group bear more effects from diseases related to climate change. That is, they have higher rates of complications and death from diseases that proliferate in response to global temperature fluctuations (e.g., the increase in mosquito-borne illnesses such as malaria or the zika virus that result because warmer temperatures are favorable for the insect carriers) (Burke et al. 2018, pp. 1–2), or to climate disaster-related pathogens (e.g., diseases linked to infectious agents in unclean water) (Currie and Deschênes 2016, p. 4). Nutritional deficits related to climate-related famine have a decidedly greater impact on children's developing bodies (Garcia and Sheehan 2016, p. 87).

In addition to such physical vulnerabilities, children face an array of socially-mediated effects from climate change (Gislason et al. 2021). They are more dependent upon others to mitigate climate change's difficult effects (Sheffield and Landrigan 2011, p. 291). Children experience particularly strong consequences from climate-related disruptions to family, community, education, and place because of the limited power they have to negotiate these environments independently. Such disruptions can happen through displacement/forced migration caused by extreme weather events (Kousky 2016). These adverse experiences may result from the need to flee conflicts and war that happen when land, water, and other resources become scarce as tensions are exacerbated by environmental factors (Garcia and Sheehan 2016, p. 86).

A primary climate change-related phenomenon such as a fire, for example, might result in a child's loss of their home, with the subsequent disruption to their ability to attend school. However, beyond this are many secondary and tertiary effects: the disruption in education brings with it a sudden change in social networks, including not only a child's peer group but also daily access to a significant group of professionals such as teachers, school nurses, chaplains, food services workers, and others who are suddenly removed from that child's "relational web". The destruction of the home represents a significant economic setback for the family, which may impact the child's access to food, clothing, healthcare, and other resources. If the family is already economically vulnerable, such stressors most certainly are compounded, amplified by intersectional features such as race. On top of these material and relational losses, a child in these circumstances will undoubtedly contend with emotional distress. Climate change thus has the power to create multiple points of impact in the lives of children, including its ability to amplify existing social inequalities as "climate change intensifies and complexifies vulnerability in the lives of children and youth" (Gislason et al. 2021, p. 2). In other words, for children already experiencing existential crises from other sources of trauma and suffering, such as the collective and historical traumas of racism, climate change and the anxieties it engenders only deepen the vulnerabilities already present.

At the same time that children experience vulnerabilities particular to their age, sociocultural, and geographical contexts, they are not without agency in relation to the current climate crisis (Gislason et al. 2021). It is tempting to paint children as *only* vulnerable and dependent (i.e., having no power or agency, needing others for care) and as *solely* vulnerable and dependent (i.e., the only creatures experiencing vulnerability and dependency). In reality, while children do suffer particular vulnerabilities and dependency, they are more than these elements alone and should not be reduced to them. Climate activism among children and youth is an important source of resiliency (Gislason et al. 2021, p. 9). Children mobilized for climate action comprise a leading voice in the growing acceptance of climate change and of the need for urgent action.[9] And while I highlight children's contingent status, this is not to ignore the interdependent and co-vulnerable reality that is a feature of *all* creatureliness. As theologian David Clough puts it, "human beings and other animals are thought of together in Christian scripture. Together they are given life by their creator as fleshly creatures made of dust and inspired by the breath of life, together they are given a common table in Eden and beyond, *"together they experience the fragility of mortal life, together they are the objects of God's providential care . . ."* (Clough 2012, p. 40, italics mine). Children's visible vulnerability and dependency bring home the often-unwanted truth that creatureliness is a precarious state for all who share this status—namely, all but God. Eco-anxiety is but another manifestation of this existential reality.

6. Critics of Eco- and Climate-Anxiety
6.1. Anthropocentrism

Not everyone acknowledges the reality of eco-anxiety, much less its occurrence among children as a problem to be addressed. One critique comes from within ecofeminism itself. While not specifically leveled against climate anxiety, this matter concerns the anthropocentric approach to climate issues within ecofeminist analysis or the tendency to "focus on the consequence to human communities" (Eaton 2021, p. 215) rather than a more expansive engagement of the wider impact beyond humans alone. A focus on climate anxiety admittedly maintains the anthropocentric approach to the climate crisis by directing attention toward the effects of ecological degradation upon humans rather than on the harm to the earth itself or non-human inhabitants (McCarroll 2020, p. 39).

It is insufficient to look at the climate crisis exclusively in terms of its impact on humans. Here, I do so self-consciously and in full awareness of the partial perspective of such an approach within ecotheology in order to foreground the situations of children as a group among earth's human population who often find themselves overlooked altogether in contemporary discussions about the planet's wellbeing. One reason to examine the climate crisis through a focus on human *children* is that until recently, literature on the climate crisis has tended to ignore children just as much as it ignores other-than-human creatures. Another more pressing reason to focus attention on human children in the current ecological situation, though, is that by virtue of children's greater proximity to the precarity and contingency experienced by other-than-human creatures in the *oikos*, concern for human children can be a way to garner greater awareness and concern for other precariously situated beings. Concern for children may function as a conduit for concern for other members of the *oikos*.

6.2. Pathologizing and Depoliticizing

Some critics of the idea of eco-anxiety contend that it "medicalizes" and pathologizes what is actually an appropriate response to a crisis in which real harm occurs (Hickman 2020, p. 414). This assessment holds that using clinical terminology such as "complicated grief" to express how children manifest their sadness over the likely extinction of loggerhead sea turtles seems unlikely to contribute to planetary healing or help children. According to those who hold this concern, a focus on eco-emotions individualizes responsibility for ecological destruction and thereby depoliticizes actions for change. That is, talk of climate grief situates action for change on the griever and on internal healing to help them feel better, rather than on collective responses to address the structures and systems that perpetuate climate destruction and serve the needs of the other-than-human species at risk. Climate anxiety, according to its critics, may be little more than a condition of privileged people who have the luxury to "feel bad about polar bears or talk to therapists", because the real problems of the climate crisis are more abstract and distant from their actual lives. Pastoral theologian Ryan LaMothe points to global capitalism as a primary culprit, inviting simultaneous care for the internal worlds of people and the systems and structures of harm, as they are co-implicated in the suffering of all (LaMothe 2020, 2021).[10]

A related critique specifies that eco-anxiety exists as a phenomenon linked to whiteness and other forms of privilege (noted by McCarroll 2020; Ray 2021a), critiquing eco-anxiety discourse with the charge that the primary people who identify with it are not the ones most vulnerable to its effects (Ray 2021a). Such claims that the children displaced by extreme weather events or who experience environmentally-related health effects are not the ones labeling their difficulties as eco-anxiety call into question the legitimacy of concern for children's eco-anxiety.

Sarah Jaquette Ray, the author of a popular 2020 book entitled *A Field Guide to Climate Anxiety*, studies the effects of climate change on people. A year after her book's publication, she wrote an opinion column in which she described being brought up short, "struck by the fact that those responding to the concept of climate anxiety are overwhelmingly white", while those most concerned about climate change are people of color who experience more negative effects from it. Ray asked, "Is climate anxiety a form of white fragility or even *racial* anxiety? Put another way, is climate anxiety just code for white people wishing to hold onto their way of life or get 'back to normal', to the comforts of their privilege?"(Ray 2021a, unpaginated text). Ray initially critiqued her own participation in a societal focus on the emotional dimensions of climate change at the expense of seeing it through a social justice lens. Her point was not to invalidate the fact that people have an emotional response to the destruction of the ecosystem. It was, rather, to recognize that "the prospect of an unlivable future has always shaped the emotional terrain for Black and brown people, whether that terrain is racism or climate change... What *is* unique [about the present moment of response to climate change] is that people who had been insulated from oppression are now waking up to the prospect of their own unlivable future" (Ray 2021a, unpaginated text).

Such critical appraisals of eco-anxiety are important and legitimate; in many ways, they parallel the historical separation between the mainstream environmental movement with its background in the creation of natural spaces for recreational use primarily by middle-class white people, and the environmental justice movement with its focus on such matters as exposing corporate toxic waste dumping in proximity to communities of color, ending colonial land-use policies on indigenous lands, or ensuring that people living in poverty have access to safe drinking water. A focus on climate anxiety may well be used to divert attention away from both the needs of an imperiled ecosphere and of BIPOC (Black, Indigenous, and People of Color) communities who often experience the most direct, negative impacts of climate change upon humans. Some will find in climate anxiety discourse an excuse to expend energy toward alleviating their anxiety and removing their discomfort rather than working to ameliorate its sources through conversion to repair the planet; some will focus on the intrapsychic idea of climate anxiety as a means of avoiding action when existing inequities are only amplified by ecological destruction.

In spite of these legitimate critiques of eco-anxiety discourse, I believe it is important to carve out space for a practical theological focus on children's climate anxiety. I do so critically, aware of the kinds of problems named above, yet equally aware that the search for purity in commitments to justice is a false pathway leading to paralysis. There is no position of innocence from which to address either the subject of the climate crisis' impact on children or the presence of racism in climate change discourse. We need to be concerned about and act to address inequities in which oppressed groups bear the greatest burdens of environmental violence and ecological degradation and to work for justice where environmental racism manifests itself while also attending to the impact of climate anxiety on all children.

It is important to address the question of the relationship between children's eco-anxiety and privilege. It simply is not the case that only privileged children experience eco or climate anxiety (Ballew et al. 2020; Garcia and Sheehan 2016). Children in BIPOC communities and others who disproportionately face the direct impact of climate degradation also experience fear, grief, and worry about the condition of the planet. When this happens, the fact that it adds onto the cumulative impact of existential crises and traumatic stress already present in the historical and contemporary narratives of these communities may mean that climate anxiety takes a less distinct role in their overall experience, not that it is absent. That is, these children too experience climate anxiety which comes as an overlay on top of other forms of struggle with which they must contend (also noted by Ray 2021a).

Seeing eco-anxiety's presence in contexts where it is not always the most salient among multiple stressors has a global dimension. It is important to resist the tendency to attribute mental health effects of the climate crisis only or primarily to children in the West or global north countries while limiting discussions of the material and physical impact of climate change on children in the global south. First, these broadly-bounded designations include children who do not fit the simple descriptor of "privileged" or "not-privileged". These social positions are shaped intersectionally. US- and North American BIPOC children living in poverty and children elsewhere living in poverty may share heightened vulnerability to climate effects related to material conditions of economic and social class, while at the same time, some among them will share certain protections with some affluent children, such as greater access to a community of support and care.

Second, for a child who undergoes extreme material and physical deprivation or experiences existential threat in the context of systemic racism's collective trauma history, these aspects of their life are likely to assume primacy in a child's everyday life, but the children are not thereby made immune from spiritual and mental health effects of ecological harm. In fact, they may be more at risk since living with chronic stress makes children more susceptible to mental health issues and, I would add, spiritual distress (Clayton et al. 2017; Doherty and Clayton 2011; Hickman et al. 2021; Kousky 2016; Macy 2013; Burke et al. 2018). Third, children whose locations make them more subject to multiple harms may also show considerable resilience and should not be identified as persons without agency or singularly constructed as victims (Davenport 2017; Nissen et al. 2021; Ojala 2012a; Ojala and Bengtsson 2019; Stanley et al. 2021; Verlie 2022; Wu et al. 2020). Thus, with Pihkala (2020b), I maintain that those suffering most directly from climate change "also suffer most heavily from the psychological impacts of environmental problems—including eco-anxiety. Thus the struggle for eco-justice and climate justice is also a struggle for more psychic and psychosocial resilience" (Pihkala 2020b, p. 183).

As it turns out, Ray (2021b) revisits her question of whether climate anxiety is found only among privileged white people. In a newer article, she takes into account the global study by Hickman et al. (2021) surveying ten thousand children in ten countries. That study reports that "respondents across all countries were worried about climate change"(p. e863). Ray, noting the study's finding that "communities of color are more worried about climate change than their white counterparts", now offers a more nuanced way of looking at the link between privilege and climate anxiety discourse that aligns with my argument here. Ray writes that climate anxiety manifests itself differently among people in different contexts, and "just because [BIPOC communities] aren't suffering from climate anxiety as it is currently defined doesn't mean they aren't deeply attuned to what is happening to the world. ... [I]t is possible to feel climate anxiety even if climate change isn't the first or worst existential threat of our lives. ... It is possible to have big feelings about other threats that may happen in relation to climate change without ever using the words 'climate change'" (Ray 2021b, pp. 4, 6).

In the long run, all of this suggests to me that one can critique the presence of diversionary tactics and of racism in the discourse on climate anxiety without abstraction from children's lived experiences. It is not helpful to pit one kind of oppression against another in the lives of children. The empathy that climate-anxious children express for other creatures communicates children's distress and has legitimacy as such.[11] So does the reality of the pain some children experience from the mental health impact of being continually bathed in a discourse of impending planetary demise. The recognition of the presence of a continual existential threat for children in BIPOC communities from systemic racism's harms remains in paramount need of transformation even as it does not erase the co-presence of eco-anxiety from the lives of BIPOC children.

Regarding the depoliticizing discourse of eco-emotions, we can generate constructive solutions to the problem of pathologizing or medicalizing what is, in reality, a normal, expectable response to the non-normal event of ecological destruction. For instance, one can add terminology that embraces the generative, life-giving impulses underlying climate anxiety instead of the language of pathology, engaging these motivations in the service of transformation. Several authors have already emphasized that eco-anxiety includes an adaptive dimension that is linked with motivation and caring (Hickman 2020; Pihkala 2020a; Hickman et al. 2021). However, rather than turning this into a simplistic optimism that ultimately translates into a practice of climate change denial, adults concerned about climate-anxious children can invoke the discursive lens variously termed "critical hope" (Ojala 2016), "active hope" (Verlie et al. 2021, p. 134), or "constructive hope" (Chawla 2020).

All of these terms point to a form of hope grounded in the sense of urgent need for change that is coupled with a vision for change and empowerment to act. In other words, it is not simply a matter of what terms are in use. The framework, cultural or otherwise, that situates *how* they are used also has relevance for the affective experiences of children, which in turn can help to empower their agency in the world.[12]

Christian theology needs to put forward a similarly critical, active, constructive vision of hope—an eschatology that links how humans inhabit God's *oikos* in the present with bold, imaginative visions of what life as creatures among others embedded in a common home might look like for all to flourish. Eschatology, writes feminist biblical theologian Barbara Rossing, "speaks about hope", and as such, is an act of imagination in which we picture a counterworld, an alternative vision to the status quo's ecological destruction. Rossing sees the current planetary crisis not as "primarily a scientific crisis, or even a moral crisis". Instead, she contends, "our crisis is a narrative crisis: it is a crisis of imagination" with very real results (Rossing 2017, pp. 328–29). The imagination Rossing calls for is active, such as the hope it engenders, as it becomes a new narrative directing our steps toward the earth's repair and restoration. It envisions what God's world with all its creatures—the whole *oikos tou Theou*—might be like in an alternative future in which practices of inhabitance promote the flourishing of all. To turn away from children's lived reality of eco-anxiety is an abdication of the Christian responsibility to nurture the eschatological imaginations of children for the sake of the planet and its many inhabitants.

Latina feminist theologian Nancy Pineda-Madrid writes of eschatological hope in an ecological framework, citing the often-repeated Spanish expression, "*somos criaturas de Dios*" (we are creatures of God). It is, for her, a way of properly locating humans within the whole of creation through a "theological anthropology of creatureliness" that puts humanity in perspective. "Our theological anthropology is doomed to distortion if considered in isolation from a healthy biology, ecology, and cosmology", she writes. However, framing human beings as creatures of God "furthers eschatological hope by foregrounding human beings' common fellowship with all other creatures of God" (Pineda-Madrid 2017, p. 312).

Nurturing an eschatological imagination among children who struggle with eco-anxiety means equipping them and all Christians with critical capacities to re-form theological ideas and practices that have "mis-sized" humanity in relation to our earth-kin. Reimagining humans—not as disproportionately significant and special above all others but as "right-sized"—as one among all of God's special and beloved creatures is a theological activity for which adults may need to look to children for leadership. Children's relatively smaller physical size gives them a kind of "epistemological privilege" to see what adults may miss about the disproportionality of human lives within the greater ecology of our inhabitance and the more finely tuned awareness among some children of both their vulnerability and their need for an interconnected, relationally rich place that is their *oikos*, may afford them a clearer view of what can go wrong when humans take an outsized view of themselves in relation to the rest of God's creatures.

Rossing and Pineda-Madrid help to further flesh out the ecofeminist retrieval of concepts of *oikos* and inhabitance found earlier in the works of Jennifer Ayres and Annalet van Schalkwyk. Such theological resources, in turn, constitute a key element within practical theological strategies for supporting children who experience eco-anxiety. The development of such strategies in their concrete forms is future work that can draw on this article's establishment of eco-anxiety among children as an important concern for practical theologians.

7. Limitations and Opportunities for Future Scholarship

This article offers a preliminary inquiry into children's eco-anxiety from the perspective of ecofeminist practical theology. Although it contributes to the literature of childhood studies and theology with its attention to eco-anxiety in children, there remains a gap in practical theology's empirical research on the subject. Research is needed with children who experience eco-anxiety. In addition, more work is needed from the perspective of pastoral and spiritual care to better understand what might be unique about climate anxiety as a specific form of distress experienced by children. Such work could provide helpful resources for caregivers regarding the most effective pastoral care interventions with eco-anxious children. Emerging self-help literature exists, addressing how to support children with climate anxiety, as does a small body of work focused upon eco-anxiety and pastoral care in general, but to my knowledge, there is no similar literature directly targeting pastoral care with children facing eco-anxiety.[13] Further work in this area would constitute a significant contribution to the field of practical theology.

8. Conclusions

Eco-anxiety is a reality in the lives of many children. Given the impact of climate destruction upon children's lives, their anxiety about the threats posed for themselves and other species and for the life of the planet is an appropriate response: *not* responding with anxiety to such grave danger would be highly problematic. However, for individual children and others, living with chronic anxiety also can be harmful. The practical theological turn toward transformation that puts care and justice side by side retrieves the ecotheological theme of the inhabitance in God's *oikos*, to support human children *and* the other-than-human members of the planetary household. Practices of care for children entail nurturing them in awareness of their embeddedness within that ecology toward the kind of deep commitment of faith that issues in wisdom—*ecosophia*—to heal the earth and live well within its diverse ecology.n the end, we are left with the practical theological question of what it would take to attend well to children experiencing eco-anxiety in the world that God created and loves? I am taken by the notion from Pope Francis' environmental manifesto, *Laudato Si* (Pope Francis 2015), that what is needed is nothing short of *ecological conversion* (See especially Ayres 2017; Calder and Morgan 2016; Hanchin and Hearlson 2020; Hearlson 2020, 2021; Helsel 2018; McCarroll 2020; Miller-McLemore 2020; Robinson and Wetochek 2021). Van Schalkwyk's "oikos cycle of care", for example, while not a prescription for "fixing" the anxiety children suffer over climate destruction, does suggest a pattern for the conversion that must take place for ecological justice to take root. Ayres' call for religious education toward inhabitance is not only for children. However, children suffering from eco-anxiety will certainly benefit from a religious education that fosters ecological kinship and invites activism on behalf of the ecosphere that is God's *oikos* (and ours). Plenty of evidence exists today that practical theology and its subfields are in the midst of an ecological turn, increasingly centering concerns over climate change and ecological consciousness in our work. It is time to bring this focus home to children with further theological reflections on childhood, ecology, and climate anxiety.

Funding: This research received no external funding.

Conflicts of Interest: The author declares no conflict of interest.

Notes

1. Some writers such as Pihkala distinguish between eco-anxiety as "any anxiety related to the climate crisis" with climate anxiety as its most common form, defined as "anxiety that is significantly related to anthropogenic climate change"(Pihkala 2020a, p. 3). Many authors use the terms interchangeably even with such distinctions. In this essay I use climate anxiety specifically in relation to climate change and planetary impacts, and eco-anxiety as the more general term.
2. Many practical theologians working on other topics that include substantive attention to ecology do relate their ecological concerns to children within the broader focus of their work. See for example (Ayres 2019; Helsel 2018; LaMothe 2021; Moore 1998; Rimmer 2020).

3   Louw (2017) provides a survey of theological meanings *oikos* in his consideration of a "practical theology of home" in the face of contemporary realities of displacement and migration. He brings these *oikos* meanings into conversation with the Zulu notion of Ekhaya, or "yearning for home." Conradie (2007) identifies "household of God" as a "theological root metaphor" wth multiple uses. He considers the metaphor's limitations as well, particularly in patriarchal contexts where it may be used to legitimize various forms of oppression. Clifford (2006) examines biblical texts connecting Divine creation and redemption. Critiquing the exclusive focus arising during the Enlightenment on humans as the object of God's redemptive work in Christ, she writes: "[A] careful look at the biblical sources shows that the neglect of *oikos* overlooks the ways in which God's work of creation providesthe cosmic purpose behind God's redemptive activity" (Clifford 2006, p. 250). Larry Rasmussen (1996) offers a theological ethics of *oikos* in relation to ecology, mining the term for its meanings of what he calls 'the story of the earth as a single, vast household" (Rasmussen 1996, p. 44). Elsewhere he defines *oikos* as "a world house"(Rasmussen 2013, p. 163) in which the *oikeloi* (household dwellers) are to "build the community and share the gifts of the Spirit for the common good... Such care requres intimate knowledge of community structures and dynamics. It requires knowing the household's logic and laws, which is exactly what 'ecology' means (*oikos* + logos), knowledge of relationships that build up and sustain" (Rasmussen 2013, p. 164).

4   Pastoral theologian Ryan LaMothe (2020) offers different language with his psychoanalytic exploration of "dwellling"that also attends to political, economic, and cultural dimensions of "experiences of being unhoused", inclusive of the reality "possibility that climate change, which human beings have caused, is likely to unhouse millions of species, includiing human beings" (p. 124).

5   Such work finds contemporary support in the decolonial biblical interpretation of Rohun Park's (2009) East Asian reading of the Parable of the Prodigal Son. Park explores the polemic of *oikos* meanings in the Gospel of Luke, in which Jesus deconstructs colonial notions of the *oikos-nomos* bound up in the imperial household with the emperor as paterfamilias. In its place, Park lifts up the *oikos tou theo* proclaimed by Jesus as an alternative economy of God constructed not for the accumulation of wealth but instead, as I would engage Park's thought for my purposes, for the wellbeing of children (and other creatures) who dwell there.

6   The theme of ecological conversion, while not new in ecotheology, has gained renewed prominance because of its engagement by Pope Francis in his recent ecological encyclical, *Laudato Si'* (Pope Francis 2015). See, for example, Elizabeth A. Johnson who bluntly admonishes humanity to repent of our harmful practices, as she asserts that "we need a deep spiritual converssion to the Earth" (Johnson 2014, p. 258).

7   Hence Rob Nixon's description of climate change as "slow violence", or "a violence that occurs gradually and out of sight, a violence of delayed destruction that is dispersed across timie and space, an attritional violence that iis typically not viewed as violence at all" (Nixon 2011, p. 2).

8   See their website for a number of resources related to children and the environment: Available online: https://www.who.int/health-topics/children-environmental-health#tab=tab_2 (accessed on 6 January 2022).

9   Ojala's (Ojala 2012a, 2012b; Ojala and Bengtsson 2019) research on how children and adolescents respond to climate change distinguished between three coping patterns. Among them, the one she calls "meaning focused coping"—using beliefs and values to help foster positive emotions in relation to the source of stress—yielded the best result in terms of diminishing negative emotions along with enhancing pro-environmental engagement. This fits with other findings (see below) that participation in youth movements around environmental activism mitigated negative mental health effects of climate anxiety. A fuller discussion of children's climate activism is beyond the scope of this essay. Current scholarship emphasizes how such activism can be an important antidote to the "climate despair" that can fuel eco-anxiety among children (Bowman and Pickard 2021; Davenport 2017; Nissen et al. 2021; Stanley et al. 2021; Trott 2021; Wu et al. 2020).

10 Elsewhere I too have interrogated the role of capitalism in constructing children into identities as excellent consumers, calling for practices with children that draw upon Christian faith as a counternarrative to consumer culture (Mercer 2004, 2005a, 2005b).

11 But see Wendy Mallette's critique as an interesting counterpoint (Mallette 2021).

12 See Susan Wardell's excellent exploration of the "names and frames for ecological distress" (Wardell 2020). She considers critiques from within the psychotherapeutic community against the framing of ecological distress in established psychgological categories that can pathologize it: "eco-anxiety discloses not the disorder of the individual, but a dis-order of ecological systems; not the nadeness of the individual, but the madness of the political, social, and economic systems that have brought us to this point" (Wardell 2020, p. 196). Wardell also reflects on the implications of how constructions of ecological distress, situated as they are in their own cultural histories, relate to activism. Ursula Heise addresses similar themes in her work. See (Heise 2016).

13 For an examples of popular literature focused on children, see (Shugarman 2020). For an example of literature on pastoral care and eco-anxiety that is not specific to children see (Pihkala 2022).

References

Albrecht, Glenn. 2005. 'Solastalgia'. A new concept in health and identity. *PAN: Philosophy Activism Nature* 3: 44–59.
Albrecht, Glenn. 2011. Chronic environmental change: Emerging 'psychoterratic'syndromes. In *Climate Change and Human Well-Being*. Berlin and Heidelberg: Springer, pp. 43–56.
Ayres, Jennifer R. 2017. Cultivating the "unquiet heart": Ecology, education, and Christian faith. *Theology Today* 74: 57–65. [CrossRef]
Ayres, Jennifer R. 2019. *Inhabitance: Ecological Religious Education*. St. Waco: Baylor University Press.

Ballew, Matthew, Edward Malbach, John Kotcher, Parrish Bergquist, Seth Rosenthal, Jennifer Marlon, and Anthony A. Leiserowitz. 2020. Which Racial/Ethnic Groups Care Most about Climate Change? In *Yale Program on Climate Change Communication: Clmate Note*. New Haven: Yale University and George Mason University.

Bowman, Benjamin, and Sarah Pickard. 2021. Peace, protest and precarity: Making conceptual sense of young people's non-violent dissent in a period of intersecting crises. *Journal of Applied Youth Studies* 4: 493–510. [CrossRef]

Burke, Susie E., Ann V. Sanson, and Judith Van Hoorn. 2018. The Psychological Effects of Climate Change on Children. *Current Psychiatry Reports* 20: 1–17. [CrossRef] [PubMed]

Calder, Andy S., and Jan E. Morgan. 2016. 'Out of the Whirlwind': Clinical Pastoral Education and Climate Change. *Journal of Pastoral Care and Counseling* 70: 16–25. [CrossRef] [PubMed]

Chawla, Louise. 2020. Childhood Nature Connection and Constructive Hope: A Review of Research on Connecting with Nature and Coping with Environmental Loss. *People and Nature* 2: 619–42. [CrossRef]

Clayton, Susan. 2020. Climate anxiety: Psychological responses to climate change. *Journal of Anxiety Disorders* 74: 102263. [CrossRef] [PubMed]

Clayton, Susan, Christie Manning, Kirra Krygsman, and Meighen Speiser. 2017. *Mental Health and Our Changing Climate: Impacts, Implications, and Guidance*. Washington: American Psychological Association and ecoAmerica.

Clifford, Anne M. 2006. From ecological lament to sustainable oikos. In *Environmental Stewardship: Critical Perspectives—Past and Present*. London: T &T Clark, pp. 247–52.

Clough, David L. 2012. *On Animals: Systematic Theology*. London: A&C Black, vol. 1.

Conradie, Ernst M. 2007. The Whole Household of God (Oikos): Some Ecclesiological Perspectives Part 1. *Scriptura* 94: 1–9.

Currie, Janet, and Olivier Deschênes. 2016. Children and climate change: Introducing the issue. *The Future of Children* 26: 3–9. [CrossRef]

Davenport, Leslie. 2017. *Emotional Resiliency in the Era of Climate Change: A Clinician's Guide*. Philadelphia: Jessica Kingsley Publishers.

Doherty, Thomas J., and Susan Clayton. 2011. The psychological impacts of global climate change. *American Psychologist* 66: 265. [CrossRef] [PubMed]

Eaton, Heather. 2021. Ecofeminist Theologies in the Age of Climate Crisis. *Feminist Theology* 29: 209–19. [CrossRef]

Garcia, Daniel Martinez, and Mary C. Sheehan. 2016. Extreme weather-driven disasters and children's health. *International Journal of Health Services* 46: 79–105. [CrossRef] [PubMed]

Gislason, Maya K., Angel M. Kennedy, and Stephanie M. Witham. 2021. The Interplay between Social and Ecological Determinants of Mental Health for Children and Youth in the Climate Crisis. *International Journal of Environmental Research and Public Health* 18: 4573. [CrossRef]

Hanchin, Timothy, and Christy Lang Hearlson. 2020. Educating for ecological conversion: An ecstatic pedagogy for Christian higher education amid climate crisis. *Religious Education* 115: 255–68. [CrossRef]

Hearlson, Christy Lang. 2020. Ecological conversion as conversion to the child: Becoming caregivers, becoming childlike. *Horizons* 47: 232–55. [CrossRef]

Hearlson, Christiane Lang. 2021. Converting the Imagination through Visual Images in Ecological Religious Education. *Religious Education* 116: 129–41. [CrossRef]

Heise, Ursula K. 2016. *Imagining Extinction: The Cultural Meanings of Endangered Species*. Chicago: University of Chicago Press.

Helsel, Philip Browning. 2018. Loving The World: Place Attachment and Environment in Pastoral Theology. *Journal of Pastoral Theology* 28: 22–33. [CrossRef]

Henriot, Peter J. 2000. *Pastoral Circle: A Strategy for Promoting Justice and Peace*. Harare: Kolbe Press Harare.

Hickman, Caroline, Elizabeth Marks, Panu Pihkala, Susan Clayton, R. Eric Lewandowski, Elouise E. Mayall, Britt Wray, Catriona Mellor, and Lise van Susteren. 2021. Climate anxiety in children and young people and their beliefs about government responses to climate change: A global survey. *The Lancet Planetary Health* 5: e863–e873. [CrossRef]

Hickman, Caroline. 2020. We need to (find a way to) talk about… Eco-anxiety. *Journal of Social Work Practice* 34: 411–24. [CrossRef]

Johnson, Elizabeth A. 2014. *Ask the Beasts: Darwin and the God of Love*. London and New York: Bloomsbury.

Kousky, Caroly. 2016. Impacts of Natural Disasters on Children. *The Future of Children* 26: 73–92. [CrossRef]

LaMothe, Ryan. 2020. On being at home in the world: A psychoanalytic-political perspective on dwelling in the Anthropocene era. *The Psychoanalytic Review* 107: 123–51. [CrossRef] [PubMed]

LaMothe, Ryan. 2021. Social and political freedom: A pastoral theological perspective—Part I. *Pastoral Psychology* 70: 255–71. [CrossRef]

Louw, Daniel J. 2017. Ekhaya: Human displacement and the yearning for familial homecoming. From Throne (Cathedra) to Home (Oikos) in a grassroots ecclesiology of place and space: Fides Quaerens Domum et Locum [Faith Seeking Home and Space]. *HTS: Theological Studies* 73: 1–11. [CrossRef]

Macy, Joanna. 2013. *Greening of the Self*. Berkeley: Parallax Press.

Mallette, Wendy. 2021. Questioning Empathetic Responsiveness to Nonhuman Animal Vulnerability: Noninnocent Relations and Affective Motivations in the Animal Turn in Religious Studies. *Journal for the Study of Religion, Nature & Culture* 15: 177–203.

McCarroll, Pamela R. 2020. Listening for the Cries of the Earth: Practical Theology in the Anthropocene. *International Journal of Practical Theology* 24: 29–46. [CrossRef]

Mercer, Joyce Ann. 2004. The child as consumer: A North American problem of ambivalence concerning the spirituality of childhood in late capitalist consumer culture. *Sewanee Theological Review* 48: 65.

Mercer, Joyce Ann. 2005a. *Welcoming Children: A Practical Theology of Childhood*. St. Louis: Chalice Press.
Mercer, Joyce Ann. 2005b. Spiritual Economies of Childhood: Christian Perspectives of Global Market Forces and Young People's Spirituality. In *Nurturing Child and Adolescent Spirituality: Perspectives from the World's Religious Traditions*. Lanham: Rowman & Littlefield Publishers, pp. 458–71.
Mercer, Joyce Ann. 2017. Environmental activism in the Philippines: A practical theological perspective. In *Planetary Solidarity: Global Women's Voices on Christian Doctrine and Climate Justice*. Edited by Grace Ji-Sun Kim and Hilda P. Koster. Minneapolis: Fortress, pp. 287–307.
Merchant, Carolyn. 1980. *The Death of Nature: Women, Ecology, and the Scientific Revolution*, 1st ed. San Francisco: Harper & Row.
Miller-McLemore, Bonnie J. 2020. Trees and the "Unthought Known": The Wisdom of the Nonhuman (or Do Humans "Have Shit for Brains"?). *Pastoral Psychology* 69: 423–43. [CrossRef]
Moore, Mary Elizabeth. 1998. *Ministering with the Earth*. Nashville: Chalice Press.
Naess, Arne. 1990. *Ecology, Community and Lifestyle: Outline of an Ecosophy*. Cambridge: Cambridge University Press.
Nissen, Sylvia, Jennifer H. K. Wong, and Sally Carlton. 2021. Children and young people's climate crisis activism–a perspective on long-term effects. *Children's Geographies* 19: 317–23. [CrossRef]
Nixon, Rob. 2011. *Slow Violence and the Environmentalism of the Poor*. Cambridge: Harvard University Press.
Ojala, Maria, and Hans Bengtsson. 2019. Young people's coping strategies concerning climate change: Relations to perceived communication with parents and friends and proenvironmental behavior. *Environment and Behavior* 51: 907–35. [CrossRef]
Ojala, Maria, Ashlee Cunsolo, Charles A. Ogunbode, and Jacqueline Middleton. 2021. Anxiety, worry, and grief in a time of environmental and climate crisis: A narrative review. *Annual Review of Environment and Resources* 46: 35–58. [CrossRef]
Ojala, Maria. 2012a. How do children cope with global climate change? Coping strategies, engagement, and well-being. *Journal of Environmental Psychology* 32: 225–33. [CrossRef]
Ojala, Maria. 2012b. Regulating Worry, Promoting Hope: How Do Children, Adolescents, and Young Adults Cope with Climate Change? *International Journal of Environmental and Science Education* 7: 537–61.
Ojala, Maria. 2016. Facing anxiety in climate change education: From therapeutic practice to hopeful transgressive learning. *Canadian Journal of Environmental Education (CJEE)* 21: 41–56.
Park, Rohun. 2009. Revisiting the parable of the prodigal son for decolonization: Luke's reconfiguration of oikos in 15: 11–32. *Biblical Interpretation* 17: 507–20. [CrossRef]
Pihkala, Panu. 2020a. Anxiety and the ecological crisis: An analysis of eco-anxiety and climate anxiety. *Sustainability* 12: 7836.
Pihkala, Panu. 2020b. Theology of "eco-anxiety" as liberating contextual theology. In *Contextual Theology*. London: Routledge, pp. 181–204.
Pihkala, Panu. 2022. Eco-Anxiety and Pastoral Care: Theoretical Considerations and Practical Suggestions. *Religions* 13: 192. [CrossRef]
Pineda-Madrid, Nancy. 2017. ¡Somos Criaturas de Dios!—Seeing and Beholding the Garden of God. In *Planetary Solidarity: Global Women's Voices on Christian Doctrine and Climate Justice*. Edited by Grace Ji-Sun Kim and Hilda P. Koster. Minneapolis: Fortress, pp. 311–24.
Plumwood, Val. 1993. *Feminism and the Mastery of Nature, Opening Out*. London/New York: Routledge.
Pope Francis. 2015. *Laudato si': On Care for Our Common Home*. Vatican City. Available online: http://w2.vatican.va/content/francesco/en/encyclicals/documents/papa-francesco_20150524_enciclica-laudato-si.pdf (accessed on 8 August 2021).
Rasmussen, Larry L. 1996. *Earth Community Earth Ethics, Ecology and Justice*. Maryknoll: Orbis Books.
Rasmussen, Larry L. 2013. *Earth-Honoring Faith Religious Ethics in a New Key*. Oxford: Oxford University Press. [CrossRef]
Ray, Sarah Jaquette. 2021a. Climate anxiety is an overwhelmingly white phenomenon. *Scientific American*. Available online: https://www.scientificamerican.com/article/the-unbearable-whiteness-of-climate-anxiety/ (accessed on 21 January 2022).
Ray, Sarah Jaquette. 2021b. Who Feels Climate Anxiety? *Cairo Review of Global Affairs* 43: 1–7.
Rimmer, Chad. 2020. Ecology and Christian education: How sustainability discourse and theological anthropology inform teaching methods. *Consensus* 41: 10.
Robinson, David S, and Jennifer Wotochek. 2021. Kenotic Theologies and the Challenge of the 'Anthropocene': From Deep Incarnation to Interspecies Encounter. *Studies in Christian Ethics* 34: 209–22. [CrossRef]
Rossing, Barbara R. 2017. Reimagining eschatology: Toward healing and hope for a world at the Eschatos. In *Planetary Solidarity: Global Women's Voices on Christian Doctrine and Climate Justice*. Edited by Grace Ji-Sun Kim and Hilda P. Koster. Minneapolis: Fortress, pp. 325–47.
Russell, Letty M. 1987. *Household of Freedom: Authority in Feminist Theology (The 1986 Annie Kinkead Warfield Lectures)*, 1st ed. Philadelphia: Westminster Press.
Sheffield, Perry E., and Philip J. Landrigan. 2011. Global climate change and children's health: Threats and strategies for prevention. *Environmental Health Perspectives* 119: 291–98. [CrossRef]
Shugarman, Harriet. 2020. *How to Talk to Your Kids about Climate Change: Turning Angst into Action*. Gabriola Island: New Society Publishers.
Stanley, Samantha K., Teaghan L. Hogg, Zoe Leviston, and Iain Walker. 2021. From anger to action: Differential impacts of eco-anxiety, eco-depression, and eco-anger on climate action and wellbeing. *The Journal of Climate Change and Health* 1: 100003. [CrossRef]
Trott, Carlie D. 2021. What difference does it make? Exploring the transformative potential of everyday climate crisis activism by children and youth. *Children's Geographies* 19: 300–8. [CrossRef]

Van Schalkwyk, Annalet. 2012. Welfare, wellbeing and the oikos cycle: An ecofeminist ethical perspective of care. *Journal of Theology for Southern Africa* 142: 98–119.

Vergunst, Francis, and Helen L. Berry. 2021. Climate Change and Children's Mental Health: A Develmental Perspective. *Clinical Psychological Science*. [CrossRef]

Verlie, Blanche, Emily Clark, Tamara Jarrett, and Emma Supriyono. 2021. Educators' Experiences and strategies for responding to ecological distress. *Australian Journal of Environmental Education* 37: 132–46. [CrossRef]

Verlie, Blanche. 2022. *Learning to Live with Climate Change: From Anxiety to Transformation*. Milton Park: Taylor & Francis

Wardell, Susan. 2020. Naming and framing ecological distress. *Medicine Anthropology Theory* 7: 187–201. [CrossRef]

Wijsen, Frans, Jozef Servaas, Peter Henriot, and Rodrigo Mejia. 2005. *The Pastoral Circle Revisited. A Critical Quest for Truth and Transformation*. Nairobi: Paulines Publications Africa.

Wu, Judy, Gaelen Snell, and Hasina Samji. 2020. Climate anxiety in young people: A call to action. *The Lancet Planetary Health* 4: e435–e436. [CrossRef]

Zhang, Ying, Peng Bi, and Janet E. Hiller. 2007. Climate Change and Disability–Adjusted Life Years. *Journal of Environmental Health* 70: 32–38. [PubMed]

MDPI
St. Alban-Anlage 66
4052 Basel
Switzerland
Tel. +41 61 683 77 34
Fax +41 61 302 89 18
www.mdpi.com

Religions Editorial Office
E-mail: religions@mdpi.com
www.mdpi.com/journal/religions

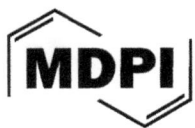

www.ingramcontent.com/pod-product-compliance
Lightning Source LLC
LaVergne TN
LVHW070735100526
838202LV00013B/1237